Cei

MW00610290

Introduction to
Hospital & Health-System
PHARMACY
PRACTICE

David A. Holdford, R.Ph., M.S., Ph.D., FAPhA
Associate Professor
Department of Pharmacotherapy and Outcomes Science
Virginia Commonwealth University School of Pharmacy
Richmond, Virginia

Thomas R. Brown, M.S., Pharm.D., FASHP
Professor Emeritus
University of Mississippi School of Pharmacy
Oxford, Mississippi

American Society of Health-System Pharmacists®
Bethesda, MD

Any correspondence regarding this publication should be sent to the publisher, American Society of Health-System Pharmacists, 7272 Wisconsin Avenue, Bethesda, MD 20814, attention: Special Publishing.

The information presented herein reflects the opinions of the contributors and advisors. It should not be interpreted as an official policy of ASHP or as an endorsement of any product.

Because of ongoing research and improvements in technology, the information and its applications contained in this text are constantly evolving and are subject to the professional judgment and interpretation of the practitioner due to the uniqueness of a clinical situation. The editors, contributors, and ASHP have made reasonable efforts to ensure the accuracy and appropriateness of the information presented in this document. However, any user of this information is advised that the editors, contributors, advisors, and ASHP are not responsible for the continued currency of the information, for any errors or omissions, and/or for any consequences arising from the use of the information in the document in any and all practice settings. Any reader of this document is cautioned that ASHP makes no representation, guarantee, or warranty, express or implied, as to the accuracy and appropriateness of the information contained in this document and specifically disclaims any liability to any party for the accuracy and/or completeness of the material or for any damages arising out of the use or non-use of any of the information contained in this document.

Director, Special Publishing: Jack Bruggeman
Acquisitions Editor: Rebecca Olson
Senior Editorial Project Manager: Dana A. Battaglia
Project Editor: Bill Fogle
Page Layout: Carol A. Barrer
Cover Design: David Wade

©2010, American Society of Health-System Pharmacists, Inc. All rights reserved.

No part of this publication may be reproduced or transmitted in any form or by any means, electronic or mechanical, including photocopying, microfilming, and recording, or by any information storage and retrieval system, without written permission from the American Society of Health-System Pharmacists.

ASHP is a service mark of the American Society of Health-System Pharmacists, Inc.; registered in the U.S. Patent and Trademark Office.

ISBN 978-1-58528-237-1

Dedications

To my love, Diane—nurse, daredevil, cowgirl.

—David A. Holdford

To my grandsons, Andrew Reaves Brown and Bennett James Brown, and my granddaughter, Piper Mackenzie Brown.

—Tom Brown

Preface

When I was a child living in Mount Vernon, Ohio, I visited my father at his workplace in the pharmacy of Mercy Hospital, a small catholic hospital serving the rural community.

My Dad, Arthur A. Holdford, R.Ph., was the director of pharmacy services. In fact, he was the only pharmacist employed by Mercy Hospital at the time. Large pharmacy staffs were not common when he first took the job at the hospital. Over time, he was able to hire employees to support the expansion of pharmacy services.

The hospital where my father worked was very different from hospitals of today. Back then, there were no computers, no Internet, and no automated dispensing cabinets. Handling, storage, and administration of sterile products and other medicines were primitive compared to today. Intravenous drugs were often prepared by nurses on the floors using less than aseptic technique. Oral medications were typically sent in bulk bottles to nursing units to be administered with little pharmacy oversight or input. Medication use systems were neither very safe, nor were they really systems.

Clinical pharmacy, as we now know it, was in its infancy back then. Clinical pharmacists were rarely seen in hospitals. Today's most commonly used drugs had not yet been invented. Major diseases including AIDS were not known either.

The hospital where my father worked was not part of an integrated health system. The hospital did not coordinate its care with a network of outpatient clinics, physicians' offices, pharmacy benefits management, long-term care facilities, home health agencies, and the like. My father worked in a hospital, not a health system.

Medicare and Medicaid were just in their infancy at that time. Pharmacy benefits managers and many other forms of managed care were virtually nonexistent. Pharmacists were not well paid compared to the salaries given to pharmacists of today. Pharmacist training was also different back then. Pharmacists needed fewer years of schooling and their education revolved around the product, not the patient. In short, a lot has changed since my father's days.

Individuals entering the pharmacy profession today are going to see some truly amazing changes in health care and pharmacy practice during their career. It is impossible to accurately predict what those changes will be exactly, just as it would have been impossible for my father to imagine the changes that would occur over his lifetime. The only certainty, however, is that change will continue. And pharmacists will be a part of that change.

Origin of this Text

The genesis of this introductory textbook came from the *Handbook of Institutional Pharmacy Practice*, first published in 1979 by Drs. Thomas Brown and Mickey Smith. The handbook was designed to achieve ASHP practice competencies and standards for pharmacists and evolved as it went through four editions. The fourth edition, edited by Thomas Brown, consists of 40 chapters covering a broad range of topics including information systems and informatics, the integrity of the U.S. drug supply, hospice and palliative care, and evidence-based medicine. Over the more than 30 years the *Handbook*

of Institutional Pharmacy Practice has been the only text available for students and practitioners, it has documented the changes in practice that have been required for clinical
and management advancement in the profession. The text has been the one reference for
students and practitioners who wished to pursue a career in institutional pharmacy.

Many chapters from the handbook served as the basis for this new text, *Introduction
to Hospital and Health-System Pharmacy Practice* (HHPP). New content and pedagogy
have been added to focus the content more on student needs and current practice. The
book provides learning tools for students (e.g., review questions, discussion questions,
and additional reading) to assist educators in building on the text's basic terminology and
concepts.

Approach and Organization

This text presents an overview of essential terms, concepts, and processes in health-
systems pharmacy in a concise, practical, and understandable way. Content comes from
recognized experts in institutional pharmacy practice. Emphasis is on explaining, developing comprehension, and encouraging application.

The book consists of nineteen chapters divided into seven sections. The first section, *Introduction*, answers the question, "What is Institutional Pharmacy Practice?" It
provides an overview of IPP, describes its history, and discusses key legal and regulatory
issues. The next section, *Managing Medication Use,* describes how the medication use
process is controlled through formularies, clinical pharmacy practice, and medication
safety practices. *Managing Medication Distribution* describes systems for managing the
distribution of medications (including controlled substances) throughout institutions.
Using Technology discusses the role of automation, technology, and information systems
in health systems. *Financial Management* reviews key management responsibilities of the
pharmacy department including inventory control, budgeting, and cost control. *Sterile
Product Preparation and Administration* discusses key systems, practices, and terms in
preparing and administering sterile products. *Managing People* addresses leadership and
human resources management in institutions. Finally, *Careers in Institutional Pharmacy
Practice* discusses different training options for careers in health systems.

Prior knowledge of health-systems practice is not necessary to use this text, because
it is written in an easy-to-read style and provides definitions for unfamiliar vocabulary.
Some of the major highlights of this book include:

- Learning objectives for each chapter
- Key terms are highlighted and defined within chapters
- Key points are highlighted and then explained by answering "so what?"
- Graphics and visual aids are used throughout to illustrate key concepts
- Review questions are provided at the end of each chapter for self-assessment
- Discussion questions are provided in each chapter to initiate dialogue and debate

Additional resources are available online at www.ashp.org/pharmacypractice including:

- Supplementary exercises that offer potential hands-on application of chapter
content
- A comprehensive glossary of all key terms used in the text

Intended Readers

This book is written for any pharmacy student interested in institutional pharmacy practice. For students interested in institutional practice, this book provides a foundation for introductory and advanced pharmacy practice experiences and on-the-job training in hospitals and health systems. Mastery of the book's terms and concepts will be particularly useful for students who plan to seek residencies.

The book can also be useful for students who plan to practice in community settings by helping them understand how health systems work. Not all community pharmacists understand institutional practice, although a general understanding of health systems can be valuable when interacting with institutional pharmacists. Interactions often occur as patients move in and out of hospitals and other settings. Greater contact and understanding will also be needed across practice settings if integrated therapeutic interventions such as disease management are going to succeed in achieving positive patient outcomes.

In addition, practicing pharmacists who read this book can gain insight into institutional practice. Non-institutional pharmacists working in community settings or other jobs will learn about the various financial, clinical, technological, and distributional systems in health care institutions. This can be especially useful for individuals seeking a career.

For Educators

This book can be used as the core text around which an elective or required course in institutional pharmacy practice can be built. It can also serve as a text for the integration of institutional pharmacy across the curriculum.

For a standalone elective or required course, educators can build learning experiences around individual chapters. The textbook offers a selection of readings that can form the backbone of the course. Faculty members can supplement the readings with presentations by practitioners, classroom assignments, and active learning projects. A textbook would also help guide the presentations of different faculty involved in team-taught courses. For instance, the first section, *Introduction*, can be used to provide an overview of health systems and pharmacy practice within them. Faculty and guest speakers can describe common types of institutional settings and the types of patients treated in each, discuss pharmacist's roles and models of practice, the history of hospital pharmacy, and the various accreditation, regulation, practice standards, and institutional policies and procedures influencing practice. Clarification of concepts within the related chapters can occur and problem based learning activities can be used to apply and synthesize ideas covered in the book and class.

Use of the text could also occur across the curriculum as part of integrated, multi-disciplinary education. This could be accomplished by mapping institutional pharmacy topics across curriculum, identifying the desired learning objectives for various courses, and matching book chapters to the learning objectives. For instance, chapters from the *Managing Medication Use* and *Managing Medication Distribution* sections of the book could be assigned as part of hospital introductory pharmacy practice experiences (IPPEs). The section *Sterile Product Preparation and Administration* could accompany laboratory classes that teach compounding of intravenous solutions. Financial management could be part of a pharmacy management course, while careers in institutional pharmacy practice could be part of career training. Students who complete all of the text's learning objectives would be able to have much richer institutional advanced pharmacy practice experiences (APPEs).

David A. Holdford, Co-Editor
Thomas R. Brown, Co-Editor

Contents

Preface v

Contributors xi

Part I: Introduction

Chapter 1: What is Institutional Pharmacy Practice? 1

Kasey K. Thompson and Douglas J. Scheckelhoff

Chapter 2: Overview of the History of Hospital Pharmacy in the
United States 17

William A. Zellmer

Chapter 3: Key Legal and Regulatory Issues in Health-System
Pharmacy Practice 39

*John P. Uselton, Lee B. Murdaugh, Patricia C. Kienle,
and David A. Holdford*

Part II: Managing Medication Use

Chapter 4: Medication Management 59

Kathy A. Chase

Chapter 5: Clinical Pharmacy 81

John E. Murphy

Chapter 6: Medication Safety 99

David A. Holdford

Part III: Managing Medication Distribution

Chapter 7: Medication Distribution Systems 123

Stephen F. Eckel and Fred M. Eckel

Chapter 8: Controlled Substances Management 143

George J. Dydek and David J. Tomich

Part IV: Using Technology

Chapter 9: Electronic Data Management:
Electronic Health Record Systems and
Computerized Provider Order Entry Systems 159

David A. Holdford, Stephen K. Huffines, and S. Trent Rosenbloom

Chapter 10: Informatics 179

James G. Stevenson, Scott R. McCreadie, and Bruce W. Chaffee

Chapter 11: Automation in Practice 203

Brad Ludwig and Jack Temple

Part V: Financial Management

Chapter 12: Purchasing and Inventory Control 229

Jerrod Milton

Chapter 13: The Basics of Financial Management and
Cost Control 253

Andrew L. Wilson

Part VI: Sterile Product Preparation and Administration

Chapter 14: Sterile Preparations and
Admixture Programs..277

Philip J. Schneider and E. Clyde Buchanan

Chapter 15: Parenteral Therapy 299

E. Clyde Buchanan

Part VII: Managing People

Chapter 16: Leadership and Management............................321

David A. Holdford

Chapter 17: Recruiting, Selecting, and Managing Pharmacy
Personnel 345

David A. Holdford

Part VIII: Careers in Health-System Pharmacy Practice

Chapter 18: Training for Careers in Hospitals and Health
Systems 367

Thomas P. Reinders and David A. Holdford

Chapter 19: Residency Training 383

Jill S. Burkiewicz and Carrie A. Sincak

Index..399

Contributors

E. Clyde Buchanan, M.S., FASHP
Director of Pharmacy (Ret.)
Consultant specializing
  in compounding sterile
  preparations
Atlanta, Georgia

Jill S. Burkiewicz, Pharm.D., BCPS
Professor & PGY1 Residency
  Director, Pharmacy Practice
Midwestern University Chicago
  College of Pharmacy
Downers Grove, Illinois

Bruce W. Chaffee, Pharm.D.
Clinical Pharmacist and Clinical
  Associate Professor
Informatics and Outcomes
College of Pharmacy
The University of Michigan
  Health System
Ann Arbor, Michigan

Kathy A. Chase, Pharm.D.
Director, Medication Solutions
Cardinal Health
Houston, Texas

George J. Dydek, Pharm.D., BCPS, FASHP, CACP
Clinical Pharmacist
Family Medicine Clinic
Madigan Army Medical Center
Tacoma, Washington

Fred M. Eckel, M.S., FASHP, FAAAS, DNAP
Professor of Pharmacy
Eshelman School of Pharmacy
University of North Carolina at
  Chapel Hill
Executive Director
NC Association of Pharmacists
Chapel Hill, North Carolina

Stephen F. Eckel, Pharm.D., MHA, BCPS, FAPhA
Assistant Director of Pharmacy,
  Residency Program Director
University of North Carolina
  Hospitals
Clinical Assistant Professor
Eshelman School of Pharmacy
University of North Carolina
Chapel Hill, North Carolina

David A. Holdford, R.Ph., M.S., Ph.D., FAPhA
Associate Professor
Department of Pharmacotherapy
  and Outcomes Science
Virginia Commonwealth
  University School of
  Pharmacy
Richmond, Virginia

Stephen K. Huffines, Pharm. D.
Director, Pharmacy Business
  Services
Vanderbilt University Medical
  Center
Nashville, Tennessee

Patricia C. Kienle, R.Ph., MPA, FASHP
Director, Accreditation and
  Medication Safety
Cardinal Health Pharmacy
  Solutions
Laflin, Pennsylvania

Brad Ludwig, R.Ph., M.S.
Assistant Director of Pharmacy
  Operations/Technology
University of Wisconsin Hospital
  and Clinics
Madison, Wisconsin

Scott R. McCreadie Pharm.D., MBA
President
McCreadie Group
Ann Arbor, Michigan

Jerrod Milton, BSc Pharm., R.Ph.
Vice President, Operations
Children's Hospital
Aurora, Colorado

Lee B. Murdaugh, R.Ph., Ph.D.
Director, Accreditation and
  Medication Safety
Quality and Regulatory Affairs
Cardinal Health Pharmacy
  Solutions
Houston, Texas

John E. Murphy, Pharm.D., FASHP, FCCP
Professor of Pharmacy Practice
  and Science
Associate Dean
The University of Arizona
  College of Pharmacy
Tucson, Arizona

Thomas P. Reinders, Pharm.D.
Associate Dean for Admission
  and Student Services
School of Pharmacy
Virginia Commonwealth
  University
Richmond, Virginia

S. Trent Rosenbloom, MD, MPH
Assistant Professor of
  Biomedical Informatics,
  Medicine and Pediatrics
Vanderbilt University Medical
  Center
Nashville, Tennessee

Douglas J. Scheckelhoff, M.S.

Vice President, Professional Development
American Society of Health-System Pharmacists
Bethesda, Maryland

Philip J. Schneider, M.S.

Clinical Professor and Associate Dean
University of Arizona College of Pharmacy
Phoenix, Arizona

Carrie A. Sincak, Pharm.D., BCPS

Associate Professor and Vice Chair of Acute Care
Department of Pharmacy Practice
Midwestern University Chicago College of Pharmacy
Downers Grove, Illinois

James G. Stevenson, Pharm.D., FASHP

Professor and Associate Dean for Clinical Sciences
University of Michigan College of Pharmacy
Director of Pharmacy Services
University of Michigan Health System
Ann Arbor, Michigan

Jack Temple, M.S., Pharm.D.

Pharmacy Manager Operational Improvement
University of Wisconsin Hospital and Clinics
Madison, Wisconsin

Kasey K. Thompson, Pharm.D.

Vice President, Office of Policy, Planning and Communications
American Society of Health-System Pharmacists
Bethesda, Maryland

David J. Tomich, Pharm.D., FASHP

Chief Clinical Pharmacy Services
Madigan Army Medical Center
Tacoma, Washington

John P. Uselton, R.Ph.

Vice President
Quality and Regulatory Affairs
Cardinal Health Pharmacy Solutions
Houston, Texas

Andrew L. Wilson, Pharm.D., FASHP

Managing Consultant, Pharmacy Optimization
McKesson Health Systems
Richmond, Virginia

William A. Zellmer, B.S. (Pharmacy), MPH

Independent consultant and speaker on strategic and professional issues in pharmacy
Bethesda, Maryland

CHAPTER 1

What is Institutional Pharmacy Practice?

Kasey K. Thompson and Douglas J. Scheckelhoff

■ ■ ■
Learning Objectives

After completing this chapter, readers should be able to:

1. Describe the most common types of institutional settings and the types of patients treated in each.
2. Describe the pharmacist's role in the medication use process and specifically how they improve outcomes, reduce cost, and improve safety.
3. Contrast the pharmacist's role in inpatient and outpatient settings.
4. Identify the three primary practice models seen in institutional settings.
5. List the types of automation and technology commonly used in today's institutional settings to improve safety and efficiency of medication use.
6. List the other disciplines usually present when providing interdisciplinary team-based care.

Key Terms and Definitions

■ **Accreditation:** Determination by an accrediting body that an eligible health care organization complies with the accrediting body's applicable standards.
■ **Institutional pharmacy practice:** Includes the provision of distributional and clinical pharmacy services at a broad range of institutional settings including hospitals, long-term care, hospice, correctional facilities, and others.
■ **Integrated health systems:** Integrate all care under the umbrella of a central organization, and often include inpatient/acute care, primary care/outpatient care, long-term care, home care, and other patient-care settings.
■ **Practice guidelines:** Tools that describe processes found by clinical trials or by consensus opinion of experts to be the most effective in evaluating and/or treating a patient who has a specific symptom, condition, or diagnosis, or that describe a specific procedure. Synonyms include clinical practice guideline, practice parameter, protocol, preferred practice pattern, and guideline.
■ **Practice model:** The operational structure that defines how and where pharmacists practice, including the type of drug distribution system used, the layout and design of the department, how pharmacists spend their time, practice functions, and practice priorities. The three predominant practice

models include the drug-distribution-centered model, the clinical-pharmacist-centered model, and the patient-centered integrated model.

- **Privileging:** The process by which an oversight body of a health care organization or other appropriate provider body, having reviewed an individual health care provider's credentials and performance and found them satis-

factory, authorizes that individual to perform a specific scope of patient care services within that setting.

- **Regulation:** Governmental order having the force of law.
- **Smart pumps:** Infusion devices with clinical decision support software and drug libraries that perform a test of reasonableness at the point of medication administration.

■ ■ ■

Introduction

This chapter will describe the unique and diverse practice of pharmacy in the institutional environment. Emphasis will be placed on hospitals and integrated health systems. The purpose of this chapter is to introduce the concept of institutional pharmacy practice and key issues that will be discussed throughout this book.

What is Institutional Pharmacy Practice?

Institutional pharmacy practice includes the provision of distributional and clinical pharmacy services at a broad range of institutional settings including hospitals, long-term care, hospice, correctional facilities, and others. Typically, the institutions that pharmacists serve are linked together formally or informally into integrated health systems. As the term implies **integrated health systems** integrate all care under the umbrella of a central organization, and often include inpatient/acute care, primary care/outpatient care, long-term care, and home care. Health systems are a collection of organizations and institutions whose mission is to positively impact health outcomes. Although health systems are made up of independent entities, they are systems because the entities are interdependent and unified. The integrated model creates the potential to provide enhanced levels of patient-care continuity through access to medical records and patient care providers. At the completion of this chapter the student will have a general understanding of the unique attributes that comprise the practice of pharmacy in hospitals and health systems, including the various factors that influence practice in these settings.

Types of Hospitals

At one time, institutional pharmacy practice referred almost exclusively to service in hospital pharmacies, and hospitals are still the biggest component of institutional practice. There are approximately 5,800 hospitals in the U.S.[1]

Key Point . . .

There are approximately 5,800 hospitals in the U.S.

. . . So what?

There are hospitals in almost any location in the country—each employing pharmacists. Opportunities in institutional pharmacy practice are everywhere.

Hospitals are traditionally focused on providing care to acutely ill patients that require constant care by a team of highly skilled nurses, physicians, pharmacists, and other providers. Hospitals are often differentiated by factors such as location, size, and specialization. Location-related factors can include whether a hospital is situated in a large urban area or small rural setting. Hospitals may be located in a single building or spread across a campus complex. Some hospitals have a distinct mission to educate and train health-care professionals. These hospitals are termed university teaching hospitals. Other hospitals emphasize distinct specialties such as cardiac surgery and oncology. The following are some common labels assigned to hospitals:

- **Community hospital**—Community hospitals are what most people think of when they hear the term "hospital." They are the most common type and are designed to deal with an assortment of diseases and injury. Community hospitals typically have emergency services for treating trauma and other imminent threats to health. They also have inpatients that need surgical, intensive care, obstetrics, long-term care, medical, and other services to treat a broad group medical conditions.
- **Specialized hospital**—Specialized hospitals serve the needs of patients suffering from some particular disease (e.g., cancer, psychiatric illness), or affecting a specific organ system (e.g., eyes, lungs) or type of patient (e.g., children, seniors).
- **Teaching hospital**—Teaching hospitals have two missions—serving patients' needs and training future health-care professionals. Teaching hospitals often have some association with medical schools and sometimes conduct medical research.
- **For-Profit hospital**—For-profit hospitals are differentiated from nonprofit hospitals by their ownership. For-profit hospitals are owned by corporations or groups of private investors. They differ from **non-profit hospitals** which do not seek a return on investment for owners. Nonprofit hospitals often operate under religious, volunteer (e.g., Shriners), community, or other voluntary patronages. Any additional revenue generated after expenses is put back into the hospital.
- **Government hospitals**—These hospitals are owned or heavily supported by federal, state, county, or other governmental entities. Federal hospitals include those run by the Veterans Administration, United States Public Health Service (e.g., Bureau of Prisons, Indian Health Service), and the Armed Services (e.g., Army, Air Force, and Navy). Various states, counties, and cities have hospitals for underserved populations such as indigent and psychiatric patients.

Pharmacy's Roles in the Medication Use Process

The role of pharmacists is to lead and influence the safety and quality of all aspects of the medication-use process.

Key Point . . .

Pharmacists have important direct or indirect roles in prescribing, transcribing, dispensing, administration, and monitoring.

. . . So what?

The pharmacist's role in drug use control does not end once a medication leaves the pharmacy. However, that role often consists of influencing others in their roles within the drug use process. Indeed, a pharmacist's greatest impact often lies in influencing the prescribing of physicians and the administration of medications by nurses.

This means that pharmacists should be involved in controlling or influencing any step of the medication-use process that can impact patient health outcomes or costs. Therefore, pharmacists have important direct or indirect roles in prescribing, transcribing, dispensing, administration, and monitoring.

Prescribing

Prescribing medications is often viewed as something that only physicians are authorized to do. However, the reality is that many other health-care professionals are authorized to prescribe by state law (e.g., dentists, nurse practitioners, optometrists, podiatrists, and others) or through a formalized process in hospitals known as **privileging**. "Privileging is the process by which an oversight body of a health care organization or other appropriate provider body, having reviewed an individual health care provider's credentials and performance and found them satisfactory, authorizes that individual to perform a specific scope of patient care services within that setting."[2] Pharmacists who have prescribing privileges in hospitals are typically authorized to do so through the formalized privileging process. A more common role for pharmacists beyond actually prescribing is the pharmacists duty to influence the prescribing of other health professionals. Pharmacists indirectly influence prescribing by acting as information resources about medications, providing feedback about the quality of prescribing, and developing prescribing protocols through the formulary system.

Transcribing

Transcribing is the process by which a prescriber's written order is copied and either manually or electronically entered into pharmacy records. The transcribing process represents an opportunity for error, especially when done manually. Pharmacists must understand potential breakdowns in the transcribing process and help find ways to minimize errors. In time, the problem of manual transcription will diminish because of the movement toward computerized prescriber order entry. However, that time is not here yet because manual transcribing of written orders is still the most common.[3]

Dispensing

Dispensing is the act of physically transferring the drug product following review and approval of the prescription to the area responsible for administering the medication to the patient. Dispensing is also an area where medication errors can occur, including, but not limited to wrong drug, wrong dose, or wrong dosage form errors.

Administration

Medication administration to the patient in hospitals is typically managed by nurses. This phase of the medication-use process is the last step before patients are given their medications, and errors at this point cannot be corrected. Errors in the administration phase have been reported as being upwards of 34%.[4] Nurses usually serve as the final check in the medication-use process. Pharmacists help improve the safety of medication administration by clearly labeling medications, using bar-coding systems and unit dose packaging, reducing the time and effort involved in accessing drugs (e.g., through the use of decentralized automated dispensing devices), and using technology that reduces administration errors (e.g., smart infusion pumps).

Monitoring. Monitoring the patient's response to the medication is a critical phase where pharmacists play a vital role. Monitoring includes reviewing laboratory values that are correlated with the expected medication-therapy outcomes, as well as other objective and subjective factors that indicate whether the therapy is effective, or may be having a toxic effect.

Practice Models

Institutional pharmacists comprise their roles in practice models. A **practice model** can be defined as the "operational structure that defines how and where pharmacists practice, including the type of drug distribution system used, the layout and design of the department, how pharmacists spend their time, practice functions, and practice priorities. The practice model is probably the most important factor determining the role and effectiveness of the pharmacy department. It sets the stage and defines the roles.[5]" The term practice model describes how pharmacists, pharmacy technicians and automation inter-relate to provide pharmacy services. Practice models used vary based on the hospital type (e.g., community vs. academic), institution size (e.g., large vs. small), patient population (e.g., chronic vs. critical care) or philosophy of how pharmacy services should be delivered.

There are three major pharmacy practice models[6]:

1. *Drug-distribution-centered model.* In this model, pharmacists primarily distribute drugs and process new medication orders. The pharmacist's role is reactive, in that he or she responds to requests of physicians and nurses but rarely initiates major changes in therapy. In this model, the pharmacist is not actively involved with the health care team or in development of therapeutic plans for the patient. Consequently, pharmacists are not accountable for the health outcomes of patients and exert little leadership in influencing the medication-use process.
2. *Clinical-pharmacist-centered model.* There are two primary types of pharmacists in pharmacy departments utilizing this model: clinical pharmacists and distributive pharmacists. Clinical pharmacists are chiefly involved in clinical activities associated with medical teams on the nursing units. In its extreme form, clinical pharmacists in this model accept little or no responsibility for the medication-use or delivery systems. Their primary responsibility is assisting physicians and other health professionals in avoiding and solving clinical problems exclusive of the distribution process. The second group are those who spend most of their time in drug distribution, reviewing orders and verifying the accuracy of medication preparation by technician. Little or no collaboration occurs between clinical and distributive pharmacists in the extreme of this model, so these pharmacists are selectively accountable for the medication-use process.
3. *Patient-centered integrated model.* In this model, all pharmacists in the department accept responsibility for all elements of the medication-use process and therefore spend their time on both clinical and distributive functions. Pharmacists' roles in drug distribution are often limited, because many distribution tasks are delegated to well-trained pharmacy technicians. Therefore, pharmacists are able to expand their clinical roles to more active engagement in medication selection and drug use as part of an interdisciplinary team. In this model, pharmacists exhibit a high degree of ownership of and accountability for the entire medication-use process.

The three models above are generalizations of what might be seen in practice, but they do describe the tension between clinical and distributional roles of pharmacists. The degree to which an institutional pharmacy resembles any model depends on a variety of factors including its leadership; the relationships it develops with medicine, nursing, and the hospital administration; its involvement with colleges of pharmacy; the drug distribution model; variations in regional practice and work force; the presence or absence of pharmacy residency training programs; and department culture (e.g., staff members' willingness to accept responsibility for patient outcomes).[6]

The culture of the department influences the success of any particular practice model. The individuals who make up a pharmacy department will ultimately determine the delivery of services. Therefore, practice models must be understood and accepted by everyone within the organization. Pharmacists, technicians, and other individuals must appreciate how their individual efforts contribute to the mission of the department. Unless the members develop a common vision, they will not work well as a team. And without teamwork, factions can develop within the pharmacy leading to "us-versus-them" attitudes.

Whatever the model of pharmacy practice, several common features are likely to emerge as key.[7]

- Practice will need to be interdisciplinary and team based. Education and training of pharmacists will need to be also.
- Medication preparation and distribution will need to be made more efficient with automation, centralization, and the use of trained technicians.
- Pharmacists' contributions to the medication-use process will be increasingly in direct patient care and less in medication distribution.
- Health information technology will give pharmacists much greater ability to positively influence the medication-use process.
- Pharmacists will need to justify their value because allocation of health care resources will be heavily driven by metrics. The benefits of pharmacy services will need to be justified against their costs. The value of services in terms of medication therapy outcomes, medication safety, and total care costs related to medication therapy will need to be defended.
- A pharmacotherapy plan should be developed for every patient. That plan should be comprehensive, multidisciplinary, accessible, and transferable to any provider or location. Primary responsibility for this plan should rest with the pharmacist.
- Pharmacists will need continuous training to practice pharmacy. Credentialing and privileging of pharmacists may be requirements for practice in general and specialty practice areas.
- Institutional pharmacists will need to collaborate better with community pharmacists to coordinate care as patients transition from one practice setting to the next.

> **Key Point . . .**
>
> The culture of the department influences the success of any particular practice model.
>
> **. . . So what?**
>
> The ability to advance the practice of pharmacy often is hindered by a culture where individuals are discouraged from trying new things. In many instances, a change in culture is necessary for evolution to a new practice model.

While there are institutional pharmacists who have purely distributional responsibilities, many are increasingly involved in direct-patient care. Direct patient care typically occurs with the pharmacist being part of an interdisciplinary patient-care team, where diverse professionals are each responsible for patient care within their scope of practice and expertise. Teams typically include physicians, nurses, and pharmacists, and may also include others such as respiratory therapists, and social workers. These teams are synergistic in that they allow the patient to benefit from their individual and collective skills in the most efficient way possible. The team concept has contributed to the pharmacist's clinical role through providing a portal for pharmacist recommendations on drug therapy and monitoring, and puts the pharmacist into daily contact with the patient. Because these models are becoming integral to experiential education models, most new graduates feel comfortable moving into these roles and often seek out these types of positions upon graduation.

Key Individuals

Pharmacists

Pharmacists can play a number of different roles in institutional settings. The most traditional role is that of the dispensing pharmacist. These individuals are responsible for preparation of medications, either directly or through supervising the preparatory work of pharmacy technicians. Dispensing pharmacists play an important role in verifying that medications are prepared correctly and are dispensed accurately. But because of the increasing use of technicians, coupled with greater use of automation and technology and more dosage forms being commercially available, positions for dispensing pharmacists are declining in some institutions. While the dispensing pharmacist is less common, pharmacist oversight over the dispensing and preparation process remains critical. Fortunately, pharmacy education is preparing new pharmacy graduates to fulfill both dispensing and non-dispensing roles.

Clinical pharmacy practice is another role for pharmacists. Clinical pharmacists are likely to serve on interdisciplinary patient-care teams, and interact directly with patients. Clinical pharmacists usually have clinical pharmacy training and often have completed a pharmacy residency. Clinical pharmacists may be "generalists" and provide clinical pharmacy services to a wide range of patients, or they may be "specialists" who have a defined expertise in one or more areas (e.g., critical care, oncology). The prevalence of these clinical pharmacy roles continues to increase and this trend will likely continue.

The most prevalent role in institutional practice is one where the pharmacist has both dispensing and clinical roles, usually referred to as an integrated practice.[3] This type of role may involve the pharmacist spending a designated amount of time in each area (e.g., 1 month dispensing alternating with a month of clinical practice) or time split in a given day (e.g., mornings spent in patient care areas rounding and providing or-

Key Point . . .

Pharmacy education is preparing new pharmacy graduates to fulfill both dispensing and non-dispensing roles.

. . . So what?

Educators still struggle with the decision about the exact role of pharmacists within institutional practice. Some advocate for the clinical-pharmacist-centered practice model, while other educators emphasize drug-distribution-centered or integrated practice models. This textbook takes the position that regardless of the preferred practice model, both dispensing and non-dispensing roles are important.

der review followed by afternoons in the pharmacy verifying technician prepared medications). For the most part, these pharmacists are considered generalists in both dispensing and clinical activities.

Pharmacists in management usually serve as the supervisor for pharmacy activities or as the director for the pharmacy department. These roles require an understanding of the practice of pharmacy and how medications are used; a good knowledge of regulations and laws that govern pharmacy practice; and basic skills in human resource management, leadership, budget management, and ensuring quality of medication use. Good managers are especially important since the effectiveness of pharmacy services often depends on how well pharmacy managers are able to manage and lead the department.

Other pharmacist roles are evolving. Examples include pharmacists who are responsible for informatics, investigational drug services, research, sterile compounding, and emergency care.

Pharmacy Technicians

Pharmacy technicians continue to play an expanding role in virtually all practice models. Technicians have been integral in the purchasing, stocking, preparation and compounding of medications. This has been and continues to be under the direct supervision of the pharmacist. The scope of this role varies, depending on the experience, training and skills of the pharmacy technician. The scope and responsibility often varies because technicians do not have consistent and standardized training requirements. Because technicians play an increasingly important role in drug preparation and dispensing, technician training standards are being established. This will allow greater responsibility to be transferred to pharmacy technicians since each will meet a defined training and certification standard.

Pharmacy technicians are also taking on new and expanded roles beyond preparation and dispensing. Some technicians are assuming roles that involve the maintenance of automated dispensing technology and other information technology systems. Others are assuming roles that assist clinical pharmacists in the collection of laboratory values or other clinical data. In some organizations, pharmacy technicians are interviewing patients and reconciling medication regimens at home with those ordered during their hospital stay. Regardless of whether technicians are in traditional medication preparation roles or in one of these new capacities, their importance in freeing the pharmacist for more direct patient care responsibilities is increasing, and so is the need for training and certification.

Importance of Automation and Technology

Automation and technology have been used in pharmacy since the before the 1990s, but are becoming increasingly used in hospitals. Pharmacy automation serves to increase efficiency and accuracy of dispensing. Medication-related technology used outside of the pharmacy (e.g., bar coded medication administration, smart pumps, computerized prescriber order entry) is usually focused on safety. Pharmacy automation is important to the practice model because utilization of many of the available technologies can influence what the pharmacist and pharmacy technician do in support of medication dispensing. Full use of automation can re-direct staff time away from routine technical tasks and towards more direct patient care activities.

The most common type of pharmacy automation is the unit-based cabinet (e.g., Pyxis®, Omnicell®). These cabinet-based technologies are usually located strategically in the patient care area and contain compartments where individual medications are stored. The compartments only open and give access to the medication when the user is authorized to do so. Usually this authorization is based on the computer in the cabinet verifying that the medication has been approved through an interface with the pharmacy computer system. These systems have been successful because they place medications much closer to the user, but still allow electronic verification that the medication and dose is correct for the patient. They also simplify billing and documentation of medication administration.

The second most common type of pharmacy automation is the pharmacy robot (e.g., McKesson Robot-Rx®). These systems contain hundreds of bar coded packages placed in designated spaces on long rods. The robot moves to the designated space, verifies that it is the correct medication using the bar code, and removes the number of doses needed. The robot is usually used to prepare a 24-hour supply of oral and prepackaged injectable medications. Pharmacist and technician time needed to prepare and check these medications is greatly reduced when this technology is used.

Automation used in sterile compounding ranges from small pumps used to fill syringes and prepare parenteral nutrition solutions to large systems with robotic arms capable of preparing all types of sterile IV solutions and infusions. These systems improve the efficiency of sterile product preparation while improving the accuracy of the preparation and minimization of potential contamination.

There are a number of medication-related technologies that are used outside of the pharmacy to improve safety. These systems have a direct impact on the pharmacy and require active involvement by the pharmacy in making sure that systems are designed and used optimally to realize their safety benefits. Examples include:

- Bar coded medication administration (BCMA) systems (see Chapter 10 for more information on BCMA), requiring pharmacy involvement in assuring that drug packages have appropriate, readable bar codes and that information systems capture and document information.
- Computerized prescriber order entry systems (CPOE) (see Chapter 9 for more information on CPOE) require an interface or integration with pharmacy information systems so that medication ordering information is able to transfer between the prescriber and the pharmacy. Standard order sets and verification mechanisms also require pharmacy involvement for these systems.
- **Smart pumps** are programmable pumps that allow the user to predefine minimum and maximum rates of administration, preventing errors where

patients are under- or over-dosed with medication. Pharmacy plays an important role in making sure that the limits contained in the "drug library" are clinically appropriate.

Key Point . . .

There has been a shift to treat patients in the home or non-hospital setting whenever possible.

. . . So what?

Inpatient pharmacists now take care of sicker patients who require increasingly complex and intense services. Inpatient pharmacists require extensive training and expertise like that acquired from accredited residency programs.

Unique Aspects of Different Patient Care Areas

Inpatient Care

Most institutional care is provided to inpatients. Since health care reimbursement models changed in the 1980s, there has been a shift to treat patients in the home or non-hospital setting whenever possible. These shifts have moved healthier patients to outpatient settings while focusing hospital care on treating only the sickest patients.

There are two primary categories of inpatient patient care areas: critical care units and general care units. Subsets exist for each which varies by the types of patients treated within and reflecting the expertise of the staff assigned. Examples of critical care units include surgical, medical, neurosurgery, pediatrics, coronary care, neonatal, burn, and others. General care units include medical, surgical, pediatrics, cardiology, orthopedics, post-partum, obstetrics and gynecology, oncology, and others. The number and mix of units is usually determined by the size and location of the hospital, which determines the number and types of patients who are admitted.

The pharmacist's role in a critical care unit is different than other settings because the patients are of a higher acuity level, meaning that they have greater needs for care. Patients in critical care are, by definition, critically ill and therefore their clinical status is constantly changing. They must be monitored closely and their drug therapy is often changed or adjusted. Typically, these patients are on multiple intravenous medications, thereby creating a high potential for incompatibilities, drug interactions, and errors. These patients also may have declining organ function, such as kidneys or liver, which affects drug dosing. The pharmacist plays a critical role in making sure that patients are receiving the right drugs, in the dose that is appropriate for their condition, and without error. The pharmacist usually participates in medical rounds with the rest of the health-care team, providing advice and information on drug therapy. After rounds, there are often follow-up on questions and responses to new treatment needs that arise throughout the day. There have been numerous studies that have documented the impact of having a pharmacist in the critical care unit on patient outcomes.[8]

The pharmacist's role in general inpatient care units is different from critical care patients primarily because the acuity of patients is less. Drug therapy is more likely to be stable and many times is a combination of oral and intravenous medications, depending on the patient's treatment regimen. The general inpatient care unit has unique issues related to medications, such as assuring that the patients orders upon admission accurately reflects those medications being taken at home (a process called medication reconciliation) and making sure that discharge orders are appropriate and that patients are going to be able to continue their medications upon arriving home. These handoffs on admission and discharge are important so that the patient has continuity of care. The pharmacist may attend medical rounds with a health-care team, depending on the nature of the hospital (some smaller and community-based hospitals do not use traditional medical rounds with a team).

Pharmacists also are responsible for the drug distribution to all inpatients. This is supported by pharmacy technicians and automation, with a goal of providing safe, efficient, and cost-effective drug therapy.

Outpatient Care

A variety of outpatient care settings are commonly associated with institutional care. The most common and perhaps most visible is the outpatient dispensing pharmacy, similar to community pharmacies without general merchandise. Many hospitals have at least one outpatient dispensing pharmacy which cater to clinic patients, patients being discharged from inpatient settings, and patients with prescriptions written in emergency departments.

Other outpatient settings are less traditional and can vary widely in the types of patients served and the nature of services provided. Pharmacists are increasingly working in emergency departments because of a growing recognition of the value they can provide in medication use. The pharmacist's role in the emergency department usually includes drug therapy consultation with providers, error prevention and patient safety, monitoring adherence to practice guidelines, medication counseling, reviewing patient profiles, and participating in resuscitation efforts.[9,10]

Another growing area of outpatient services includes ambulatory care clinics. Clinics may be general in nature (e.g., primary care, medication adherence) or specialized (e.g., anticoagulation, palliative care). In these settings, medication therapy is managed by a pharmacist and usually patients see the pharmacist one-on-one by appointment. Pharmacists have great potential to improve medication-therapy outcomes, reduce errors, and reduce readmissions in outpatient clinic settings.

Another unique outpatient care setting includes home health care. Home health care services, most specifically home infusion services, have evolved as a way for patients to be treated in a non-hospital setting, usually their home. These pharmacy services are unique in that they provide infusion therapy for both short term and long-term chronic conditions. Common therapies include antimicrobial therapy, pain management, parenteral nutrition, and chemotherapy administration. Since there is not a nurse administering the drug or monitoring the patient, considerations for training, storage, labeling, administration, and disposal must all be taken into consideration. Pharmacists play an important role in making sure that patients receive their medications appropriately under these less controlled conditions.

Accreditation and Standards of Practice

Institutional pharmacy practice is governed by a variety of requirements and guidance including, respectively, accreditation and practice standards. **Accreditation** is a voluntary process by which the quality of care provided by a hospital is assessed by an outside accrediting body on a routine basis. Groups that accredit hospitals in the United States include The Joint Commission, American Osteopathic Association, and DMV. Accreditation organizations are different from regulatory bodies in that their primary purpose is to assess and improve the quality of patient care (i.e., when they identify a quality of care problem they work with the hospital to make improvements).

Accreditation organizations have no authority to impose fines or bring forth legal action. **Regulatory bodies** such as the Food and Drug Administration, Centers for Medicare & Medicaid Services, Drug Enforcement Administration, state and local departments of health, and state boards of pharmacy are law enforcement bodies whose purpose is public protection, and are therefore tasked with imposing fines and taking other legal actions.

Practice standards or practice guidelines are those practices that a profession develops and imposes on itself. Practice standards should be based on the best scientific evidence, and should ideally strive to surpass minimum requirements established by law or regulation. Although elements of practice standards may be adopted or adapted into law or regulation, they are still considered different from laws and regulations due to the fact that they are developed by the profession that is engaged in the practice for which the standards are developed, they are voluntary, and they surpass minimums. Standards for the practice of pharmacy in hospitals and health systems are developed by the American Society of Health-System Pharmacists,[2] and are termed *Best Practices*.

The details of accreditation, regulation, and practice standards are beyond the scope of this chapter, so they are discussed in greater detail in Chapter 3: Key Legal and Regulatory Issues in Institutional Pharmacy Practice. The important thing to recognize is that hospitals and health systems are highly regulated organizations that can be subjected to voluntary accreditation and are always subjected to regulatory oversight.

Importance of Pharmacy Leadership

Possessing good leadership skills and providing leadership is important for virtually all pharmacist roles, but it is especially crucial for those individuals responsible for the oversight of pharmacy services. This includes the primary pharmacist in charge and other pharmacy managers who have responsibility for specific aspects of pharmacy services.

The primary pharmacist in charge, usually referred to as the Director of Pharmacy, has ultimate responsibility and accountability for all aspects of the pharmacy service. This includes the safety of medication use, quality of drug information provided, financial budgeting and management, human resources, drug procurement, technology implementation, education and qualifications of their staff, regulatory compliance and adherence to accreditation standards.[11,12] The quality of services depends on strong leadership in these types of positions, as well as the advancement of pharmacy practice.

Summary

The practice of pharmacy in the institutional setting, namely, hospitals and health systems, is a unique and diverse setting that requires pharmacists to have skills and expertise beyond which are generally gained through pharmacy education. However, the nature and diversity of the institutional pharmacy environment present opportunities for pharmacists to provide patient-care services as integrated members of the health-care team. The integrated health-system model by which acute care, ambulatory care, long-term care, home care, and other patient-care settings are integrated under one organization provide additional opportunities to create an interconnected continuum of care in which all health-care providers have information about the patient from all other settings in which care was provided. Having access to patient information throughout the continuum of care creates opportunities to streamline and improve care, and minimizes the potential for medication errors and other adverse events.

The practice model in pharmacy continues to evolve, as do the skills required to manage complex medication therapies. Many changes have occurred over the past 20 years that have positioned pharmacists who work in hospital and health-system settings as the medication therapy and medication-use system experts. This recognition of the

Key Point . . .

The quality of pharmacy services depends on strong leadership.

. . . So what?

Good leadership can make the difference between excellent pharmaceutical care and that which is deficient. Institutions need pharmacists to take both formal and informal leadership roles within hospitals and other practice settings.

pharmacist as an integral member of the patient-care team brings the pharmacy profession closer to a patient-centric practice model.

Suggested Reading

English DE, II. Removing the self-imposed labels of pharmacists. *Am J Health-Syst Pharm*. 2008;65:2153-2155.

Joint Commission Report: Health Care at the Crossroads: Guiding Principles for the Development of the Hospital of the Future. January 2008. Available at: http://www.jointcommission.org/NR/rdonlyres/1C9A7079-7A29-4658-B80D-A7D-F8771309B/0/Hosptal_Future.pdf. Accessed June 4, 2009.

References

1. Fast Facts on U.S. Hospitals. American Hospital Association. Chicago, IL. Available at: http://www.aha.org/aha/resource-center/Statistics-and-Studies/fast-facts.html. Accessed January 2, 2010.

2. Best Practices for Hospital and Health-System Pharmacy. ASHP Policy 0905. Bethesda, MD: American Society of Health-System Pharmacists. Available at: http://www.ashp.org/DocLibrary/BestPractices/HRPositions09.aspx Accessed November 27, 2009.

3. Pedersen CA, Schneider PJ, Scheckelhoff DJ. ASHP national survey of pharmacy practice in hospital settings: Dispensing and administration 2008. *Am J Health-Syst Pharm*. 2009; 66:926-946.

4. Leape LL, Bates DW, Cullen DJ, Cooper J, Demonaco HJ, Gallivan T, et al. Systems analysis of adverse drug events: ADE prevention study group. *JAMA*. 1995 July 5; 274(1):35-43.

5. Breland B. Believing what we know: Pharmacy provides value. *Am J Health-Syst Pharm*. 2007;64:1284-1291.

6. Woods TM. Practice model challenge. *Am J Health-Syst Pharm*. 2009;66:1167.

7. Abramowitz PW. The evolution and metamorphosis of the pharmacy practice model. *Am J Health-Syst Pharm*. 2009;66:1437-1446.

8. Bjornson DC, Hiner WO, Jr., Potyk RP, Nelson BA, Lombardo FA, Morton TA, Larson LV, Martin BP, Sikora RG, Cammarata FA. Effect of pharmacists on health care outcomes in hospitalized patients. *Am J Health-Syst Pharm*. Sep 1993;50:1875-1884.

9. Pedersen CA, Schneider PJ, Scheckelhoff DJ. ASHP national survey of pharmacy practice in hospital settings: monitoring and patient education—2006. *Am J Health-Syst Pharm*. 2007;64(5):507-520.

10. ASHP Statement on Pharmacy Services to the Emergency Department. *Am J Health-Syst Pharm*. 2008;65:2380-2383.

11. Ivey MF. Rationale for having a chief pharmacy officer in a health care organization. *Am J Health-Syst Pharm*. May 2005;62:975-978.

12. ASHP Statement on the Roles and Responsibilities of the Pharmacy Executive. Available at: http://www.ashp.org/DocLibrary/BestPractices/Mgmt_St_Exec.aspx Accessed June 23, 2009.

Chapter Review Questions

1. **Which of the following are NOT steps in the medication-use process?**
   a. Transcribing
   b. Diagnosis
   c. Monitoring
   d. Dispensing
   e. Prescribing

   Answer: b. Diagnosis. Diagnosing illnesses and injuries is the one of the primary tasks of physicians. It falls outside of the pharmacist's responsibility, although some pharmacists are involved in some diagnosis of minor illnesses as part of collaborative practice plans. The medication-use process describes all steps involved in the use of medications in inpatients, including prescribing, transcribing, dispensing, administration, and monitoring. It is important that the pharmacist be involved in assuring the safety and quality of each step.

2. **The pharmacy practice model is one where pharmacists are chiefly involved in clinical activities associated with medical teams on the nursing units.**
   a. True
   b. False

   Answer: b. False. There is no single pharmacy practice model. A practice model can be defined as the "operational structure that defines how and where pharmacists practice, including the type of drug distribution system used, the layout and design of the department, how pharmacists spend their time, practice functions, and practice priorities." There are many practice models with the three predominant models consisting of the drug-distribution-centered model, the clinical-pharmacist-centered model, and the patient-centered integrated model.

3. **Which of the following key components influence the type of pharmacy practice model utilized in an institution?**
   a. The culture of the department
   b. The pharmacists working in the pharmacy
   c. The technicians
   d. Availability of automation and technology
   e. All of the above

   Answer: e. All of the above. Many different factors influence the type of pharmacy practice model in an institution. One important factor is the culture of the department and vision for practice, including the pharmacists role in providing direct patient care vs. distribution. Also, the role of pharmacy technicians in providing drug distribution is a key component. The use of automation and technology can impact the safety and efficiency of drug distribution and free up the pharmacist to provide direct patient care. The pharmacy's commitment to team based care can also be a factor in how the practice model is structured and how it functions.

4. **The practice of pharmacy in institutions consists of clinical pharmacists working alone to identify and resolve drug related problems within the drug use system.**
   a. True
   b. False

   Answer: b. False. Pharmacists need to work in teams to identify and resolve drug related problems. Working alone will not allow them to achieve their professional role. Team based care is based on the notion that members of the team are each responsible for patient care within their scope of practice and expertise. Teams are synergistic in that they allow the patient to benefit from their individual and collective skills in the most efficient way possible. The team concept has contributed to the pharmacist's clinical role through providing a portal for pharmacist recommendations on drug therapy and monitoring, and puts the pharmacist into daily contact with the patient.

5. **Describe the types of automation and technology commonly used in hospitals that support safe and effective medication use.**

Answer: Commonly used technologies include unit-based cabinets for medication dispensing, robotic dispensing systems, bar coded medication administration, smart pumps, and computerized prescriber order entry.

6. **The pharmacist role in an inpatient critical care unit differs from a general inpatient care unit because the acuity level is higher in a critical care unit.**
   a. True
   b. False

Answer: a. True. The pharmacist's role in a critical care unit is different than other settings because the patients are of a higher acuity level. Patients must be monitored closely and their drug therapy is often changed or adjusted. The pharmacist plays a crucial role in making sure that patients are receiving the right drugs, in the dose that is appropriate for their condition, and without error. The pharmacist usually participates in medical rounds with the rest of the health-care team, providing advice and information on drug therapy. After rounds, there are often follow-up on questions, and response to new treatment needs that arise throughout the day. The pharmacist's role in general inpatient care units is different from critical care patients primarily because the acuity of patients is less. Drug therapy is more likely to be stable and many times is a combination of oral and intravenous medications, depending on the patient's treatment regimen. The pharmacist may attend medical rounds with a health-care team, depending on the nature of the hospital (some smaller and community-based hospitals do not use traditional medical rounds with a team).

7. **Which of the following are developed by the pharmacy profession and imposed on pharmacy professionals voluntarily?**
   a. Regulations
   b. Policies and procedures
   c. Laws
   d. Practice standards
   e. None of the above

Answer: d. Practice standards. Practice standards or practice guidelines are those practices that a profession develops and imposes on itself. Practice standards should be based on the best scientific evidence, and should ideally strive to surpass minimum requirements established by law or regulation. Although elements of practice standards may be adopted or adapted into law or regulation, they are still considered different from laws and regulations due to the fact that they are developed by the profession that is engaged in the practice for which the standards are developed, they are voluntary, and they surpass minimums. Standards for the practice of pharmacy in hospitals and health systems are developed by the American Society of Health-System Pharmacists,[1] and are termed *Best Practices*.

8. **Who usually has ultimate responsibility and authority for all aspects of a pharmacy service?**
   a. The chief executive officer of the institution

b. The pharmacy staff

c. The medical staff

d. The institution's board of directors

e. The director of pharmacy

Answer: e. The director of pharmacy. The director of pharmacy has ultimate responsibility and accountability for the pharmacy service. This includes the safety of medication use, quality of drug information provided, financial budgeting and management, human resources, drug procurement, technology implementation, education and qualifications of their staff, regulatory compliance and adherence to accreditation standards.

9. **The difference between a "for-profit hospital" and a "non-profit hospital" is that non-profit hospitals do not make any money.**

a. True

b. False

Answer: b. False. Non-profit hospitals bring in a lot of revenue, often exceeding their expenses by a healthy margin. In reality, for-profit hospitals are differentiated from nonprofit hospitals by their ownership. For-profit hospitals are owned by corporations or groups of private investors. They differ from non-profit hospitals which do not seek a return on investment for owners. Nonprofit hospitals often operate under religious, volunteer, community, or other voluntary patronage. Any additional revenue generated after expenses is put back into the hospital.

10. **What are some of the traditional and non-traditional roles of pharmacists in outpatient settings within institutional or health-system settings?**

Answer: The most common and most traditional role is within the outpatient dispensing pharmacy, similar to community pharmacies without general merchandise. There is a growing number of pharmacists, though, that practice in new areas. For example, pharmacists are increasingly working in emergency departments because of a growing recognition of the value they can provide in medication use. Another growing area of outpatient services includes ambulatory care clinics. Clinics may be general in nature (e.g. primary care, medication adherence) or specialized (e.g., anticoagulation, palliative care). Another unique outpatient care setting includes home health care. Home health care services, most specifically home infusion services, have evolved as a way for patients to be treated in a non-hospital setting, usually their home.

Chapter Discussion Questions

1. What is the current pharmacy practice model in most U.S. hospitals, and how will it change in the future? Why?

2. How do the roles of pharmacists and technicians differ?

3. In the future, will automation replace the pharmacist or enhance their practice?

4. Are practice and accreditation standards good or bad for pharmacy practice? Why?

CHAPTER 2

Overview of the History of Hospital Pharmacy in the United States

William A. Zellmer

■ ■ ■

Learning Objectives

After completing this chapter, readers will be able to:

1. Describe how hospital pharmacy developed in the U.S.
2. Analyze the forces that shaped the hospital pharmacy movement.
3. Use history to discuss challenges to the future of institutional practice.
4. Discuss how professional organizations such as ASHP advanced the practice of institutional pharmacy practice.
5. Define key terms associated with the history of hospital pharmacy.

Key Terms and Definitions

■ *Mirror to Hospital Pharmacy:* A publication documenting the state of pharmacy services in hospitals in the late 1950s.

■ **ASHP Hilton Head conference:** A conference of hospital pharmacy leaders and pharmacy educators conducted in 1985 in Hilton Head, South Carolina, that emerged with the idea that hospital pharmacies should function as clinical departments with the mission of fostering the appropriate use of medicines.

■ **Practice standard:** An authoritative advisory document, issued by an expert body, that offers advice on the minimum requirements or optimal method for addressing an important issue or problem. It does not typically have the force of law.

■ **Pharmacy and therapeutics (P&T) committee:** A committee of the medical staff of a hospital or health system with oversight for medication management. The committee establishes a formulary, assesses medication use, and makes recommendations on policies and procedures associated with medication management. It is made up of representatives of the medical staff, administration, pharmacy, nursing, and other parties interested in the medication use process; a pharmacist often serves as secretary of the committee.

■ **Full time equivalent:** A method for standardizing the number of full and part-time employees working in an institution. A full time employee working a 40 hour week is equal to one full-time equivalent (FTE) and an employ who works for 20 hours per week is equal to 0.5 FTEs.

■ **Formulary system:** A structure whereby the medical staff of a hospital or health system, working through the P&T committee, evaluates, appraises, and selects from among the drug products available those that are considered most useful in patient care. It is also the framework in which medication-use policies are established and implemented.

■ **Formulary:** A list of drugs approved for use within the hospital or health system by the P&T Committee.

■ ■ ■

Introduction

Hospitals and other institutional practice settings today offer immense opportunities for pharmacists who want to practice in an environment that draws on the full range of their professional education and training. It was not always so.

This chapter tells the story of how hospital pharmacy developed in this country, analyzes the forces that shaped the hospital pharmacy movement, and draws lessons from the changes in this area of pharmacy practice. The historical facets discussed here are highly selective, reflecting the author's judgment about the most important points to cover within the limits of one chapter.

Hospital Pharmacy's Nascence[a,1-4]

Pharmacists have been associated with hospitals as long as there have been hospitals in America. When the Pennsylvania Hospital (the first hospital in Colonial America) was established in 1752, Jonathan Roberts was appointed as its apothecary. At that time, medicine and pharmacy were commonly practiced together in the community, with drug preparation often the responsibility of a medical apprentice.[7]

However, hospital pharmacy practice in the United States never developed into a significant movement until the 1920s. Although there were important milestones before that era (including the pioneering hospital pharmacy practices of Charles Rice [1841–1901][5]—see Figure 2-1—and Martin Wilbert [1865–1916]), many factors kept hospital pharmacy at the fringes of the broader development of pharmacy practice and pharmacy education.[6]

For much of the nation's history, hospital pharmacists were rare because there were few hospitals. In 1800, with a population of 5 million, the nation had only two hospitals. Even by 1873, with a population of 43 million, the United States had only 178 hospitals with fewer than 50,000 beds.[2] This might have not been a bad thing, because

[a]Well-documented accounts of the development of hospital pharmacy practice in the United States were published by the American Society of Health-System Pharmacists (ASHP) in conjunction with anniversaries of its 1942 founding. Particularly noteworthy are the "decennial issue" of the Bulletin on the American Society of Hospital Pharmacists and articles that marked ASHP's 50th anniversary.(1–3) Readers who have an interest in more detail are encouraged to seek out those references and others. (4) This section of the chapter is based closely on reference 2.

Figure 2-1. Hospital Pharmacy Department, Bellevue Hospital, New York City, Late 1800s.[a]
Source: AJHP.

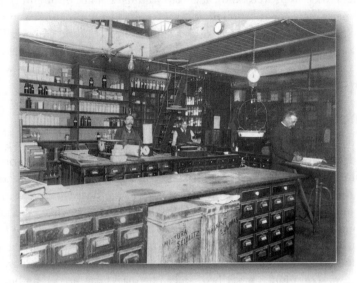

[a]The bulk medicine area, where medicines were packaged for use on the wards, at Bellevue Hospital, New York City, in the late 1800s. Standing on the right is Charles Rice, the eminent chief pharmacist at Bellevue, who headed three revisions of the United States Pharmacopeia.

hospitals were "places of dreaded impurity and exiled human wreckage" and physicians seldom had anything to do with them.[8] Hospitals played a small role in health care, and pharmacists played a very small role in hospitals.

1800s

In the early to mid-1800s, drug therapy consisted of strong cathartics, emetics, and diaphoretics. Clean air and good food rather than medicines were the treatments emphasized in hospitals. The medical elite avoided drug use or used newer alkaloidal drugs such as morphine, strychnine, and quinine. An organized pharmacy service was not seen as necessary in hospitals, except in the largest facilities. The situation changed somewhat during the Civil War when hospital directors sought out pharmacists for their experience in extemporaneous manufacturing and in purchasing medical goods.[2]

In the 1870s and 1880s, responding to the influx of immigrants, the number of hospitals in cities doubled. Most immigrants in this period were Roman Catholic, and they built Catholic hospitals. This

Key Point . . .

Catholic hospitals were important to the progress of hospital pharmacy because they charged patients a small fee (which allowed services to be improved), and they were willing to train, or obtain training for, nuns in pharmacy.

. . . So what?

It might surprise some students and young pharmacists of the critical importance of religious organizations in the progress of the pharmacy profession. Look at pictures of hospital pharmacy leaders in the 20th Century, and it will be common to see nuns prominent among that group.

was significant for two reasons—Catholic hospitals charged patients a small fee (which allowed services to be improved) and they were willing to train, or obtain training for, nuns in pharmacy. This era of hospital expansion coincided with reforms in nursing, development of germ theories, and the rise of scientific medicine and surgery. The general adoption of aseptic surgery in the 1890s made the hospital the center of medical care. Advances in surgery led to growth of community hospitals, most of which were small and relied on community pharmacies to supply medicines.[2]

Early 1900s

By the early twentieth century, hospitals had developed to the point of having more division of labor, more specialization in medical practice, a greater need for professional pharmaceutical services for handling complex therapies, and recognition that it was more economical to fill inpatient orders in-house. Hospital pharmacists retained the traditional role of compounding, which fostered a sense of camaraderie among them and an impetus to improve product quality and standardization. The advent of the hospital formulary concept persuaded many hospital leaders about the value of professional pharmaceutical services. An important reason for hiring a hospital pharmacist in the 1920s was Prohibition—alcohol was commonly prescribed, and a pharmacist was needed for both inventory control and to manufacture alcohol-containing preparations, which were expensive to obtain commercially.[2]

By the 1930s, pharmacy-related issues in hospitals had coalesced to the point that the American Hospital Association (AHA) created a Committee of Pharmacy to analyze the problems and make recommendations. The 1937 report of that committee was considered so seminal by hospital pharmacy leaders that even a decade later they saw value in republishing it.[9] The aim of the committee was to develop minimum standards for hospital pharmacy departments and to prepare a manual of pharmacy operations. The committee characterized pharmacy practices in hospitals at the time as "chaotic" and commented, "Few departments in hospital performance have been given less attention by and large than the hospital pharmacy." In the committee's view, "… any hospital larger than one hundred beds warrants the employment of a registered pharmacist…. Unregistered or incompetent service should not be countenanced, not only because of legal complications but to insure absolute safety to the patient."[9] The proliferation of unapproved and proprietary drug products in hospitals was the target of extensive criticism by the committee.

> **Key Point . . .**
>
> It was not until the 1930s that hospital leaders explicitly recognized the need for pharmacy services.
>
> **. . . So what?**
>
> Pharmacy may have a long history, but it was only 80 years ago that hospital leaders recognized a need for pharmacists.

A 50-Year Perspective

There is much that can be learned by comparing contemporary hospital pharmacy with practice of 50 years ago. Fifty years is a comprehensible period of time for most people and, in hospital pharmacy's case, the past half century was a period of astonishing advancement.

The data sources for making such a comparison are remarkably good. A major study of hospital pharmacy was conducted between 1957 and 1960—the Audit of Pharmaceutical Services in Hospitals—and published in a book, *Mirror to Hospital Pharmacy,* which remains a reference of monumental importance.[10] In more recent times, ASHP has documented the progress of health systems pharmacy through its annual surveys of hospital practice, yielding contemporary data for comparison with the figures of an earlier era.

Four major themes emerge from an examination of changes over this period:

1. Hospitals have recognized universally that pharmacists must be in charge of drug product acquisition, distribution, and control.
2. Hospital pharmacy departments have assumed a major role in patient safety.
3. Hospital pharmacy departments have assumed a major role in promoting rational drug therapy.
4. Hospital pharmacy departments have come to see their mission as fostering optimal patient outcomes from medication use.

It is important to keep in mind what was happening over this 50- to 60-year period in the United States as a whole. Since 1950, the U.S. population has grown 86%. Expenditures for health care services have grown from about 5% of gross domestic product to 14%. This growth has fostered an endless stream of public and private initiatives to curtail health care spending. Average daily hospital census, on a per-population basis, has declined by 24% during this period as a result of public and private initiatives to reduce hospital use. Nonfederal, short-term general hospitals in 1950 numbered 5,031 and rose to a zenith of 5,979 in 1975; in 2003 the number stood at 4,918, nearly 18% fewer than the peak of three decades before. On a per-capita basis, the number of inpatient hospital beds has declined 65% since 1950. Since 1965 (the first year AHA reported these data), hospital outpatient visits have increased more than fourfold.[11]

Drug Product Acquisition, Distribution, and Control

Sixty to seventy years ago, pharmaceutical services were of marginal importance to hospitals. The 1949 hospital standards of the American College of Surgeons had only three questions related to pharmacy in its point-rating system, and responses to those questions contributed only 10% to the overall rating. Pharmacy was perceived as a complementary service department, not as an essential service.[12]

Fewer than half the hospital beds in the nation (47%) in the late 1950s were located in facilities that had the services of a full-time pharmacist.[10] Fewer than 4 out of 10 hospitals (39%) had the services of a pharmacist. Hospital size was an important determinant of the availability of a pharmacist. All larger short-term institutions—those with 300 beds or more—employed a full-time pharmacist. This performance declined sharply with

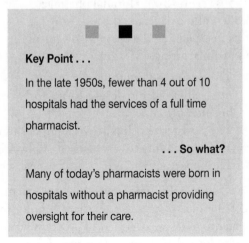

Key Point . . .

In the late 1950s, fewer than 4 out of 10 hospitals had the services of a full time pharmacist.

. . . So what?

Many of today's pharmacists were born in hospitals without a pharmacist providing oversight for their care.

decreasing hospital size—for hospitals of 200–299 beds, 96% employed pharmacists; 100–199 beds, 72%; 50–99 beds, 18%; and under 50 beds, 3.5%.

Today, the vast majority of hospitals in the United States have the services of one or more pharmacists. Important exceptions are small rural hospitals that still rely on the services of local community pharmacists. About 7% of the nation's hospitals have fewer than 25 beds; it is not known how many of them employ a pharmacist.

In 1957, the total number of hospital pharmacists was 4,850 full time and about 1,000 part-time.[10] Today, there are about 50,000 **full-time equivalent (FTE)** pharmacists providing inpatient services in nonfederal short-term hospitals.[13] (Hospitals employ an equal number of pharmacy technicians.) About one fourth of all actively practicing pharmacists in the U.S. today are in hospitals.

Today's hospitals employ approximately thirteen FTE pharmacists per 100 occupied beds.[13] The comparable figure for 1957 was approximately 0.4 FTE pharmacists per 100 occupied beds. In other words, pharmacist staffing in hospitals is 30-fold more intensive today. During the same interval, the intensity of hospital staffing as a whole increased approximately sevenfold.[11] Reflective of more intensified pharmacist staffing, many hospitals offer 24-hour inpatient pharmacy services.[13]

In the middle of the 20th century, nurses and community pharmacists—not hospital pharmacists—were responsible for hospital drug product acquisition, distribution, and control in many hospitals. At the time, *Mirror to Hospital Pharmacy* estimated that 4,000 nurses were engaged in pharmacy work. In 1957, drug product control in many hospitals was the realm of non-pharmacists (generally nurses) sometimes assisted by community pharmacists.

Two types of services—bulk compounding and sterile solution manufacturing—were a major element of the hospital pharmacists' professional identity in the 1950s (Figure 2-2). Hospital pharmacy leaders of the day cited the following factors in explaining the heavy involvement in manufacturing:

■ The unsuitability of many commercially available dosage forms for hospital use
■ The close relationship between physicians and pharmacists in hospitals
■ The opportunity to serve a need of physicians and patients
■ The opportunity to offer a professional service and build interprofessional relations[10]

Key Point . . .

Today, approximately one fourth of all actively practicing pharmacists in the U.S. work in hospitals.

. . . So what?

The public image of the pharmacist is one working in an independent or chain pharmacy in the community. The public is generally unaware of the large number of pharmacists providing innovative services in hospitals and other institutional settings.

Today, bulk compounding or manufacturing is no longer a significant activity in U.S. hospital pharmacies. In sharp contrast to 50 years ago, hospital pharmacists now prefer to purchase commercial products whenever they are available, in the interests of appropriate deployment of the workforce and of using products of standard commercial quality. Changes in the laws and regulations that govern drug product manufacturing

Figure 2-2. Sterile Solution Laboratory, Cardinal Glennon Memorial Hospital for Children, St. Louis, Missouri, circa 1950s.[a] *Source:* ASHP Archives.

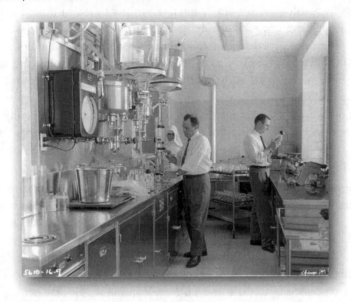

[a]Production of distilled water and the manufacture of large-volume sterile solutions were major pharmacy activities in medium and large hospitals in the 1950s and 1960s.

and distribution, the development of a well-regulated generic pharmaceutical industry, and a shift in the perceived mission of pharmacy practice were among the factors that led to the relegation of manufacturing to hospital pharmacy's past.

In summary, from mid-twentieth century to today, hospital pharmacy in the United States moved from an optional service to an essential service. It used to be that the administrator, the physicians, and the nurses in many institutions, especially smaller facilities, believed that they could function adequately with a drug room controlled by nurses. Today it is beyond question by anyone in the hospital field that medications need to be controlled by a pharmacy department that is managed by qualified pharmacists. Moreover, as pharmacists have become firmly established in hospitals, they have been recognized for their expertise beyond drug acquisition, distribution, and control functions, which has led to greatly intensified pharmacy staffing. The growing opportunities in hospitals have attracted more practitioners to the field, which has made hospital practice a major sector of the profession.

> ## Key Point . . .
>
> From the mid-twentieth century to today, hospital pharmacy in the United States has moved from an optional service to an essential service.
>
> ### . . . So what?
>
> Over the years, pharmacists have identified opportunities in health care institutions and carved out roles in managing the medication use process. This has taken leadership, hard work, building strong professional relationships, and caring for the patient.

Patient Safety

The clarion call to professionalism in hospital pharmacy in recent times has been the patient safety imperative. Hospital pharmacists have made immense progress in this arena. Initially, that progress was tied to greater accuracy in dispensing and administration of medications, but it has evolved to also focus on improving prescribing and monitoring the results of therapy. But it all started with a desire to improve drug product distribution for inpatients.

In 1957, drug products were distributed to hospital inpatients using floor stock or patient prescription systems.[10] See chapter 7 for more information on these distribution systems. The authors of the *Mirror to Hospital Pharmacy* highlighted a critical limitation of medication systems of that era:

> From the viewpoint of patient safety, one of the major advances in dispensing procedures would be the interpretation by the pharmacist of the physician's original ... order for the patient. In many hospitals, the pharmacist never sees the physician's original order. In cases where the physician does write an original prescription, he does so only for a limited number of drugs, the other drugs being stock items on the nursing units. In many cases the pharmacist receives only an order transcribed by a nurse or even more commonly by a lay person such as a ward clerk. As a result, errors made by the prescribing physician and errors made in transcribing his orders often go undetected, while the patient receives the wrong drug, the wrong dosage form, or wrong amount of the drug, or is given the drug by injection when oral administration was intended, and vice versa.[14]

Concerns about medication errors and about overall efficiencies and best use of hospital personnel led to the development of improved drug distribution systems.[15] Studies of unit dose drug distribution using centralized and decentralized systems (see Chapter 7 for more information on these distribution systems) were conducted that documented important benefits to unit dose drug distribution, including greater nursing efficiency, better use of the pharmacist's talents, cost savings, and improved patient safety.[16,17]

The key elements of unit dose drug distribution, as the system has evolved from the original studies, are as follows:

1. The pharmacist receives the physician's original order or a direct copy of the order.
2. A pharmacist reviews the medication order before the first dose is dispensed.
3. Medications are contained in single-unit packaging.
4. Medications are dispensed in as ready-to-administer form as possible.
5. Not more than a 24-hour supply of doses is delivered or available at the patient-care area at any time.
6. A patient medication profile is concurrently maintained for each patient.[18]

These precepts for state-of-the-art drug distribution are met widely in U.S. hospitals today.[19]

There has been much debate in hospital pharmacy over the years about the virtues of centralized versus decentralized drug distribution. In centralized systems, preparation and distribution of medications is more efficient—making it easier to do more with less when dispensing drugs to patients. In decentralized systems, pharmacists come in contact more regularly with physicians, nurses, and patients and are in a better position to influence the entire medication-use process, which is consistent with contemporary views about how the profession should be practiced. Among all hospitals, approximately one-fourth use a decentralized system.[19]

U.S. hospitals have shown a remarkable rate of adoption of point-of-use automated storage and distribution devices. Eighty-three percent of hospitals use automated dispensing cabinets, 10.1% use robots for dispensing, and 12.7% use carousel systems to manage inventory.[19]

There is immense interest in U.S. hospitals in applying computer technology to improve the safety of medication prescribing, dispensing, and administration, although adoption has been slow. Nearly half of hospitals have components of an electronic medical record (EMR) but only 5.9% of hospitals are fully digital (without paper records).[19] An estimated 12.0% of hospitals use computerized prescriber-order-entry systems with decision support, 24.1% use bar-code medication administration, and 44.0% use intelligent infusion devices (smart pumps).[19] However, many of these technologies are not optimally configured, and hospitals have yet to fully realize the benefits of these technologies.[19]

Because of the concerns of groups such as the Institute of Medicine and various federal agencies, improving patient safety is now a major national priority.[21] Since that general interest in patient safety embraces medication-use safety, hospital pharmacists have cheered and felt "it's about time!" Further breakthrough advances in medication-use safety will depend on a fundamental reengineering of the entire medication-use process, a shift toward a true team culture in providing care, and wider application of computer technology.[22] As new technologies or new patterns of health professional behavior evolve, history suggests that hospital pharmacists will be at the leading edge of those advances.

Promoting Rational Drug Use

In U.S. hospitals, the concept of a **pharmacy and therapeutics (P&T) committee**, as a formal mechanism for the pharmacy department and the medical staff to communicate on drug-use issues, was first promulgated in 1936 by Edward Spease (dean of the School of Pharmacy at Western Reserve University) and Robert Porter (chief pharmacist at the University's hospitals).[23] Subsequently, the American Hospital Association and the American Society of Hospital Pharmacists jointly developed guidance on the P&T committee and on the operation of a hospital formulary system. The **formulary system** is a method whereby the medical staff of a hospital, working through the P&T committee, evaluates, appraises, and selects from among the drug products available those that are considered most useful in patient care. The formulary system is also the framework in which a hospital's medication-use policies are established and implemented.

A major imperative for the advocates of the formulary system in the mid-1900s was to manage the proliferation of drug products. In just one year, 1951, the number of market entries consisted of 332 new drug products, 35 new drug entities, 74 duplications of drug entities, and 221 combination products.[24] In 1957, slightly more than half of all hospitals operated under the formulary system.[10] Today, essentially all hospitals do so.[13] In 1957, 58% of hospitals had an active P&T committee, and a similar percentage of hospitals had a **formulary** or approved drug list. However, about one fourth of the P&T committees were inactive.[10] Today, nearly all hospitals in the U.S. have an active P&T committee that meets an average of seven times a year.[13]

In the late 1950s, the functions of P&T committees focused on very basic activities such as delegating to the chief pharmacist responsibility for preparing product specifications and selecting sources of supply (66% of committees) and approving drugs by nonproprietary name (50%).[10] In most hospitals today, the P&T committee has authorized pharmacists to track and assess adverse drug events (ADEs), conduct retrospective drug-use evaluations, and identify and monitor patients on high-risk therapies.[13]

In summary, concepts first advanced in the 1930s regarding a formal communications linkage between the hospital pharmacy department and the medical staff with respect to drug-use policy have taken hold firmly. Hospital pharmacists are heavily engaged in helping the medical staff establish drug-use policies, in implementing those policies, in monitoring compliance with those policies, and in taking corrective action. The invention of the pharmacy and therapeutics committee and the hospital formulary system has facilitated the deep involvement of pharmacists in promoting rational drug use in hospitals.

Key Point . . .

The invention of the pharmacy and therapeutics committee and the hospital formulary system has facilitated the deep involvement of pharmacists in promoting rational drug use in hospitals.

. . . So what?

The pharmacist's role on the pharmacy and therapeutics committee has allowed pharmacists to build their professional standing in institutions. If they had never accepted leadership in establishing and maintaining these committees, their influence might have been diminished.

Fostering Optimal Patient Outcomes

U.S. hospital pharmacists have evolved markedly in their self-concept over the past 50 years. As recently as 20 years ago, the traditional pharmacist mission prevailed, a mission that was captured in the words, *right drug, right patient, right time,* connoting a drug-product-handling function. *Right drug* in this context meant whatever the physician ordered. Today's philosophy about the mission of pharmacists focuses on achieving optimal outcomes from medication use. The overarching question for the hospital pharmacist is whether the right drug is being used in the first place. A popular phrase used to summarize this philosophy is, "The mission of pharmacists is to help people make the best use of medicines." These words reflect a profound paradigm shift with respect to the primary purpose of pharmacy practice.[25,26]

In the 1950s, hospital pharmacy's Spartan staffing levels did not leave much time for work beyond the basics of acquiring, storing, compounding, and distributing medications. Nevertheless, chief pharmacists of the time were called upon frequently by physicians and nurses to answer drug information questions related to dosage, dosage forms, and pharmacology. Somewhat less frequently, pharmacists were asked for advice on adverse drug reactions and clinical comparisons of products. In analyzing pharmacist consultations, the authors of the *Mirror to Hospital Pharmacy* suggested that both weakness in the pharmacist's scientific knowledge and lack of time contributed to limited progress in this realm.

The transformation of the hospital pharmacy department from a product orientation to a clinical orientation was stimulated by active consensus-building efforts by hospital pharmacy leaders. One important example of such efforts was the ASHP Hilton Head conference.[25]

Hilton Head refers to a consensus-seeking invitational conference conducted in 1985 in Hilton Head, South Carolina, officially designated as an invitational conference on Directions for Clinical Practice in Pharmacy. The purpose of the meeting was to assess the progress of hospital pharmacy departments in implementing clinical pharmacy. What emerged from the event was the idea that clinical pharmacy should not be thought of as something separate from pharmacy practice as a whole. Rather, hospital pharmacies should function as clinical departments with a mission of fostering the appropriate use of medicines. This was a very important idea because most hospital pharmacists thought in terms of adding discrete clinical services (such as pharmacokinetic monitoring) rather than conceptualizing the totality of the department's work as a clinical enterprise.

Working through its affiliated state societies, ASHP supported repetitions of the conference on a regional basis. ASHP leaders spoke at meetings around the country about the ideas of Hilton Head, and the *American Journal of Hospital Pharmacy* published numerous papers on the subject.

As a result, many individual pharmacy departments began to hold retreats of their staffs to reassess the fundamental mission of their work. It was common for departments to adopt mission statements that, for the first time, framed their work not in terms of drug distribution but in terms of achieving optimal patient outcomes from the use of medicines. They were supported by a growing body of scientific evidence, published in both the medical and pharmacy literature, about the positive outcomes achieved through pharmacist involvement in direct patient care.[27-30]

In summary, U.S. hospital pharmacists today are engaged in extensive clinical activity, which is a major change from practice of 50 years ago. We are not yet at the point where a majority of hospital patients who are on medication therapy receive the benefit of clinical oversight by the pharmacist, but progress in this direction continues to be made.

Key Point . . .

After the Hilton Head conference, hospital pharmacy departments began to frame their work not in terms of drug distribution but in terms of achieving optimal patient outcomes from the use of medicines.

. . . So what?

The Hilton Head Conference changed the practice model in institutions away from the process of drug distribution to a system of care that attempts to achieve optimal health outcomes. Many of the profession's initiatives in hospital practice have their origin in this conference.

Recap of Major Themes

Thus we have a picture of the major thrust of changes in hospital pharmacy over the past 50 years. The four major themes have been, first, the universal recognition by hospitals that pharmacists must be in charge of drug product acquisition, distribution, and control; second, hospital pharmacy departments have assumed a major role in patient safety; third, pharmacy departments have assumed a major role in promoting rational drug therapy; and, finally, pharmacy departments have defined their mission in terms of optimal patient outcomes from medication use. Taken together, these changes signify that pharmacy practice in U.S. hospitals over the past 50 years has become more intensive in its professional staffing, more directly focused on patient care, and more directly influential on the quality and outcome of patient care. In short, hospital pharmacy has been transformed from a marginal, optional activity into a vital profession contributing immensely to the health and well being of patients and to the stability of the institutions that employ them.

Explaining the Transformation

A combination of indirect and direct factors helps explain this transformation in hospital pharmacy. Indirect factors are those forces external to hospital pharmacy that fostered development of the field. These factors include the following:

- Shift of national resources into health care, especially hospital care (stimulated immensely by implementation of Medicare in 1965 and expansion of other health insurance coverage)
- Expanded clinical research and drug product development
- Greater complexity and cost of drug therapy accompanied by sophisticated pharmaceutical product marketing
- Growing interest in improving the quality of health care services

More important for this chapter's discussion are the internal factors within hospital pharmacy that precipitated the changes discussed above. In this category, five points merit discussion:

1. Visionary leadership
2. Professional associations
3. Pharmacy education
4. Postgraduate residency education and training
5. Practice standards

Visionary Leadership

One cannot read the early literature of hospital pharmacy in the U.S. without being impressed by the clear articulation of an exciting, uplifting vision by that era's practice leaders. These views were being expressed at a time when pharmacy was a marginal profession in the U.S.; when most pharmacists were engaged primarily in retail, mercantile activities; when hospital pharmacy had little visibility and respect; and when hospital pharmacy was a refuge for pharmacists who preferred minimal interactions with the public. Out of this environment emerged a number of hospital pharmacists, many of them at university teaching hospitals, who expressed an inspiring vision about the development of hospital pharmacy and about the role of hospital pharmacy in elevating the status of pharmacy as a whole.

These were leaders such as Arthur Purdum, Edward Spease, Harvey A. K. Whitney, and Donald E. Francke (to mention only a few) who were familiar with the history of pharmacy and had a sense of pharmacy's unfulfilled potential. Many of them had seen European pharmacy firsthand and decried the immense gap in professional status and scope of practice between the two continents.

A sense of the deep feelings of these leaders may be gained from the following comment by Edward Spease, a retired pharmacy dean speaking in 1952 about his initial exploration of hospital pharmacy 40 years earlier:

I expected to see true professional pharmacy in hospitals and was much disappointed that it did not exist there. The more I observed and heard about the growing tendency towards commercialism in drugstores, the more I felt that if professional pharmacy was to exist, let alone grow to an ideal state, it would have to be in the hospital where the health professions were trained.... Good pharmacy is as important in hospitals away from teaching centers as it is in the teaching and research hospital. It can be developed to a high degree of perfection there, too, *if the pharmacist can get the picture in his mind.*[31]

"...if the pharmacist can get the picture in his mind." Those are key words that reflect that early hospital pharmacy leaders were trying to create a new model for pharmacy practice in hospitals and not allow this practice setting to become an extension of the type of practice that prevailed in community pharmacies. These leaders were change agents with a missionary zeal, and they were blessed with the ability to infect others with their passion.

It is noteworthy that the *Mirror to Hospital Pharmacy* framed the entire Audit project in the context of professional advancement. The report laid out the essential characteristics of a profession and articulated goals for hospital pharmacy that would bring pharmacy as a whole into better alignment with those characteristics.

Professional Associations

The national organization of hospital pharmacists—American Society of Health-System Pharmacists (ASHP)—has had a profound effect on the advancement of the field. The visionary hospital pharmacists of the early 1900s focused much of their energies on the creation of an organizational structure for hospital pharmacy. One landmark event was the creation of the Hospital Pharmacy Association of Southern California in 1925. On a national level, organizational efforts were funneled through the American Pharmaceutical Association (APhA), the oldest national pharmacist organization in the country. For years, hospital pharmacists participated in various committee activities of APhA focused on their particular interest. Then, in 1936, a formal APhA subsection on hospital pharmacy was created. This modest achievement evolved to the creation of ASHP in 1942 as an independent organization affiliated with APhA.[32]

There are two essential things that ASHP has done for the advancement of hospital pharmacy. One is to serve as a vehicle for the nurturing, expression, and actualization of the professional ideals and aspirations of hospital pharmacists. In its early years, ASHP conducted a series of educational institutes that were very influential in enhancing

Key Point . . .

One cannot read the early literature of hospital pharmacy in the U.S. without being impressed by the clear articulation of an exciting, uplifting vision by that era's practice leaders.

. . . So what?

Hospital pharmacy has not always been the way it is now. It was built by pharmacists who led change in practice. In order for institutional pharmacy practice to thrive in the future, pharmacy students and newly graduated pharmacists will need to accept leadership positions vacated by pharmacy leaders who retire or leave the profession for other opportunities. They will need to provide a new vision for the profession for the 21st Century.

knowledge and skills and in building esprit de corps among hospital pharmacists.[33] Also noteworthy, especially as the organization has grown in size and diversity, is ASHP's efforts to develop consensus about the direction of practice.[25,26]

The second essential act of ASHP has been its creations of resources to assist practitioners in fostering the development of hospital pharmacy practice. One example is the *AHFS Drug Information* reference book (and, in recent times, electronic versions for central information systems, desktop computers, and handheld devices), which is widely used independent source of drug information in U.S. hospitals. Another example is the *American Journal of Health-System Pharmacy*. These two publications, and other ASHP activities such as the Midyear Clinical Meeting, have produced a source of funds beyond membership dues that ASHP has used to develop a broad array of services that help members advance practice.

The original objectives of ASHP were as follows:

- Establish minimum standards of pharmaceutical service in hospitals
- Ensure an adequate supply of qualified hospital pharmacists by providing standardized hospital pharmacy training for 4-year pharmacy graduates
- Arrange for interchange of information among hospital pharmacists
- Aid the medical profession in the economic and rational use of medicines

The core strengths of ASHP today are as follows:

- Practice standards and professional policy
- Advocacy (government affairs and public relations)
- Residency and technician training accreditation
- Drug information
- Practitioner education
- Publications and communications

One of the reasons for ASHP's success has been its clarity about objectives and its concentrated focus on a limited number of goals. It is a testament to the wisdom of ASHP's early leaders that the goals expressed in 1942 still serve to guide the organization, although different words are used today to express the same ideas, and some other points have been added. The organization continues as a powerful force in the ongoing efforts to align pharmacists with the needs that patients, health professionals, and administrators in hospitals have related to the appropriate use of medicines.

Pharmacy Education

There are three important points about the role of pharmacy education in transforming hospital pharmacy. First, as pharmacy education as a whole has been upgraded over the years, hospital pharmacy has benefited by gaining practitioners who are better educated and better prepared to meet the demands in hospital practice. Second, hospital pharmacy leaders have put considerable pressure on pharmacy educators to upgrade the pharmacy curriculum, to make it more consistent with the needs in hospital practice. This is significant because practice demands have always been far more intense in hospitals than in community pharmacy, so pressure to meet the demands in hospitals served to elevate education for all pharmacists. Also, beginning in the 1970s, corresponding with increased emphasis on clinical pharmacy in the curriculum, hospital pharmacies played a much larger role in pharmacy education as clerkship rotation sites for pharmacy students. Third, in the early days of clinical education, faculty members from schools of pharmacy began establishing practice sites in hospitals, which often had a large impact on the nature of the hospital's pharmacy service.

Table 2-1 shows how the minimum requirements for pharmacy education have evolved over the years. It took a very long time for pharmacy in the U.S. to settle on the Pharm.D. as the sole degree for pharmacy practice. Many bitter fights—between educators, between practitioners, among educators and practitioners, and among educators and the retail employers of pharmacists—occurred over this issue. Now that the matter is settled, everyone seems to be moving on with the intention of making the best application of the pharmacist's excellent education.

Over the past 20 years, pharmacy education in the U.S. has been transformed completely from teaching primarily about the science of drug products to teaching primarily about the science of drug therapy. Transformation of hospital pharmacy practice from a product orientation to a patient orientation could not have occurred without this change in education.

Postgraduate Residency Education and Training

Stemming from its early concerns about the inadequacy of pharmacy education for hospital practice, ASHP leaders advocated internships in hospitals and worked for years to establish standards for such training. This led to the concept of residency training in hospital pharmacy and a related ASHP accreditation program.[33–35]

Early hospital pharmacy leaders noted the following imperatives for hospital pharmacy residency training[36]:

- Hospitals were expanding, thereby creating a growing unmet need for pharmacists who had been educated and trained in hospital pharmacy
- Pharmaceutical education was out of touch with the needs in hospital pharmacy
- The internship training required by state boards for licensure was not adequate preparation for a career in hospital pharmacy practice
- Hospital pharmacists required specialized training in manufacturing, sterile solutions, and pharmacy department administration
- Organized effort was needed to achieve improvements in hospital pharmacy internships or residencies

Table 2-1.

Evolution of Minimum Requirements for Pharmacist Education in the United States

Year	Minimum Requirement (Length of Curriculum and Degree Awarded)
1907	2 years (Graduate in Pharmacy)
1925	3 years (Graduate in Pharmacy or Pharmaceutical Chemist)
1932	4 years (B.S. or B.S. in Pharmacy)
1960	5 years (B.S. or B.S. in Pharmacy)[a]
2004	6 years (Pharm.D.)

[a]Transition period; some schools offered only the B.S. or the Pharm.D. degree; many schools offered both degrees, with the Pharm.D. considered an advanced degree.

There are well over 10,000 pharmacists in practice who have completed accredited residency training. These individuals have been trained as change agents and practice leaders. Early in their careers, they came to understand the complexity of hospital pharmacy, including inpatient operations, outpatient services, drug product technology and quality, and medication-use policy. Residency training is the height of mentorship in professionalism in American pharmacy. Dreams are fostered in residency training of the profession becoming an ever more vital force in health care; dreams of patients improving their health status more readily because pharmacists are there to help them.

Practice Standards

Numerous legal and quasi-legal requirements affect hospital pharmacy practice. On the legal end of the spectrum are various federal laws governing drug products and state practice acts governing how the pharmacist behaves and how pharmacies are operated. At the opposite end of the spectrum are voluntary practice standards promulgated by organizations such as ASHP.

A **practice standard** is an authoritative advisory document, issued by an expert body, that offers advice on the minimum requirements or optimal method for addressing an important issue or problem. A practice standard does not generally have the force of law. Methods used to foster compliance with practice standards include education and peer pressure. ASHP's practice standards have been very important in elevating hospital pharmacy in the United States.

The origins of hospital pharmacy practice standards go back to 1936 when the American College of Surgeons adopted the *Minimum Standard for Pharmacies in Hospitals*. This document was semi-dormant for a number of years, but it served as a rallying point for hospital pharmacists[3] and revision and promulgation of the Standard became a priority for ASHP.[37]

The revision pursued by ASHP in the 1940s specified the following minimum requirements:

- An organized pharmacy department under the direction of a professionally competent, legally qualified pharmacist
- Pharmacist authority to develop administrative policies for the department
- Development of professional policies for the department with the approval of the pharmacy and therapeutics committee
- Ample number of qualified personnel in the department
- Adequate facilities
- Expanded scope of pharmacist's responsibilities:
  - Maintain a drug information service
  - Nurse and physician teaching
  - File periodic progress reports with administrator
- P&T committee must establish a formulary

From this modest beginning, ASHP has developed more than 60 practice standards that deal with most aspects of hospital pharmacy operations and several major controversies in therapeutics.[38]

ASHP practice standards have been used effectively over the years as a lever for raising the quality of hospital pharmacy services. The standards have been used in the following ways:

- Requirements for pharmacy practice sites that conduct accredited residency programs
- Guidance to practitioners who desire to voluntarily comply with national standards
- Guidance to The Joint Commission, the major hospital-accreditation organization, in developing standards for pharmacy and the medication-use process
- Tools for pharmacy directors who are seeking administrative approval for practice changes
- Guidance to regulatory bodies and courts of law
- Guidance to curriculum committees of schools of pharmacy

Summary of Internal Factors

In summary, five internal factors have played a large role in transforming U.S. hospital pharmacy over the past 50 years: (1) visionary leadership, (2) a strong professional society, (3) reforms in pharmacy education, (4) residency training, and (5) practice standards. The common element among these forces has been dissatisfaction with the status quo and burning desire to bring hospital pharmacy in better alignment with the needs of patients and the needs of physicians, nurses, other health professionals, and administrators in hospitals.

Summary

From the author's perspective, colored to be sure by participation in the hospital pharmacy movement for many years, four tentative lessons may be drawn from the history of U.S. hospital pharmacy:

1. Fundamental change of complex endeavors requires leadership and time. Hospital pharmacists are sometimes frustrated by the slow pace of change. Wider study of history might help practitioners dissolve that discouragement.
2. It is important to engage as many practitioners as possible in assessing hospital pharmacy's problems and identifying solutions, so that a large number of individuals identify with the final plan and are committed to pursuing it.
3. It is critical to recognize and capitalize on changes in the environment that may make conditions more favorable to the advancement of hospital pharmacy. This requires curiosity about the world at large.
4. It is important to regularly and honestly assess progress and embark on a new approach if the existing plan for constructive change is not working or has run its course. This requires open-mindedness and a good sense of timing.

Today's challenges in hospital pharmacy are no more daunting than those that faced hospital pharmacy's leaders and innovators in the past. Fortunately, hospital pharmacy is imbued with a culture of taking stock, setting goals, making and executing plans, measuring results, and refining plans. If hospital pharmacy sticks to this time-tested formula, it will continue to be a beacon for the profession as a whole.

Suggested Reading

Francke DE, Latiolais CJ, Francke GN, et al. *Mirror to Hospital Pharmacy—A Report of the Audit of Pharmaceutical Services in Hospitals.* Washington: American Society of Hospital Pharmacists; 1964.

Higby G. American hospital pharmacy from the colonial period to the 1930s. *Am J Hosp Pharm.* 1994;51:2817-2823.

Williams WH. Pharmacists at America's first hospital, 1752–1841. *Am J Hosp Pharm.* 1976;33:804-807.

References

1. Niemeyer G, Berman A, Francke DE. Ten years of the American Society of Hospital Pharmacists, 1942–1952. *Bull Am Soc Hosp Pharm.* 1952;9:279-421.

2. Higby G. American hospital pharmacy from the colonial period to the 1930s. *Am J Hosp Pharm.* 1994;51:2817-2823.

3. Harris RR, McConnell WE. The American Society of Hospital Pharmacists: a history. *Am J Hosp Pharm.* 1993;50(suppl 2):S3-S45.

4. Berman A. Historical currents in American hospital pharmacy. *Drug Intell Clin Pharm.* 1972;6:441-447.

5. Wolfe HG. Charles Rice (1841–1901), an immigrant in pharmacy. *Am J Pharm Educ.* 1950;14:285-305.

6. Burkholder DF. Martin Inventius Wilbert (1865–1916): hospital pharmacist, historian, and scientist. *Am J Hosp Pharm.* 1968;25:330-343.

7. Williams WH. Pharmacists at America's first hospital, 1752–1841. *Am J Hosp Pharm.* 1976;33:804-807.

8. Starr P. The reconstitution of the hospital. In: Starr P. *The Social Transformation of American Medicine.* New York: Basic Books; 1982:145-179.

9. Hayhow EC, Amberg G, Dooley MS, et al. Report of committee on pharmacy, American Hospital Association, 1937. *Bull Am Soc Hosp Pharm.* 1948;5:89-96.

10. Francke DE, Latiolais CJ, Francke GN, et al. *Mirror to Hospital Pharmacy—A Report of the Audit of Pharmaceutical Services in Hospitals.* Washington: American Society of Hospital Pharmacists; 1964.

11. *AHA Hospital Statistics, 2005.* Chicago: Health Forum; 2005.

12. Purdum WA. Minimum standards and the future. *Bull Am Soc Hosp Pharm.* 1951;8:114-117.

13. Pedersen CA, Schneider PJ, Scheckelhoff DJ. ASHP national survey of pharmacy practice in hospital settings: Prescribing and transcribing—2007. *Am J Health Syst Pharm.* 2008 May 1;65(9):827-843.

14. Francke DE, Latiolais CJ, Francke GN, op. cit. p. 115.

15. Barker KN, McConnell WE. The problems of detecting medication errors in hospitals. *Am J Hosp Pharm.* 1962;19:361-369.

16. Barker KN, Heller WM. The development of a centralized unit dose dispensing system, part one: description of the UAMC experimental system. *Am J Hosp Pharm.* 1963;20:568-579.

17. Black HJ, Tester WW. Decentralized pharmacy operations utilizing the unit dose concept. *Am J Hosp Pharm.* 1964;21:344-350.

18. ASHP technical assistance bulletin on hospital drug distribution and control. *Am J Hosp Pharm.* 1980;37:1097-1103.

19. Pedersen CA, Schneider PJ, Scheckelhoff DJ. ASHP national survey of pharmacy practice in hospital settings: Dispensing and administration—2005. *Am J Health Syst Pharm.* 2006 February 15;63(4):327-345.

20. Holysko Sr, MN, Ravin RL. A pharmacy centralized intravenous additive service. *Am J Hosp Pharm.* 1965;22:266-271.

21. Committee on Quality of Health Care in America (Institute of Medicine). *Crossing the Quality Chasm: New Health System for the 21st Century.* Washington: National Academy Press; 2001.

22. Re-engineering the medication-use system—proceedings of a national interdisciplinary conference conducted by the Joint Commission of Pharmacy Practitioners. *Am J Health-Syst Pharm.* 2000;57:537-601.

23. Francke DE, Latiolais CJ, Francke GN, op. cit. p. 139.

24. Francke DE. Hospital pharmacy looks to the future. In: *Harvey A. K. Whitney Award Lectures (1950–2003).* Bethesda, MD: ASHP Research and Education Foundation; 2004:19-25.

25. Directions for clinical practice in pharmacy—proceedings of an invitational conference conducted by the ASHP Research and Education Foundation and the February 10–13, 1985, Hilton Head Island, South Carolina. *Am J Hosp Pharm.* 1985;42:1287-342.

26. Implementing pharmaceutical care. Proceedings of an invitational conference conducted by the American Society of Hospital Pharmacists and the ASHP Research and Education Foundation. *Am J Hosp Pharm.* 1993;50:1585-656.

27. Leape LL, Cullen DJ, Clapp MD, et al. Pharmacist participation on physician rounds and adverse drug events in the intensive care unit. *JAMA.* 1999;282:267-270.

28. Kucukarslan SN, Peters M, Mlynarek M, et al. Pharmacists on rounding teams reduce preventable adverse drug events in hospital general medicine units. *Arch Intern Med.* 2003;163:2014-2018.

29. Boyko WL, Yurkowski PJ, Ivey MF, et al. Pharmacist influence on economic and morbidity outcomes in a tertiary care teaching hospital. *Am J Health-Syst Pharm.* 1997;54:1591-1595.

30. Bjornson DC, Hiner WO, Potyk RP, et al. Effect of pharmacists on health care outcomes in hospitalized patients. *Am J Hosp Pharm.* 1993;1875-1884.

31. Spease E. Background to progress. *Bull Am Soc Hosp Pharm.* 1953;10:362-364.

32. Niemeyer G. Founding and growth. *Bull Am Soc Hosp Pharm.* 1952;9:299-338.

33. Niemeyer G. Education and training. *Bull Am Soc Hosp Pharm.* 1952;9:363-375.

34. Francke DE. Contributions of residency training to institutional pharmacy practice. *Am J Hosp Pharm.* 1967;24:193-203.

35. ASHP residency and accreditation information. Available at: http://www.ashp.org/rtp/index.cfm?cfid=4992632&CFToken=35717293. Accessed February 1, 2005.

36. Francke DE, Latiolais CJ, Francke GN, op. cit. p. 157-167.

37. Niemeyer G. Establishment of minimum standard. *Bull Am Soc Hosp Pharm.* 1952;9:339-346.

38. ASHP policy positions, statements, and guidelines. Available at: http://www.ashp.org/Import/PRACTICEANDPOLICY/PolicyPositionGuidelinesBestPractices.aspx Accessed June 9, 2009.

Chapter Review Questions

1. **When was the first hospital pharmacist employed in the U.S.?**
    a. 1752
    b. 1813
    c. 1854
    d. 1895

    Answer: a. 1752. In that year, Jonathan Roberts was appointed as the apothecary at the first hospital in Colonial America, the Pennsylvania Hospital.

2. **Which of the following events furthered the progression of hospital pharmacy in the U.S.?**
    a. An influx of immigrants in the late 1800s
    b. The Civil War
    c. Prohibition
    d. All of the above

    Answer: d. All of the above. All of these events led to changes in hospital pharmacy. The influx of immigrants to cities increased the number of Catholic hospitals and nuns trained as pharmacists. The Civil War increased the demand for pharmacists who could provide compounding and distribution expertise. Prohibition required pharmacists to provide greater oversight of alcohol-containing medical preparations.

3. **Hospital leaders explicitly recognized the need for pharmacy services in the:**
    a. 1920s
    b. 1930s

c. 1940s

d. 1950s

Answer: b. 1930s. In 1937, the American Hospital Association (AHA) created a Committee of Pharmacy which found that pharmacy practice at that time was "chaotic" and that "…any hospital larger than one hundred beds warrants the employment of a registered pharmacist…"

4. **Approximately what percent of U.S. pharmacists in practice today work in hospitals?**

   a. 5 percent

   b. 10 percent

   c. 15 percent

   d. 25 percent

   Answer: d. 25%. Today, there are about 50,000 pharmacists providing inpatient services in nonfederal short-term hospitals and an equal number of pharmacy technicians. That is approximately one fourth of all actively practicing pharmacists in the U.S.

5. **The majority of hospitals in the U.S. today are fully digital (without paper records).**

   a. True

   b. False

   Answer: b. False. Digitalization of medical records in the U.S. has a long way to go before the majority of hospitals are fully digital. Nearly half of hospitals have at least some component of an electronic medical record (EMR) on at least one unit of the hospital, but only 5.9% of hospitals are fully digital (without paper records) throughout the institution.

6. **Pharmacy and Therapeutics committees (P&T) are a relatively recent phenomenon in institutional pharmacy.**

   a. True

   b. False

   Answer: b. False. The first documented report of a pharmacy and therapeutics (P&T) committee was in 1936.

7. **The _____ conference was important to the progress of institutional pharmacy because leaders in the profession agreed that hospital pharmacies should function as clinical departments with a mission of fostering the appropriate use of medicines.**

   a. Miami Beach

   b. La Jolla

   c. Las Vegas

   d. Hilton Head

   Answer: d. Hilton Head. This consensus-seeking invitational conference was officially called the conference on Directions for Clinical Practice in Pharmacy. What emerged from the event was the idea that hospital pharmacy was a clinical enterprise focusing on the appropriate use of medicines.

8. **Which of the following is NOT a professional organization associated with institutional pharmacy practice?**
    a. ASHP
    b. ASCP
    c. NACDS
    d. All of the above pharmacy organizations represent pharmacists who are associated with institutions.

    Answer: c. NACDS. National Association of Chain Drug Stores represents retail chain pharmacists.

9. **Hospital pharmacists have a significant impact on the clinical and scientific focus of curricula in U.S. pharmacy schools.**
    a. True
    b. False

    Answer: a. True. Hospital pharmacy leaders have exerted pressure on pharmacy schools to train students for the needs of hospital practice. Hospital pharmacists have also influenced education by engaging in clerkship rotations with pharmacy students and teaching students in the classroom.

10. **_____ are advisory documents developed by pharmacists that offer advice on the minimum requirements or optimal method for addressing an important issue or problem in hospitals.**
    a. Practice standards
    b. Regulations
    c. Laws
    d. Reports

    Answer: a. Practice standards. A practice standard is an authoritative advisory document, issued by expert bodies within the profession, that offers advice on the minimum requirements or optimal method for addressing an important issue or problem. Practice standards do not generally have the force of law. They have been very important in elevating hospital pharmacy in the United States.

Chapter Discussion Questions

1. How do you respond to older pharmacists who talk longingly about the "good old days" of hospital pharmacy practice?
2. Speak to a hospital pharmacist who is about half-way through his or her career (i.e., graduating a minimum of 20 years ago). Identify all of the major advances that have occurred in institutional pharmacy practice (e.g., important drugs, medical conditions, technology) that have occurred since that person has graduated. Now, try to project the changes that will occur in the next 20 years of pharmacy practice.
3. Pharmacy leaders argue that pharmacists can no longer be a product (i.e., medication) centered profession. Does this mean that pharmacists should move to relinquish their responsibilities in drug product acquisition and distribution?
4. Compare the current state of community pharmacy practice with hospital pharmacy practice. What lessons can community pharmacists learn from the history of hospital pharmacy?

CHAPTER 3

Key Legal and Regulatory Issues in Health-System Pharmacy Practice

John P. Uselton, Lee B. Murdaugh, Patricia C. Kienle, and David A. Holdford

Learning Objectives

After completing this chapter, readers should be able to:

1. Explain the complementary roles of accreditation, regulation, practice standards, and health-system policies and procedures.
2. List key certifying and accrediting agencies of institutions and their purposes.
3. Describe key federal and state regulatory agencies of institutions.
4. Identify professional associations involved with health-system pharmacy practice issues.
5. Describe the role of health-system policies and procedures in health-system pharmacy practice.

Key Terms and Definitions

A number of terms are closely associated with health-system accreditation and pharmacy guidelines. Many are defined in context in the chapter; others are defined here. Definitions of some terms vary or are evolving.

- **Accrediting body:** An organization or entity that establishes standards for accreditation and determines that a health care organization complies with the standards.
- **Certification:** Confirmation by an entity that an organization complies with the entity's predetermined standards.
- **Certifying body:** An organization or entity that establishes standards for certification and determines that a health care organization complies with the standards.
- **Compliance:** Meeting or adhering to the requirements of a standard, law, rule, or regulation.
- **Deemed status:** An accrediting organization approved by CMS that is in compliance with the Medicare Conditions of Participation.
- **Guideline:** Voluntary guidance and direction to practitioners and other audiences based on consensus of professional judgment, expert opinion, and documented evidence. Guidelines are written to establish reasonable goals, to be progressive and challenging, yet attainable as "best practices" in applicable settings.

- **Healthcare Facilities Accreditation Program (HFAP):** The American Osteopathic Association's (AOA) accrediting organization for the operation of hospitals.
- **The Joint Commission:** The principal accrediting organization for the operation of hospitals and other health care organizations.
- **Law:** A legally binding requirement imposed by a legislative body (e.g., U.S. Congress).
- **National Integrated Accreditation for Healthcare Organizations (NIAHO[SM]):** Det Norske Vertitas' (DNV) accrediting organization for the operation of hospitals.
- **Performance improvement:** The continuous measurement, analysis, and improvement of the performance of systems and processes to achieve desired outcomes.

- **Quality improvement:** A formal approach to the analysis of performance and the systematic approach to improve it.
- **Regulation:** Governmental order having the force of law.
- **Rule:** An authoritative recommendation meant to guide behaviors associated with specific, limited situations.
- **Standard:** "A statement that defines the performance expectations, structures, or processes that must be in place for an organization to provide safe and high quality care, treatment, and services."[1] Standards often reflect best practices (i.e., recognized by a majority of professionals in a particular field).
- **Survey:** "A key component in the accreditation process, whereby a surveyor(s) conducts an on-site evaluation of an organization's compliance with ... standards."[2]

■ ■ ■

Introduction

This chapter describes **standards** (including **laws**, rules, regulations, pharmacy professional standards, national codes and **guidelines**, and organization-specific requirements) that guide pharmacy practice in hospitals and health systems. Major entities that influence these standards are also identified and described. The information is an introductory overview, and individuals interested in more detailed information discussed in this chapter should visit each entity's respective website.

Health-system pharmacists and practice are directed by numerous accreditation and **certifying bodies**, federal and state government organizations, nongovernmental standards setting bodies, pharmacy professional associations, and health-system entities (Figure 3-1). Some influence through their formal legal authority and ability to punish offenders with fines and imprisonment. Others influence through persuasion and the exertion of peer and consumer pressure. Influence comes from external entities (e.g., Food and Drug Administration [FDA], **The Joint Commission**), the profession (e.g., American Society of Health-System Pharmacists [ASHP]), or the provider institution itself (e.g., Pharmacy Department). All health-system pharmacists should have a working knowledge of various bodies that influence how they practice.

Influence by External Bodies

Health-system pharmacy practice is highly regulated by accrediting bodies, governmental agencies, professional organizations, and other standard-setting entities external to the

Figure 3-1. Numerous demands are placed on pharmacists by entities internal and external to the institution where they practice. *Source:* D. A. Holdford

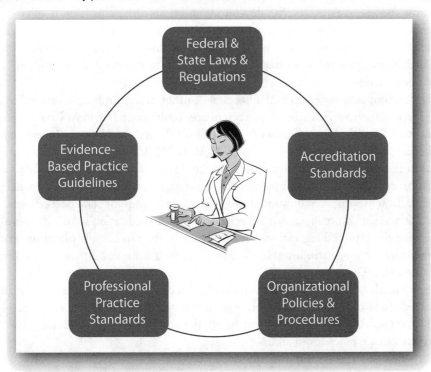

institution in which pharmacists practice. They hold pharmacists accountable for maintaining minimum standards of practice.

Health-system Certification and Accreditation Programs

Health care organizations obtain certification to meet the terms of participation in governmental (e.g., Medicare, Medicaid) or private (e.g., Kaiser) reimbursement programs. For instance, institutions must be certified by the Centers for Medicare and Medicaid Services (**CMS**) to participate in the federal Medicare program. CMS is a federal agency that administers health-related programs such as the Medicare program and works in partnership with the states to administer Medicaid, the Children's Health Insurance Program (CHIP), and the Health Insurance Portability and Accountability Act (HIPAA).[3] CMS maintains oversight of the survey and certification of "acute and continu-

Key Point . . .

Some entities influence pharmacists through their formal legal authority while others influence through persuasion and the exertion of peer and consumer pressure.

. . . So what?

Many of the rules and standards influencing pharmacy practice have been established within the profession by pharmacists, not imposed by external regulatory bodies. These rules and standards are followed by pharmacists because the profession agrees that they are the best thing for our patients and the public.

ing care providers (including hospitals, nursing homes, home health agencies [HHAs], end-stage renal disease [ESRD] facilities, hospices, and other facilities serving Medicare and Medicaid beneficiaries)…"[4] CMS develops Conditions of Participation (CoPs) that health care organizations must meet to participate in the Medicare and Medicaid programs. Each CoP consists of one or more standards that define the requirements for compliance. These standards are used to improve quality and protect the health and safety of beneficiaries.[5]

Accreditation acknowledges that a hospital or other health care organization has met or exceeded the requirements of an **accrediting body** (e.g., The Joint Commission, the **Healthcare Facilities Accreditation Program [HFAP],** and the **National Integrated Accreditation for Healthcare Organizations [NIAHO**SM**]**). Health care organizations stress the importance of maintaining their accredited status for several reasons. Loss of accreditation can severely affect an organization's prestige and make it difficult to attract qualified staff. Achieving accreditation in many states is helpful for state licensure and may exempt accredited organizations from inspections. Accreditation standards sometimes become the expected legal standards of care and failure to comply might present legal difficulties for an organization. It also affects an institution's ability to receive funding from health care insurers.

The standards take into consideration that health care organizations are subject to state and federal laws and undergo substantial state inspection through licensure programs (hospital, pharmacy, fire and safety, health department, etc.). Therefore, CMS standards encourage practices in accordance with generally recognized principles and avoid conflict with state and federal laws, state licensure requirements, and Joint Commission, HFAP, and NIAHO standards. Although CMS conditions and standards are uniform throughout the country, interpretation and stringency of application vary considerably from state to state or between regions. However, one is typically in **compliance** if state board of pharmacy rules and regulations and standards of an accrediting body are met. CMS confers **deemed status** on a health care organization when that organization is judged or determined to be in compliance with relevant Medicare requirements. An organization is in compliance when it has been accredited by a voluntary organization whose standards and survey process are determined by CMS to be equivalent to those of the Medicare program.[6] Joint Commission, HFAP, and NIAHO accredited organizations are eligible automatically to participate in the Medicare program. Joint Commission accreditation, HFAP

Key Point . . .

The Centers for Medicare and Medicaid Services (CMS) certify. The Joint Commission, HFAP, and NIAHO accredit.

. . . So what?

CMS decides the standards needed for participating in the Medicare and Medicaid programs—standards followed by private insurers and other payers. Thus, CMS determines the quality standards needed to receive compensation for a major portion of the health care market. Compliance with these standards is determined by accrediting agencies like The Joint Commission, HFAP, and NIAHO. Recommendations by any of these nongovernmental agencies should be seen as having the support of CMS and the Federal Government.

accreditation, NIAHO accreditation, or CMS certification qualifies an organization to participate in the Medicare program.

The Joint Commission (formerly known as the Joint Commission on Accreditation of Healthcare Organizations) is "an independent, not-for-profit organization dedicated to improving the safety and quality of health care" in organized health care settings. Founded in 1951, its members represent the American College of Physicians, the American College of Surgeons, the American Dental Association, the American Hospital Association, the American Medical Association, the public, and the nursing profession. The Joint Commission engages in issues and activities concerning the advancement of health care safety and quality, including public policy initiatives, standards development, and accreditation and certification programs.[2] The Joint Commission is the principal accrediting body for the operation of hospitals and other health care organizations.

The Joint Commission sets continually evolving standards for acute care hospitals and other health care organizations. By definition, standards establish performance expectations for entities. Standards describe what needs to be done and provide enough detail for professionals to make decisions on how best to accomplish any given standard in their individual organizations. They are not instruction manuals or cookbooks and do not typically provide step-by-step instructions on how every step in the process gets accomplished and by whom. Rather, they outline common expectations by suggesting a framework.

The Joint Commission standards that are relevant to pharmacy include those for medication management, infection control, patient care, medical records, safety and security, education, performance improvement and environment of care (i.e., facilities). In addition to the standards, The Joint Commission has developed National Patient Safety Goals (NPSGs) that address specific patient safety issues.[7] Some of these goals are medication related. Each standard and NPSG includes one or more elements of performance (i.e., "the specific performance expectations and/or structures or processes that must be in place in order for an organization to provide safe, high-quality care, treatment, and services"[8]). Accreditation is for three years.

The American Osteopathic Association's (AOA) Healthcare Facilities Accreditation Program (HFAP) is the principal accreditation agency for osteopathic medical colleges and health care facilities. HFAP accreditation is not limited to osteopathic hospitals and some health care organizations are accredited by both HFAP and The Joint Commission. HFAP standards address all departments and functions including pharmacy services and medication use.[9] Some HFAP standards are more prescriptive than other accreditation standards and CMS standards. Therefore, compliance with other accreditation standards or CMS standards is not necessarily sufficient to meet HFAP standards and vice versa. If HFAP finds an organization compliant with its standards, it lists the organization as accredited. Accreditation is for three years.

Det Norske Veritas Healthcare's (DNV) National Integrated Accreditation for Healthcare Organizations (NIAHO) is another option for accreditation. The NIAHO standards integrate requirements based on the CMS Conditions of Participation with International Organization for Standardization (ISO) 9001 Standards.[10] The ISO 9001 standards are global principles designed to provide assurance that quality is imbedded in supplier-customer relationships (i.e., health care systems-patients). NIAHO is designed to facilitate the development and implementation of a Quality Management System for health care organizations. The NIAHO standards require that a hospital become compliant with ISO 9001 within 3 years of the first NIAHO accreditation. If NIAHO finds an organization compliant with its standards, it lists the organization as accredited. Accreditation is for three years.

Health care organizations undergo surveys (i.e., evaluations) to determine their level of compliance with accreditation standards and goals. Surveyors review key systems, assess compliance with relevant standards, and determine how well the organization provides care, treatment, and services. If the accrediting agency finds an organization compliant with the standards (and, if surveyed by The Joint Commission, the NPSGs), it lists the organization as accredited. Accreditation is typically awarded for 3 years. Note that The Joint Commission, HFAP, and NIAHO accredit health care organizations—not departments and services. Pharmacists must work with other departments and professionals in their organization to ensure that their organization complies with the standards.

Preparing for an Accreditation Survey Visit

ASHP's *Assuring Continuous Compliance with Joint Commission Standards: A Pharmacy Guide* provides complete guidelines for compliance with standards relating to pharmacy and guidance in preparing for survey visits from The Joint Commission, as well as CMS, HFAP, and NIAHO.[11] The Joint Commission's *Healthcare Activity Survey Guide* helps hospitals understand the Joint Commission's accreditation process, what to expect during a survey, and other information needed to assure a smooth survey experience.[12] The Joint Commission publishes its standards in the *Comprehensive Accreditation Manual for Hospitals: The Official Handbook (CAMH)*. The *CAMH* includes accreditation policies and procedures, accreditation participation requirements, the latest standards, compliance information, how to gauge compliance, and a glossary of terms.[13] The Joint Commission also publishes standards for ambulatory care, behavioral health care, home care, long-term care, and other health care organizations. AOA publishes the HFAP standards in *Accreditation Requirements for Healthcare Facilities*.[14] DNV publishes the NIAHO standards in *National Integrated Accreditation for Healthcare Organizations (NIAHO^{SM}) Accreditation Requirements: Interpretive Guidelines and Surveyor Guidance*.[15]

> **Key Point . . .**
>
> To be accredited by The Joint Commission, HFAP, or NIAHO, pharmacists must work cooperatively with other departments and professionals.
>
> **. . . So what?**
>
> Deficiencies within the medication use system are the responsibility of pharmacists, no matter where they occur in an institution. Meeting accreditation standards for medication use requires pharmacists to understand where medications go, how they are used, the individuals involved, and the outcomes achieved. This can only be done by collaborating with physicians, nurses, and other health care professionals.

Federal and State Laws and Regulations

Laws, regulations, and rules are legal requirements that govern action. **Laws** are often imposed by an authority (e.g., federal or state government), **regulations** are governmental orders having the force of law, and **rules** address specific, limited situations. The legal requirements of federal and state entities may directly or indirectly affect the practice of pharmacy. Detailed discussions of these authorities are beyond the scope of this chapter. Short descriptions of key authorities are provided below only to illustrate the complicated sets of laws and regulations governing health-system pharmacy practice.

Food and Drug Administration (FDA)

The Federal Food and Drug Administration (FDA) "…is responsible for protecting the public health by assuring the safety, efficacy, and security of human and veterinary drugs, biological products, medical devices, our nation's food supply, cosmetics, and products that emit radiation. The FDA is also responsible for advancing the public health by helping to speed innovations that make medicines and foods more effective, safer, and more affordable; and helping the public get the accurate, science-based information they need to use medicines and foods to improve their health."[16] The FDA implements and enforces the federal Food, Drug, and Cosmetic Act, sets labeling requirements for food, prescription and over-the-counter drugs and cosmetics, sets standards for investigational drug studies and product approval, and regulates and oversees the manufacturing and marketing of drugs.[17]

Drug Enforcement Administration (DEA)

The Drug Enforcement Administration (DEA) enforces the federal controlled substances laws and regulations. The DEA investigates and prepares for the prosecution of those who violate controlled substances laws and regulations and enforces provisions of the controlled substances act relating to the manufacture, distribution, and dispensing of legally produced controlled substances.[18] Most states have a similar agency that enforces controlled substances laws at the state level. Security and accountability for controlled substances are significant challenges for health care organizations.

Occupational Safety and Health Administration (OSHA)

The mission of the Occupational Safety and Health Administration (OSHA) "… is to assure safe and healthful working conditions for working men and women; by authorizing enforcement of standards … by assisting and encouraging the States in their efforts to assure safe and healthful working conditions, by providing for research, information, education, and training in the field of occupational safety and health."[19] OSHA conducts periodic workplace inspections to ensure that workers are kept safe in their jobs. OSHA standards affecting health-system pharmacies include those dealing with workplace accidents and exposure to hazardous materials. ASHP's *Competence Assessment Tools for Health-System Pharmacies* contains materials for assessing pharmacy staff competence in handling hazardous materials.[20]

National Institute for Occupational Safety and Health (NIOSH)

"The National Institute for Occupational Safety and Health (NIOSH) is the federal agency responsible for conducting research and making recommendations for the prevention of work-related injury and illness."[21] This differs from OSHA which sets and enforces safety standards for workers. NIOSH originated from the same legislation as OSHA (i.e., Occupational Safety and Health Act of 1970) and the differences between the two agencies can be somewhat obscure. Some NIOSH recommendations are of concern to health-system pharmacies. For example, a NIOSH alert "Preventing Occupational Exposure to Antineoplastic and other Hazardous Drugs in Healthcare Settings" warns of the health risks to workers exposed to these drugs and recommends protection procedures for minimizing the potential adverse health effects.[22] Pharmacies should ensure that their policies and procedures for handling these drugs reflect the NIOSH recommendations.

Centers for Disease Control and Prevention (CDC)

The Centers for Disease Control and Prevention (CDC) is "dedicated to protecting health and promoting quality of life through the prevention and control of disease, injury, and disability."[23] CDC guidelines address hand-hygiene, standard (or universal) precautions, and other infection control issues that must be considered when developing organization and department practices.

Office of Inspector General (OIG)

The mission of the Office of Inspector General (OIG) is to protect the integrity of certain governmental programs, as well as, the health and welfare of the beneficiaries of those programs. OIG duties are fulfilled through a nationwide network of audits, investigations, inspections, and other related functions.[24]

Environmental Protection Agency (EPA)

The Environmental Protection Agency (EPA) is responsible for developing and enforcing regulations pertaining to environmental laws and issues. It also conducts research and provides information and education on environmental issues and works with state and local governments and businesses to protect the environment.[25] The EPA enforces the Resource Conservation and Recovery Act (RCRA) which regulates the handling and disposal of hazardous waste from the point of generation to final disposal.[26] The RCRA applies to hazardous pharmaceutical waste discarded by health care organizations.

Office for Civil Rights (OCR)

The responsibilities of the Office for Civil Rights (OCR) include enforcing Title VI of the Civil Rights Act of 1964 and its amendments and certain provisions of the Health Insurance Portability and Accountability Act of 1996 (HIPAA).[27] The Civil Rights Act of 1964 deals primarily with human relations management—prohibiting discrimination in employment hiring, promotion, compensation, and treatment of protected employee groups. Protected groups are those who might be discriminated against based on their gender, race, age, religion, sexual preference, height, weight, arrest record, national origin, financial status, military record, or disability.

HIPAA aims to assure health insurance portability, reduce health care fraud and abuse, enforce standards for health information, and guarantee security and privacy of health information. Compliance with the security and privacy provisions of the act may be particularly challenging for pharmacies.

State Boards of Pharmacy

States regulate pharmacy practice through their state boards of pharmacy (although the actual name of the agency may vary). Boards of pharmacy responsibilities include setting licensure requirements for individuals, pharmacies, and some health care organizations. Boards of pharmacy also establish and enforce the rules and regulations of the state's pharmacy practice act and discipline pharmacists and pharmacies. Some boards of pharmacy enforce their state's controlled substances act. Specific responsibilities differ from state to state. State requirements may be less stringent or more stringent than accreditation and certification requirements. In all cases, the most stringent requirements take precedence. Pharmacists should contact their state board of pharmacy for specific information relating to licensure and pharmacy practice in their state.

Other Agencies

Some government agencies share responsibilities associated with certain legal requirements. For example, the Department of Health and Human Services, Department of Justice, Department of Labor, Department of Transportation, Equal Opportunity Employment Commission, Federal Communications Commission, and other government agencies share responsibilities associated with the Americans with Disabilities Act (ADA). The ADA protects the rights of Americans with physical and mental disabilities.[28] Pharmacy departments must be aware of the provisions of the act and be prepared to make reasonable accommodations for disabled individuals. Pharmacy standards of performance must not impose an undue hardship on these individuals.

Key Point . . .

Boards of pharmacy establish and enforce the rules and regulations of state pharmacy practice acts and set licensure requirements for pharmacists and pharmacies.

. . . So what?

Some state boards of pharmacy seem to focus on issues of interest to community pharmacy rather than hospital pharmacy practice. Indeed, many of the rules and regulations set by state boards of pharmacy are seen as obstacles to innovative institutional pharmacy practice. For instance, some boards have established rigid technician to pharmacist ratios (e.g., two technicians for every pharmacist). This hinders the ability of institutional pharmacies to delegate distributional duties to highly trained technicians and free pharmacists for clinical activities.

Nongovernmental Standards-Setting Entities

Nongovernmental organizations often set standards that are enforced by government agencies (e.g., FDA and boards of pharmacy) and other entities (e.g., The Joint Commission). Three examples are described below.

United States Pharmacopeia (USP)

The United States Pharmacopeia (USP) is a nongovernmental, standards-setting organization that advances public health by ensuring the quality of medicines, food ingredients, and other health care products, promoting the safe and proper use of medications, and verifying ingredients in dietary supplements.[29] The USP provides standards for drugs, dietary supplements, and health care products. These standards are published in the *United States Pharmacopeia and National Formulary.* USP Chapter <795> sets standards for non-sterile compounding.[30] USP Chapter <797> sets standards for pharmaceutical compounding of sterile preparations (including personnel competence, design of facilities, beyond-use dating, storage conditions, environmental monitoring, and suggested standard operating procedures).[31] Further discussion of USP Chapter <797> regulations is provided in Chapter 14 of this text on Sterile Preparations and Admixture Programs.

National Fire Protection Association (NFPA)

The National Fire Protection Association (NFPA) aims "… to reduce the worldwide burden of fire and other hazards on the quality of life by providing and advocating consensus codes and standards, research, training and education."[32] Health-system pharmacies are subject to fire risks because of the large number of flammable materials (e.g., alcohol) stored there. Organization and department standards must be compliant with NFPA's Life Safety Code®[33] and other provisions.

Institute of Medicine (IOM) of the National Academies

The Institute of Medicine (IOM) of the National Academies is a nongovernmental, not-for-profit organization that provides a vital service by working outside the framework of government to ensure scientifically informed analysis and independent guidance. Although they do not set standards, they provide standard-setting entities with unbiased, evidence-based, and authoritative information and advice. The IOM's many notable contributions include their ground-breaking reports, *To Err is Human: Building a Safer Health System* (1999) and *Crossing the Quality Chasm: A New Health System for the 21st Century* (2001).[34]

Pharmacy Professional Organizations

Pharmacy professional organizations have established standards of practice, guidelines, and codes for their specialty areas. Through their efforts, these organizations have raised the expectations for pharmacy practice. Pharmacy organizations are prepared to educate pharmacists about the standards and assist them in implementing and maintaining practices that meet the standards. When necessary, pharmacy organizations work with accrediting bodies, governmental agencies, and other groups to assure consistency and currency.

American College of Clinical Pharmacy (ACCP)

"The American College of Clinical Pharmacy (ACCP) is a professional and scientific society that provides leadership, education, advocacy, and resources enabling clinical pharmacists to achieve excellence in practice and research."[35] ACCP practice resources are the foundation of clinical pharmacy standards.

American Pharmacists Association (APhA)

The American Pharmacists Association (APhA) is a national professional society of pharmacists. It "provides information, education, and advocacy to empower its members to improve medication use and advance patient care."[36] The APhA's Code of Ethics for Pharmacists states the principles that "… guide pharmacists in relationships with patients, health professionals, and society."[37]

American Society of Consultant Pharmacists (ASCP)

The American Society of Consultant Pharmacists (ASCP) is a professional association representing senior care pharmacists. ASCP's Web site provides resources and links to federal standards relating to optimum provision of pharmaceutical care to patients residing in health-system and residential settings.[38]

American Society of Health-System Pharmacists (ASHP)

The American Society of Health-System Pharmacists (ASHP) is a professional organization for pharmacists practicing in health-systems. ASHP has adopted professional policy positions, statements, and guidelines that foster improvement in pharmacy practice and patient care. They "… represent a consensus of professional judgment, expert opinion, and documented evidence."[39] Since ASHP policy positions, statements, and guidelines are often more stringent, more explicit, and less subject to misinterpretation than Joint Commission, HFAP, NIAHO, and CMS standards, they can help an organization meet or exceed accreditation and certification requirements.

ASHP is also the accrediting body for practice sites that conduct pharmacy residency programs and technician training programs. ASHP standards are available on the ASHP Web site.[40] Meeting ASHP requirements for residency accreditation and technician training can help pharmacies raise the quality of their services.

ASHP develops standards to help pharmacists who practice in hospitals and health systems improve medication use and enhance patient safety. These standards have served a vital role through the provision of a national evidence-based framework that has helped to guide local, state, and federal regulators and national accrediting bodies in their enforcement activities, as well as providing pharmacy practitioners, hospitals and health systems, and other health care professionals with a strong sense of direction on the best approaches to ensuring patient safety, quality, and optimal medication-use outcomes.

The 1999 Institute of Medicine (IOM) report, *To Err is Human: Building a Safer Health System,* recognized ASHP as an organization that publishes extensively on safe medication practices. The IOM noted that ASHP has developed many standards and guidelines and has widely disseminated a list of top priority actions for preventing adverse drug events in hospitals.[41] The point to be made is that by the time the IOM published its seminal report on medical errors that essentially launched the "patient safety movement," ASHP had, in fact, been publishing and developing standards on safe medication practice for nearly 60 years.

Adaptability of standards is important because services and the types of patients served differ from one organization to another. Differences, for example, might include the types of services a large university hospital provides (e.g., transplant and other complex procedures, etc.,) with 24-hour pharmacy services as compared to a small rural hospital that might only have a pharmacist on duty for a limited number of hours. However, adaptability does not imply that standards should be different or do not apply to one setting but not another. The endpoint of the standard remains the same, but the methods and intervening steps to achieving the standard may differ. For example, it is essential to have a pharmacist review all medication orders against the patient's profile for appropriateness before the medication is administered to the patient. However, in the case

> **Key Point . . .**
>
> ASHP policy positions, statements, and guidelines are often more stringent, more explicit, and less subject to misinterpretation than Joint Commission, HFAP, NIAHO, and CMS standards.
>
> **. . . So what?**
>
> ASHP helps to establish and clarify expectations of performance for health-systems pharmacists. In many instances, ASHP policy positions, statements, and guidelines provide better guidance than standards of accreditation agencies.

of some small and rural hospitals that do not have 24-hour services, the order might be reviewed through the use of technology that allows a pharmacist in a remote location (from another hospital or remote-order entry service) to access the patient record and review and approve the order. In this example the standard is the same, but the approach to achieving the standard is different.

Ideally, consistency associated with evidence-based practices is enhanced, and patient care outcomes are ultimately improved through standardization. The practice standards, *Best Practices for Hospital and Health-System Pharmacy: Position and Guidance Documents of ASHP*, developed by ASHP represent a rich source of information on virtually every area in hospital and health-system pharmacy practice. This valuable resource is available free on the Web to anyone who seeks to design safer and more effective medication-use systems.[42] Topics include the following:

- Automation and Information Technology
- Drug Distribution and Control
- Education and Training
- Ethics
- Formulary Management
- Government, Law, and Regulation
- Medication Misadventures
- Medication Therapy and Patient Care
- Pharmaceutical Industry
- Pharmacy Management
- Practice Settings
- Research

Standards development occurs in a variety of ways depending on the type of standard being developed and the processes employed by the developing organization. The following process is used by ASHP to develop guidance documents and serves as a good example of how an organization that represents a distinct group of professionals approaches standards development.

Step 1: An ASHP member council or commission recommends the development of a guidance document after considering whether the topic has the following:

- Generates a need among practitioners for authoritative advice
- Achieves some stability and there is sufficient experience upon which to base a guideline
- Is relevant to the practice of a significant portion of ASHP's members
- Is within the purview of pharmacy practice in hospitals and health systems
- Is without other sufficient guidance
- Does not pose significant legal risks to ASHP
- Is determined by ASHP leadership that there is room for improvements in practice and that an ASHP document would foster that improvement[43]

Step 2: A group of experts (usually ASHP members) on a given topic volunteer to develop a preliminary draft. Drafters are selected based on demonstrated knowledge of the topic and their practice settings.

Step 3: The draft is sent by ASHP to reviewers who have interest and expertise in the given topic. Reviewers consist of hospital and health-system pharmacists and selected individuals, such as other health care professionals, who are knowledgeable in the content area, representatives of various ASHP bodies, and other professional organizations. The draft is posted on the ASHP Web site to allow time for public comment. A strength of ASHP's guidelines resides in this public comment process that allows anyone who is interested in commenting to do so, as well as active outreach by ASHP to other interested individuals and organizations.

Step 4: Based on the comments, a revised draft is submitted to the appropriate ASHP policy-recommending body for action. When the draft meets the established criteria for content and quality, that body recommends that the ASHP Board of Directors approve the document.

The guidance documents developed by ASHP are voluntary and do not have the force of law or regulation. However, it is sometimes the case that a state board of pharmacy or federal regulator such as the FDA or national accrediting body such as The Joint Commission, might look to ASHP guidelines to provide a framework for the development of laws, regulations, and enforceable standards, respectively. When one compares ASHP guidelines to Joint Commission Medication Management standards published in the *Comprehensive Accreditation Manual for Hospitals: The Official Handbook,* it is evident how ASHP practice standards provide a framework for the development of enforceable standards by other organizations.

Standards for the practice of pharmacy in hospitals and health systems are, and continue to be, integral to the safe and effective use of medications. More important than gaining an understanding of how practice standards are developed and used, is for individual pharmacy practitioners to contribute to the practice standards development process throughout their entire careers, remembering that the best standards are those that are developed by the professionals who are engaged in the practice and will be most affected by the standards once they are implemented.

ASHP dedicates significant resources to the development of practice standards to advance overall public health related to medication use and the practice of pharmacy in hospitals and health systems. It can be difficult to judge at the time a standard is conceptualized and developed whether that standard will ultimately have an impact on improving patient care or advancing pharmacy practice. However, evidence to date suggests that most issues rising to the level of standards development are ones that either immediately, or over a period of time, have made a measurable difference in the lives of the patients we serve.

Influence by Internal Bodies

Although accrediting bodies, regulatory agencies, professional organizations, and other standards setting entities define external requirements and expectations, health care organizations must develop internal requirements (i.e., standards) that are specific to their needs. Important health-system bodies influencing pharmacy practice are the pharmacy and therapeutics (P&T) committee and medical executive committee of each institution. They provide oversight and approval of standards of performance for the organization and each department. Other health-system bodies that play a role in pharmacy practice include the infection control, quality/performance improvement, and safety committees and the institutional review board.

Organization and Department Standards

Organization and department standards must establish the management framework to ensure compliance and quality of care. External and internal requirements must be integrated into organization and department policies and procedures, competence requirements, performance evaluations, and performance improvement programs. Pharmacy assessments should include compliance with their organization and department standards.

Bylaws, Rules, Regulations, Policies and Procedures

An institution's medical staff bylaws, rules, and regulations provide the framework for governing the organization. Policies and procedures are the formal, approved description of how a process is defined, organized and carried out. Pharmacy departments must comply with their institution's bylaws, rules, and regulations. Departmental policies and procedures must be consistent with the organization's requirements and should be developed with the input of pharmacists and support staff. Policies and procedures should be used in orientation, education and training of staff and competence assessment.

Key Point . . .

The pharmacy and therapeutics and medical executive committees are the two primary bodies influencing pharmacy practice within institutions.

. . . So what?

In most institutions, the levers of influence over pharmacy practice lie within these two bodies. Initiatives designed to improve medication use must be supported by individuals within these committees. Good professional relationships are needed with these individuals in order to advocate and lead change.

Competence Assessment and Performance Evaluation Programs

Health care organizations should have programs for determining that individuals are competent (i.e., have the skills, knowledge, and ability to perform a job according to defined expectations). [44] The Joint Commission requires its accredited organizations to define the competencies that are required and how they will be assessed, use appropriately qualified individuals to assess competence, assess competence at defined intervals, and take action when a person does not meet the competency requirements. [45]

Performance evaluation programs are ongoing processes for providing feedback on job performance to staff and students as well as volunteers. Some organizations conduct performance evaluations concurrently with competence assessments. Performance expectations must be reasonable, achievable, measurable, and reflect the person's job responsibilities, adherence to policies, and predefined behavioral requirements. Pharmacy leadership and staff should work together to develop expectations that are mutually agreeable. ASHP's *Competence Assessment Tools for Health-System Pharmacies* contains job descriptions, performance evaluations, study materials, tests, skills assessment checklists, and guidelines for assessing the competence of pharmacists and support staff. [46]

Performance Improvement Programs

Most health care organizations have active **performance improvement (PI)** programs designed to improve processes related to care, treatment, and services. PI programs are evolving. Although approaches vary, most contain elements of quality control and **quality improvement**.

The Joint Commission's approach to PI includes outcome, process, and structure measures and reflects current standards of practice. The Joint Commission's PI standards require a proactive, organization-wide program that includes the following:

- monitoring performance and collecting data
- aggregating and analyzing data
- analyzing undesirable patterns and trends in performance
- identifying and managing sentinel events
- using information from data analysis, to identify and prioritize opportunities for improvement
- improve performance by taking action on improvement opportunities
- evaluating those actions for effectiveness and taking further action when improvement is not achieved or sustained[47]

Many organizations coordinate their PI program with their risk management activities (i.e., determining, identifying, and preventing adverse patient and employee events).

Summary

Health-system certification and accreditation requirements and pharmacy guidelines form a basis for setting pharmacy standards. Compliance with accreditation and certification standards, while voluntary, is essential for an organization. Meeting the minimum requirements of state and federal legal entities is mandatory. Certain nongovernmental organizations set standards that are enforced by governmental agencies or other entities. Standards established by pharmacy professional organizations are often optimal and may be more challenging than accreditation and legal requirements. Internal requirements (e.g., organization and department standards) must be consistent with external requirements. Whatever the source and whether voluntary or mandatory, compliance with these requirements raises the level of pharmacy services and improves the quality of patient care.

Suggested Reading

Boyle CJ, Beardsley RS, Holdford DA, eds. *Leadership and Advocacy for Pharmacy.* American Pharmacists Association Publications, Washington, DC. 2007.

Uselton JP, Kienle PC, Murdaugh LB. *Assuring Continuous Compliance with Joint Commission Standards: A Pharmacy Guide.* 8th ed. Bethesda, MD; American Society of Health-System Pharmacists: 2010.

Murdaugh LB. *Competence Assessment Tools for Health-System Pharmacies.* 4th ed. Bethesda, MD: American Society of Health-System Pharmacists; 2008.

References

1. The Joint Commission. *Comprehensive Accreditation Manual for Hospitals: The Official Handbook.* Oakbrook Terrace, IL: The Joint Commission; 2009:GL-18.

2. The Joint Commission. *Comprehensive Accreditation Manual for Hospitals: The Official Handbook.* Oakbrook Terrace, IL: The Joint Commission; 2009:GL-19.

3. Centers for Medicare and Medicaid Services. About CMS. Available at: http://www.cms.hhs.gov/home/aboutcms.asp. Accessed July 2, 2009.

4. Centers for Medicare and Medicaid Services. Survey and certification. Available at: http://www.cms.hhs. govSurveyCertificationGenInfo. Accessed July 2, 2009.

5. Centers for Medicare and Medicaid Services. Conditions for coverage (CfCs) and Conditions of participation (CoPs) . Available at: http://www.cms.hhs.gov/CFCsAndCoPs. Accessed July 2, 2009.

6. The Joint Commission. *Comprehensive Accreditation Manual for Hospitals: The Official Handbook.* Oakbrook Terrace, IL: The Joint Commission; 2009:GL-6.

7. The Joint Commission. Facts about the National Patient Safety Goals. Available at: http://www.joint-commission.org/PatientSafety/NationalPatientSafetyGoals/npsg-facts.htm. Accessed July 3, 2009.

8. The Joint Commission. *Comprehensive Accreditation Manual for Hospitals: The Official Handbook.* Oakbrook Terrace, IL: The Joint Commission; 2009:GL-7.

9. Healthcare Facilities Accreditation Program. About HFAP - overview. Available at http://www.hfap.org/about/overview.aspx. Accessed July 3, 2009.

10. NIAHO Accreditation Program Frequently Asked Questions (February 10, 2009). Available at http://www.dnv.com/binaries/FAQs-021009%20_tcm4-329532.pdf. Accessed July 7, 2009.

11. Uselton JP, Kienle PC, Murdaugh LB. *Assuring Continuous Compliance with Joint Commission Standards: A Pharmacy Guide.* 8th ed. Bethesda, MD; American Society of Health-System Pharmacists: 2010

12. The Joint Commission Healthcare Activity Survey Guide. Available at http://www.jointcommission.org/NR/rdonlyres/481CE5EA-D02C-46C3-AA5F-DF328FE13174/0/HealthCareOrganizationSAG2009_Feb09Update.pdf. Accessed July 7, 2009.

13. The Joint Commission. *Comprehensive Accreditation Manual for Hospitals: The Official Handbook.* Oakbrook Terrace, IL: The Joint Commission; 2009.

14. American Osteopathic Association. *Accreditation Requirements for Healthcare Facilities.* Chicago, IL: American Osteopathic Association; 2008.

15. Det Norske Veritas Healthcare. National Integrated Accreditation for Healthcare Organizations (NIAHO^SM) Accreditation Requirements: Interpretive Guidelines and Surveyor Guidance, Rev. 8.0. Cincinnati, OH: Det Norske Veritas Healthcare; 2010.

16. U.S. Food and Drug Administration. FDA's mission statement. Available at: http://www.fda.gov/opacom/ morechoices/mission.html. Accessed July 3, 2009.

17. U.S. Food and Drug Administration. What FDA regulates. Available at: http://www.fda.gov/AboutFDA/WhatWeDo/WhatFDARegulates/default.htm. Accessed July 3, 2009.

18. U.S. Drug Enforcement Administration. DEA mission statement. Available at: http://www.usdoj.gov/dea/agency/mission.htm. Accessed July 3, 2009.

19. Occupational Safety and Health Administration. OSHA mission statement. Available at: http://www.osha.gov/oshainfo/mission.html. Accessed July 3, 2009.

20. Murdaugh LB. *Competence Assessment Tools for Health-System Pharmacies.* 4th ed. Bethesda MD: American Society of Health-System Pharmacists; 2008:153-176.

21. National Institute for Occupational Safety and Health. About NIOSH. Available at: http://www.cdc.gov/niosh/ about.html. Accessed July 3, 2009.

22. National Institute for Occupational Safety and Health. NIOSH alert: preventing occupational exposures to antineoplastic and other hazardous drugs in healthcare settings. Available at: http://www.cdc.gov/niosh/ docs/2004-165. Accessed July 1, 2009.

23. Centers for Disease Control and Prevention. About CDC. Available at: http://www.cdc.gov/about. Accessed July 3, 2009.

24. Office of Inspector General. About OIG. Available at: http://oig.hhs.gov/organization.asp. Accessed July 8, 2009.

25. Environmental Protection Agency. About EPA - What We Do. Available at: http://www.epa.gov/epahome/whatwedo.htm. Accessed July 3, 2009.

26. Environmental Protection Agency. RCRA Cleanup. Available at: http://epa.gov/oecaerth/cleanup/rcra/index.html. Accessed July 3, 2009.

27. United States Department of Health and Human Services (HHS). Medical privacy—national standards to protect the privacy of personal health information. Available at: http://www.hhs.gov/ocr/privacy/index.html. Accessed July 3, 2009.

28. U.S. Department of Justice. ADA home page. Available at: http://www.ada.gov. Accessed July 3, 2009.

29. United States Pharmacopeia. About USP - an overview. Available at: http://www.usp.org/aboutusp. Accessed July 3, 2009.

30. The United States Pharmacopeial Convention. Pharmaceutical compounding – nonsterile preparations. In: *The United States Pharmacopeia* 32nd revision and the *National Formulary* 27th edition, 2009: page 314. Available at http://www.uspp2.com. Accessed July 7, 2009.

31. The United States Pharmacopeial Convention. Pharmaceutical compounding—sterile preparations. In: *The United States Pharmacopeia.* 32nd revision, and the *National Formulary,* 27th edition, 2009: page 318. Available at: http://www.uspp2.com. Accessed July 7, 2009.

32. National Fire Protection Association. About NFPA. Available at: http://www.nfpa.org/categoryList. asp?categoryID=143&URL=About%20NFPA. Accessed July 3, 2009.

33. NFPA 101: Life Safety Code®, Available at: http://www.nfpa.org/aboutthecodes/aboutthecodes. asp?docnum=101&cookie%5Ftest=1.Accessed July 7, 2009.

34. Institute of Medicine of the National Academies. About the IOM. Available at: http://www.iom.edu/ CMS/3239.aspx. Accessed July 8, 2009.

35. American College of Clinical Pharmacy. About ACCP. Available at: http://www.accp.com/about/index. aspx. Accessed July 3, 2009.

36. American Pharmacists Association. About the APhA. Available at: http:www.pharmacist.com. Accessed July 3, 2009.

37. American Pharmacists Association. Code of ethics for pharmacists. Available at: http://www.pharmacist. com. Accessed July 3, 2009.

38. American Society of Consultant Pharmacists. Practice resources. Available at: http://www.ascp.com/ resources/. Accessed July 7, 2009.

39. American Society of Health-System Pharmacists. ASHP policy positions and guidelines (best practices). Available at: http://www.ashp.org/IMPORT/PRACTICEANDPOLICY/PolicyPositionsGuidelinesBest-Practices/AboutGuidelines.aspx. Accessed July 2, 2009.

40. American Society of Health-System Pharmacists. Accreditation. Available at: http://www.ashp.org/Import/ACCREDITATION.aspx. Accessed July 7, 2009.

41. Kohn LT, Corrigan JM, Donaldson MS. To err is human: building a safer health system. Committee on quality and health care in America. Washington, DC: National Academy Press; 1999.

42. American Society of Health-System Pharmacists. Practice and Policy. Available at: http://www.ashp.org/ practice-policy/. Accessed July 7, 2009.

43. *Best Practices for Hospital and Health-System Pharmacy: Position and Guidance Documents of ASHP, 2008-2009.* Bethesda, MD: American Society of Health-System Pharmacists, 2008:xxi.

44. Murdaugh LB. *Competence Assessment Tools for Health-System Pharmacies.* 4th ed. Bethesda, MD: American Society of Health-System Pharmacists; 2008:3.

45. The Joint Commission. *Comprehensive Accreditation Manual for Hospitals: The Official Handbook.* Oakbrook Terrace, IL: The Joint Commission; 2009:HR-6-7.

46. Murdaugh LB. *Competence Assessment Tools for Health-System Pharmacies.* 4th ed. Bethesda, MD: American Society of Health-System Pharmacists; 2008.

47. The Joint Commission. *Comprehensive Accreditation Manual for Hospitals: The Official Handbook.* Oakbrook Terrace, IL: The Joint Commission; 2009:PI-4-6.

Chapter Review Questions

1. **Accreditation and certification are very similar in their purpose.**
   a. True
   b. False

   Answer: a. True. Accreditation attempts to *determine* if an organization has met requirements of an accrediting body while certification attempts to *confirm* that requirements have been met by a certifying institution.

2. **The Joint Commission's mission is to improve the safety and quality of care of health care in institutions.**
   a. True
   b. False

   Answer: a. True. The Joint Commission engages in issues and activities concerning the advancement of health care safety and quality, including public policy initiatives, standards development, and accreditation and certification programs.

3. **The hospital pharmacy department can receive accreditation from The Joint Commission, HFAP, or NIAHO even when other departments in an institution do not.**
   a. True
   b. False

   Answer: b. False. One non-compliant department in an institution can lead to the entire organization losing accreditation. Pharmacists must work as part of a team with other departments and services in their organization to receive accreditation.

4. **When state and federal laws both have requirements for pharmacy practice, pharmacists can choose the least stringent requirement—either state or federal—and follow it.**
   a. True
   b. False

   Answer: b. False. In all cases, the most stringent requirements—state or federal—take precedence. Following the least stringent requirement can leave a pharmacist subject to legal action.

5. **Joint Commission accredited organizations are eligible automatically to participate in the Medicare program.**
   a. True
   b. False

   Answer: a. True. CMS deems Joint Commission standards to be equivalent or better than those of the Medicare program.

6. **_____ enforces the Federal Food Drug and Cosmetic Act.**
   a. FDA
   b. DEA
   c. OSHA
   d. The Joint Commission

   Answer: a. FDA implements and enforces the federal Food, Drug, and Cosmetic Act.

7. **Which of the following is NOT a governmental organization?**
   a. CDC
   b. USP
   c. OSHA
   d. DEA

Answer: b. The United States Pharmacopeia (USP) is a nongovernmental, standards-setting organization that advances public health by ensuring the quality of medicines, food ingredients, and other health care products, promoting the safe and proper use of medications, and verifying ingredients in dietary supplements.

8. **Any health system pharmacist can contribute to the development of ASHP standards of practice.**
   a. True
   b. False

   Answer: a. True. The process of developing ASHP practice standards provides several opportunities for pharmacists to contribute including a process for providing public comments.

9. **The IOM report,** *To Err is Human: Building a Safer Health System,* **was the stimulus for ASHP to begin developing standards on safe medication practices in institutions.**
   a. True
   b. False

   Answer: b. False. ASHP has been publishing and developing standards on safe medication practice for nearly 60 years.

10. **Which of the following professional organization's primary mission is to represent pharmacists serving senior citizens?**
    a. ASCP
    b. ASHP
    c. APhA
    d. ACCP

    Answer: a. The American Society of Consultant Pharmacists (ASCP) is a professional association representing senior care pharmacists.

Chapter Discussion Questions

1. Why is it important for health-system pharmacists to be politically active?
2. Go to the Web sites of pharmacy professional organizations listed in this chapter. How do they advocate for the profession?
3. One of the characteristics of any profession is that it be self-regulating. Do you believe that the practice of health-system pharmacy is regulated by pharmacists or by others? Explain your answer.
4. Where do you think pharmacists can have the greatest impact on the regulation of practice within their institutions?

CHAPTER 4

Medication Management

Kathy A. Chase

■ ■ ■

Learning Objectives

After completing this chapter, readers should be able to:

1. Describe the purpose of a formulary system in managing medication use in institutions.
2. Discuss the organization and role of the pharmacy and therapeutics committee.
3. Explain how formulary management works.
4. List the principles of a sound formulary system.
5. Define key terms in formulary management.

Key Terms and Definitions

■ **Closed formulary:** A list of medications (formulary) which limits access of a practitioner to some medications. A closed formulary may limit drugs to specific physicians, patient care areas, or disease states via formulary restrictions.

■ **Drug formulary:** A formulary is a continually updated list of medications and related information, representing the clinical judgment of pharmacists, physicians, and other experts in the diagnosis and/or treatment of disease and promotion of health.

■ **Drug monograph:** A written, unbiased evaluation of a specific medication. This document includes the drug name, therapeutic class, pharmacology, indications for use, summary of clinical trials, pharmacokinetics/dynamics, adverse effects, drug interactions, dosage regimens, and cost.

■ **Drug therapy guidelines:** A document describing the indications, dosage regimens, duration of therapy, mode(s) of administration, monitoring parameters and special considerations for use of a specific medication or medication class.

■ **Drug use evaluation (DUE):** A process used to assess the appropriateness of drug therapy by engaging in the evaluation of data on drug use in a given health care environment against predetermined criteria and standards.

◆ **Diagnosis-related DUE:** A drug use evaluation completed on patients with a specific disease state or diagnosis. An example is the use of antibiotics in patients with community acquired pneumonia.

- ◆ **Prescriber-related DUE:** A drug use evaluation completed on patients managed by a specific physician or physician group. For example, selected antibiotics may be limited to infectious disease specialists or drotrecogin alfa may be limited to critical care specialists.
- ◆ **Drug-specific DUE:** A drug use evaluation completed on a drug (medication).

- **FOCUS-PDSA:** A performance improvement model used by hospitals and health-systems. It includes the performance improvement elements of measuring the output of the process and modifying the process to improve the outcome.

- **Formulary restriction:** The act of limiting the use of specific formulary medications to specific physicians based on areas of expertise (e.g., cardiology), patient disease state (e.g., acute myocardial infarction), or location (e.g., operating room).

- **Formulary system:** An ongoing process whereby a health care organization, through its physicians, pharmacists, and other health care professionals, establishes policies on the use of drug products and therapies and identifies drug products and therapies that are the most medically appropriate and cost-effective to best serve the health interests of a given patient population.

- **Health-system board:** A committee of hospital and community members chosen to govern the affairs of hospital or health-system.

- **Medical executive committee:** A committee of the hospital medical staff that has the primary authority

for activities related to self governance and for performance improvement of the professional services provided by all practitioners privileged through medical staff process.

- **Medication use review:** A performance-improvement method that focuses on evaluating and improving medication-use processes with the goal of optimal patient outcomes.

- **Nonformulary agent:** A medication that is not a part of the drug formulary. This may be due to the medication not being considered for formulary addition or the medication being considered but the P&T committee choosing not to add it.

- **Open formulary:** A list of medications (formulary) which has no limitation to access to a medication by a practitioner.

- **Order entry rules:** Logic established within the hospital information system order entry module to notify prescribers of adverse effects, drug interactions, monitoring required or other actions required.

- **Outcome assessment:** A systematic process of evaluating the appropriateness, safety and efficacy of a medication. The process involves review of patient medical records to evaluate the drug use against predetermined criteria and standards.

- **Pop-ups:** Information that appears on a computer monitor when specific actions are taken. Hospital information systems often use *rules* to determine when *pop-ups* will occur. These pop-ups may contain clinical information about medication use, potential drug interactions, recommended monitoring, etc.

- **Stop orders:** Physician orders that are automatically terminated. The P&T committee may establish *stop orders* for medications that require additional evaluation after a specific time. Examples of stop orders are antibiotic therapy stopped after 7 days and nesiritide therapy stopped after 24 hours.

- **Therapeutic class review:** An evaluation of a group of medications with an established therapeutic class (e.g., first-generation cephalosporins). The review evaluates the indications for use, pharmacokinetics/dynamics, adverse effects, drug interactions, dosage regimens, and cost to determine similarities and differences.
- **Therapeutic equivalent:** Drug products with different chemical structures but of the same pharmacologic or therapeutic class and usually having similar therapeutic effects and adverse-reaction profiles when administered to patients in therapeutically equivalent doses.
- **Therapeutic interchange:** Authorized exchange of therapeutic alternatives in accordance with previously established and approved written guidelines or protocols within a formulary system.

Introduction

Medication use management describes the process used to assure the safe and effective use of drugs in a cost conscious manner. Key to medication management in the health-system environment is the formulary system. The formulary system is a mechanism for ongoing assessment of medications that are available for use. The system is managed by a committee of experts, which includes pharmacists and physicians.

This chapter will discuss the medication management system with focus on the following:

- Formulary system
- Pharmacy and therapeutics committee
- Formulary management
- Drug use evaluation
- Medication use policies
- Published formulary

The Formulary System

A drug formulary is a continually updated list of medications and related information, representing the clinical judgment of pharmacists, physicians, and other experts in the diagnosis and/or treatment of disease and promotion of health. It is often described as a list of medications routinely stocked by the health care system. The formulary was developed by hospitals in the 1950s as a management tool. It was initially used to assure that physicians had an adequate and consistent supply of medications for their day-to-day needs. A key purpose of the formulary was to discourage the use of marginally effective drugs and treatments.

Over time, the formulary has evolved beyond a simple list of medications. It is now one element of a system that includes medication use policies, a pharmacy and therapeutics committee, medication use evaluation, and formulary management. The formulary, today, can be more accurately defined as a continually updated list of medications and related information, representing the clinical judgment of pharmacists, physicians, and other experts in the diagnosis and/or treatment of disease and promotion of health.

Formularies are fundamental to the formulary system—defined as an ongoing process which methodically evaluates medications on an ongoing basis for inclusion or exclusion, establishes guidelines for optimal medication use, and develops policies and procedures for prescribing, dispensing, and administering medications. The formulary system is managed by the pharmacy and therapeutics committee or equivalent group—made up of an organized team of medication system experts.

There are advantages and disadvantages to a formulary system. The primary advantage is that it provides a systematic method to review scientific evidence on clinical effectiveness and cost effectiveness in drug selection decision, thus potentially improving health outcomes while reducing costs. A major disadvantage, however, is that an overly restrictive formulary system may potentially reduce the quality of care by limiting access to clinically indicated medications.

■ ■ ■

Key Point . . .

The formulary has evolved beyond a list of medications to a system that manages the drug use process.

. . . So what?

Standard definitions of formularies refer to them as static compilations of recommended medications in a pharmacy. In truth, they are really dynamic entities that consist of a constantly changing medication list, policies and procedures for managing that list, and tools used to encourage appropriate use of medications on that list—e.g., therapeutic substitution, drug utilization review).

The Pharmacy and Therapeutics Committee

The pharmacy and therapeutics committee (P&T committee) has oversight for medication management in the health-system. Specific regulatory or accrediting bodies may confirm this accountability. To be effective, the committee must have the support of the individual members as well as the health-system and medical staff as a whole.

Organization

The committee is generally a policy recommending body to the medical staff through the **medical executive committee**—a group of the hospital medical staff in charge of institutional governance and performance. The committee is responsible to the medical staff as a whole, and its recommendations are subject to approval by the organized medical staff as well as the routine administrative approval process. More recently, in some organizations, the P&T committee has reported directly to a non-medical staff advisory committee of hospital and community members called a **health-system board** rather than a local medical executive committee.

Because drug products and medical literature are continually changing, meetings should occur at least four to six times per year. Generally, monthly meetings are needed to keep the meeting time to 60–90 minutes.

Subcommittees or task forces have been established to facilitate meeting efficiency. Examples of subcommittees include medication safety, drug review panels, and medication use review. The medication safety task force may be charged with review of adverse drug events and medication errors, their trending, and development of plans for prevention of future events. Drug review panels may be focused on a particular specialty such as cardiology or infectious disease and review drug products and guidelines in their area of specialty. The medication use review task force may monitor one or more medications use reviews, evaluate the data and development plans to optimize specific drug use. Figure 4-1 illustrates how these subcommittees relate to the organizational structure of the P&T committee.

It is important to establish rules for a quorum to make certain that key stakeholders are represented at meetings. Such rules may establish a minimum number of members that must be present to conduct a meeting or a minimum number of member types that must be present to conduct a meeting. For example, a committee with 15 members might be required to have at least five members present of which two must be physicians and one must be a pharmacist before a quorum has been established.

Committee Membership

P&T committee membership should include pharmacists, nurses, physicians, administrators, risk or quality improvement managers, and others as appropriate. These members are selected with the guidance of the medical staff. Medication management is a multidisciplinary process. Committee

Key Point . . .

Medication management is a multidisciplinary process.

. . . So what?

Even though it is called the *Pharmacy* and Therapeutics committee, representation on the committee often includes physicians, nurses, and respiratory therapists given their roles within the medication use process. The collective efforts of all of the disciplines is needed to achieve optimal health outcomes.

Figure 4-1. Formulary management process.

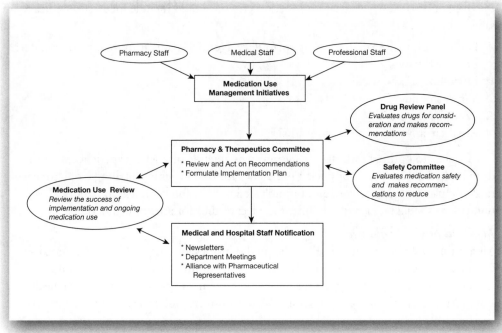

membership should include nonphysician members such as nurses, respiratory therapists, and other health care professionals. While the voting members of the P&T committee in many hospitals remains the physician members only, this is changing as the committee membership is evolving.

Responsibilities

The committee performs the following functions:

- Establishes and maintains the formulary system.
- Selects medications for formulary inclusion by considering the relative clinical, quality of life, safety, and pharmacoeconomic outcomes. Decisions should be balanced to all of the above. Decisions should include consideration of continuity of care (e.g., local health plan formularies).
- Evaluates medication use and related outcomes.
- Prevents and monitors adverse drug reactions and medications errors.
- Evaluates or develops and promotes use of drug therapy guidelines.
- Develops policies and procedures for handling medications to include their procurement prescribing, distribution, and administration.
- Educates health professionals to the optimal use of medications.

Formulary System Maintenance

The committee develops a list of medications for use in the organization. They may also develop guidelines for the optimal use of the medications and/or for specific disease management. They review the medication list and guidelines on a regular basis to assure that it is current and meets the needs of the medical staff and patients.

Medication Selection and Review

The committee should have established methods for medication selection and review. A written medication review is prepared from available literature. The review should be unbiased, as should the discussion of the review. Meeting participants (committee members and guests) should be required to discuss any conflict of interests prior to discussion of the drug or drug class. Medication selection criteria should include medication efficacy, safety, and cost.

- Is it a duplication of an existing formulary agent? If so, is it more effective? Safer? Less costly?
- How should it be used?
- When should it be used?
- Who should use it?
- Are there any other special concerns?

Barriers to optimal formulary decisions may include physician experience with the drug under consideration, physician preference for other agents, detailing by pharmaceutical company representatives, and unpublished or anecdotal studies and reports. Selection criteria should be such to minimize the effect of the aforementioned barriers.

Medication Use Evaluation

Medication use evaluation (MUE) is the method for evaluating and improving medication-use processes with the goal of optimal patient outcomes. The P&T committee should establish a regular process for reviewing how medications are used in the health-system (i.e., medication use evaluation). Medications may be considered for review based on their use, safety, cost or a combination of factors. For example, antibiotics represent a high use item; overuse of a particular antibiotic may place patients at risk for the development of resistant infections; and some antibiotics may also be costly. Establishment of specific criteria for use, review for compliance to the criteria, and routine review of the data is the foundation of the medication use process. Key to the process is timely data to review, action plan development, and follow-up.

Medication Safety Evaluation

Medication safety is evaluated through adverse drug reaction reports and medication error reports. Such reports may be local (i.e., from the health-system) or global (i.e., literature, press releases). The impact of such reports should be considered relative to the health-system population, resources, and alternatives. A report of increased bleeding in patients over the age of 65 may not be critical in a pediatric hospital. However, reports of infusion rate reactions may require changes in nursing procedures in drug administration. Such reports should be used in considering whether a drug should be added to the formulary, retained on the formulary, or deleted from the formulary.

Drug Therapy Guidelines

Drug therapy guidelines are a listing of the indications, dosage regimens, duration of therapy, mode(s) of administration, monitoring parameters and special considerations for use of a specific medication or medication class. In a hospital or health-system, these guidelines are developed with the oversight of practitioners with expertise in the use of a specific medication or management of a disease state. The guidelines are often put into practice via a pre-printed physician order sheet placed in the patient chart or computerized order set.

The development of drug therapy guidelines is often the result of a medication use review or medication safety evaluation. A review of this data may indicate that the drug is not being used in an optimal manner with regard to patient selection, dosage, frequency, route, length of therapy, or a combination. The development and implementation of drug therapy guidelines may foster the safe, efficacious and cost effective use of selected drug products. Education of the professional and medical staff to these guidelines is critical to their success. Just as important is a method for routine review of the guidelines to assure they are current.

Policy and Procedure Development

The P&T committee is responsible for medication use in the hospital. This includes the development of guidelines on historically pharmacy related topics of medication procurement, selection, and distribution. In addition, they are responsible for the medication administration process. This may include determining what medications are administered in specific locations for the hospital (i.e., intensive care unit) or under specific conditions (i.e., by chemotherapy certified nurse). Finally, they define the formulary management process, specifically, guidelines for the evaluation of medications by the P&T committee, frequency of such review, maintenance of the medication list, et cetera.

Education

The P&T committee must communicate its actions to health-system staff and physicians. A newsletter is often employed to communicate these decisions. The newsletter may also include clinical information on drugs added to the formulary, drug therapy guidelines developed, and medication safety information available. The success of a newsletter may be limited by the format and content. The newsletter should be visually pleasing, easy to follow, and succinct. Optimally, it should be limited to two to four pages in length. The audience for the newsletter is generally broad and includes physicians, nurses, pharmacists, and other health care professionals. Other methods to communicate and educate others to P&T committee actions are presentation at medical staff department meetings, nursing unit staff meetings, and pharmacy staff meetings and electronic messaging through email or the health-system website. The P&T committee may also assist in the development of programs to educate health care professionals or patients regarding medications.

Regulatory and Accrediting Bodies

Regulatory and accrediting bodies may require a P&T committee and define its membership and responsibilities. Regulatory bodies requiring such activity include the State Department of Health or Board of Pharmacy; this varies by state. Accrediting bodies requiring this activity include The Joint Commission, the American Osteopathic Association (AOA), and Commission on Accreditation of Rehabilitation Facilities (CARF). The facility type will define the accrediting body; each has a slightly different interpretation of the term *formulary*. Regulations and accreditation standards are dynamic and require vigilance by the pharmacy to assure compliance.

Pharmacist Role

Pharmacists are essential to the formulary management process. Often pharmacists will guide the P&T committee activities to assure optimal medication management. The pharmacist responsibilities may include the following:

- Establish P&T committee meeting agenda.
- Analyze and disseminate scientific, clinical, and health economic information regarding a medication or therapeutic class for review by the P&T committee.
- Conduct drug use evaluation and analyze data.
- Record and archive P&T committee actions.
- Follow-up with research when necessary.
- Communicate P&T committee decisions to other health care professionals such as pharmacy staff, medical staff, and patient care staff.

Formulary Management

The formulary is the foundation of the formulary system. In its simplest form, the formulary is a list of medications available for use at a hospital or health-system. This list includes the dosage forms, strengths and package sizes of each of the medications on it. Diligent management of this list has both patient care and financial implications. Patient care considerations include medication efficacy and safety. Financial considerations are the cost of the drug as well as the costs associated with stocking the medication such as shelf space, drug outdates, and handling.

Formularies can be categorized by their access to medications as *open* or *closed*. An open formulary has no limitation to access to a medication. **Open formularies** are generally large. A **closed formulary** is a limited list of medications. A closed formulary may limit drugs to specific physicians, patient care areas, or disease states via *formulary restrictions*.

Formulary restrictions (i.e., limits on institutional drug use) do not necessarily translate to optimal medication management. For example, limitation of an antibiotic to a *restricted* status may result in shifting to a different antibiotic. While sometimes this change is desirable, that may not always be the case. The *new agent of choice* may be more expensive or less safe than the *restricted* agent. Careful consideration of the impact of the formulary product selection and/or restriction is critical to the process. Some authors have suggested that restricting formularies has resulted in increased health care costs by increasing utilization of physician visits and hospitalizations.[1,2] While this data has been criticized, it is important to note the impact of formulary decisions in total health care costs.[3] The Institute of Medicine (IOM) evaluated the Veterans Administration (VA) *National Formulary* impact on health care costs in six closed or *preferred* class of drugs.[4] The IOM concluded that the VA National Formulary was cost saving, probably generating savings of $100 million over 2 years and did not appear to have any effect on hospital admissions for selected heart or ulcer related conditions.

Key Point . . .

Formulary restrictions do not necessarily translate to optimal medication management.

. . . So what?

Formulary restrictions often have unintended consequences. For example, strict limitations on the number of antibiotics used within a hospital may allow microbes a better chance of adapting to these few medications and developing antibiotic resistance in comparison to an institution with no restrictions on antibiotic use. The key is to carefully consider the potential impact of formulary restrictions prior to implementation and to monitor the actual impact after implementation.

Drug product selection should be based on individual chemical entities. The Food and Drug Administration (FDA) defines the equivalence of individual chemical entities or generic equivalents. A list of such equivalents can be found in the Approved Drug Products with Therapeutic Equivalence Evaluation commonly known as the *Orange Book*. Policies for the use and dispensing of generically equivalent products should be set forth in the formulary system policy.

Many health systems have also established *therapeutic equivalents* and *therapeutic interchange* programs. **Therapeutic equivalents** are drug products with different chemical structure but are of the same pharmacologic and/or therapeutic class and are expected to have similar therapeutic effects and adverse effects. Examples of therapeutic equivalents include first generation cephalosporins and histamine-2 blockers. **Therapeutic interchange** is the authorized exchange of therapeutic alternatives in accordance with previously established and approved written guidelines. Establishment of therapeutic equivalents extends beyond the chemical entity. It must include the dosage strength, dose frequency, and route of administration for the interchange. Examples of therapeutic interchanges are listed in Table 4-1.

The P&T committee should establish guidelines for generic substitution and therapeutic interchange. Such guidelines should include the following:

- The pharmacist is responsible for selecting generically equivalent products in concert with FDA regulations.
- Prescribers may specify a specific brand if clinically justified. The decision should be based on pharmacologic and/or therapeutic considerations relative to the patient.

Table 4-1.

Therapeutic Interchange Equivalence by Therapeutic Class

Therapeutic Class	Generic Name	Dosage	Dosage Frequency	Route
First generation	Cefazolin	1 g	Every 8 hr	IV
Cephalosporins	Cephalothin	1 g	Every 6 hr	IV
	Cephapirin	1 g	Every 6 hr	IV
H2 blockers	Cimetidine	300 mg	Every 6 hr	IV
	Ranitidine	50 mg	Every 8 hr	IV
	Famotidine	20 mg	Every 12 hr	IV

■ The P&T committee determines therapeutic equivalents and how they are processed.

The pharmacist is responsible for the quality, quantity, and source of all medications, chemical, biologicals, and pharmaceutical preparations used in the diagnosis and treatment of patients. Such products should meet the standards of the United States Pharmacopeia and the Food and Drug Administration.

Formulary maintenance is the ongoing process of assuring relative safety and efficacy of agents available for use in the health-system. Processes used in formulary maintenance include the following:

■ New product evaluation
■ Therapeutic class review
■ Formulary changes (rationale for retaining or deleting an agent from the formulary)
■ Nonformulary drug use review

New Product Evaluation

Pharmacists have the opportunity to assume a leadership role in the selection of agents to the formulary. The evaluation of an agent should consider the indications for use, pharmacokinetics, safety, and cost. Considerations to drug storage, mode of administration, special considerations, and drug-dispensing issues should also be included in the evaluation. Development of a standard format for new drug evaluations is useful in facilitating P&T committee discussions. Standard elements include the following:

■ *generic name*—List officially approved name of all chemical entities in the drug product.
■ *trade name*—List common trade name(s) of the drug product.
■ *therapeutic or pharmacologic class*—State the pharmaceutical or therapeutic class to which the agent belongs. Similar agents within the class may be listed.
■ *pharmacology*—Describe the mechanism of action and related pharmacologic effects of the drug. If the mechanism is unknown, state this.
■ *pharmacokinetics*—Describe how the drug is handled by the body. Include onset of effect, serum half-life, metabolic considerations, and route of excretion as appropriate.
■ *indications for use*—State the indications approved for use by the Food and Drug Administration. Include any additional uses under investigation.
■ *clinical studies*—Briefly describe clinical study data supporting the indications for use. This review should be an unbiased, comparative review of studies, which identifies

strengths and weaknesses as appropriate. Study description should include information about the patient populations, inclusion and exclusion criteria, study design and protocol, statistical analysis, outcomes, and conclusions.

- *adverse effects/warnings*—List adverse effects associated with the drug and the frequency of occurrence. Describe methods to reduce or treat adverse effects. Discuss the risks and benefits of this drug therapy. Also, list any special precautions such as drug use in pregnancy and excretion of the drug into breast milk.
- *drug interactions*—List drug-drug and drug-food interactions associated with this agent, significance of these interactions, and methods for prevention.
- *dosage range*—List a dosage range for different routes of administration and indications for the drug. Include special dosing considerations for renal disease, age, and hepatic function.
- *dosage form and cost*—List the dosage form and strengths proposed for formulary addition. Include the cost of each dosage form and strength. A table listing comparable agents may be useful in determining the value of a formulary addition or modification.
- *summary*—Summarize the information provided in a single paragraph.
- *recommendation*—State the recommendation and rationale for the recommendation. Recommended actions may include formulary addition, formulary restriction, formulary deletion, or do not add to formulary.
- *references*—List references used. Reference materials useful in preparation of the formulary monograph should be unbiased and current. Peer-reviewed primary literature is optimal whenever possible. Other resources include textbooks such as *American Hospital Formulary Service Drug Information* and *Drug Facts and Comparisons*. Electronic databases such as DrugDex (www.micromedex.com), Medline (www.ncbi.nlm.nih.gov/entrez/query.fcgi?), and National Guideline Clearinghouse (www.guideline.gov) are often useful.

In preparing the drug monograph, it is important to understand the P&T committee needs. Some committees desire a detailed analysis of the points listed above, whereas others prefer an abbreviated monograph. Critical elements to both are efficacy, safety, and cost. To assist the P&T committee membership, use of tables and comparative data within a therapeutic class or indication is useful. Knowing the cost of an agent is meaningless if the cost of comparator agents is unknown. The recommendation put forth by the pharmacist should be concise, include the rationale for the decision, any possible formulary dele-

Key Point . . .

Conditional approval allows the P&T committee to further assess the use and safety of the product before *final* formulary addition.

. . . So what?

A "wait and see" attitude often serves a P&T committee well when deciding to add a new drug. Many new drugs on the market can have insufficient evidence of safety because they only need to be tested on a limited number of patients prior to FDA approval. In addition, utilization patterns for the new drugs by physicians will also be unclear. Unexpected widespread adoption of a very expensive medication can bust the pharmacy drug budget. Conditional approval can help things from getting out of hand.

tions that might result by adding this agent, guidelines for use when appropriate, and consideration for future review. Some health systems add new agents to the formulary for a limited or *trial* period such as 3 or 6 months. This conditional approval allows the P&T committee to further assess the use and safety of the product before *final* formulary addition.

Therapeutic Class Review

The regular review of drug classes by the P&T committee is useful in assuring that optimal drug therapeutic options are available. Therapeutic class reviews should not be so broad or all inclusive so as to not be meaningful. The review of antimicrobials may be too broad whereas the review of quinolone antibiotics may prove to be more useful. The committee may set forth criteria for these reviews. Such criteria might include new medical information, adverse event profiles, purchase or use data and cost. Some P&T committees conduct a therapeutic class review with each consideration for formulary addition. The objective is to have the optimal agents within a therapeutic class in terms of efficacy, safety, and cost. The end result of a therapeutic class review may be formulary modifications (i.e., additions or deletions), implementation of a drug use review or the development of therapeutic guidelines.

Formulary Changes

A process to continually update the formulary must be established. Such a process should include a method for making additions and deletions to the formulary. This process typically involves the submission of a request for formulary addition or deletion from the pharmacy or medical staff. This request may be written or verbal. Requests generally require specific information.

- Agent to be considered for addition or deletion.
- Rationale for request. This should include the impact on the cost and quality of patient care.
- Alternative agents currently on the formulary.

Some organizations require or permit the requesting individual to attend the P&T committee to support their request.

Nonformulary Drug Review

The objective of a formulary is to have the most efficacious, safe, and cost effective agents available for routine use in the health-system. On occasion, unique patient needs may require the use of a **nonformulary** agent. To prevent the erosion of the formulary system by overuse of nonformulary agents, a process for the management of nonformulary agents should be in place. Such a process should include a policy for the use of nonformulary drugs, procedure for procurement of nonformulary drugs, and regular review of nonformulary drug use by the P&T committee. The policy for use of nonformulary drugs should include pharmacist contact with the prescribing physician to offer alternatives. It may also include the completion of a nonformulary request form by the prescribing physician or authorization by the P&T committee chair prior to dispensing. The procedure for drug procurement should be well-defined and communicated to the pharmacy, medical, and nursing staff so that expectations are appropriately understood. Such a procedure may indicate up to a 24-hour delivery time for nonformulary medications. It may also permit the use of a patient's own medications in concert with other hospital policies. The ongoing assessment of nonformulary drug use by the P&T committee is an important part in managing the medication process. Critical information for the committee to consider includes the agent used, formulary alternatives, number of times used in previous 6–12 months, patient safety, and cost impact. Understanding this information will allow the committee to determine an action plan. Such actions may include reconsideration of an agent for formulary addition, development of guidelines for use of a drug within a therapeutic class or disease state, or individual physician intervention.

A national survey of hospital pharmacy practice was conducted in 2007.[9] The authors described the various formulary techniques used in their hospitals (those aforementioned in this chapter). They noted the decline of all but two of these techniques: therapeutic interchange and nonformulary medication management. The use of clinical practice or drug therapy guidelines has become a key tool in managing drug use in the health-system.

A new and evolving method of formulary management has resulted from automating the medication prescribing process. Computerized prescriber order entry facilitates the implementation and compliance with drug therapy guidelines. Formulary management oversight includes the establishment and/or review of **order entry rules**. Such rules may include weight based dosing, required laboratory tests, and allergy checks. In addition, the responses (**pop-ups***)* to the rules may be determined by the P&T committee through the formulary management process. Review of this information will be a key element in managing and monitoring medication use throughout the health-system.

Drug Use Evaluation

Drug use evaluation (DUE) is a systematic process used to assess the appropriateness of drug therapy by engaging in the evaluation of data on drug use in a given health care environment against predetermined criteria and standards. Medication use evaluation (MUE) encompasses the goals and objectives of DUE in its broadest application, with an emphasis on improving patient outcomes. Use of *MUE* rather than *DUE* emphasizes the need for a more multifaceted approach to improving medication use.

Medication use or drug use evaluation programs were first established in the 1980s. They provide an ongoing, structured, organized approach to ensure that drugs are used appropriately. More recently, the term *outcome assessment* has been used to describe such programs. The desired endpoint is the same—safe, efficacious drug therapy.

Key Point . . .

Medication use evaluation (MUE) encompasses the goals and objectives of DUE in its broadest application, with an emphasis on improving patient outcomes.

. . . So what?

In some respects, the differences between MUE, DUE, and outcomes assessment are arbitrary. Nevertheless, these definitions have evolved in response to a tendency for some pharmacists to only see medication use as it relates to the world of pharmacy. Therefore, compliance with formulary restrictions, pharmacy policies and procedures, and other processes are sometimes emphasized over the actual outcomes achieved by patients. Redefining terminology can refocus efforts of medication use evaluation toward achieving the goal of positive patient outcomes.

Medication use evaluation programs should be incorporated into the overall hospital performance improvement process. They should employ the performance improvement model used by the health-system. There are multiple performance improvement models. A common model used in health-systems is FOCUS-PDCA or (PDSA). The acronym is described below:

Find process to improve

Organize a team that knows the process

Clarify current knowledge of the process

Understand causes of process variation

Select process improvement

Plan

Do

Check (or Study)

Act

Figure 4-2 illustrates a drug use evaluation using the PDCA model for antibiotic prophylaxis for surgery.

Pharmacists can take a leadership role in designing the drug use evaluation programs. The program should measure and compare the outcomes of patients who received drug therapy in concert with approved criteria versus those that did not. Selection of agents for drug use evaluation programs should be based on whether a drug is high-use, high-cost, or high-risk. Many drugs fall into more than one category: thrombolytic agents are high-cost and high-risk; select antibiotics may be high-use. Medication use criteria may be diagnosis-related, prescriber-related, or drug-specific.

Diagnosis-related DUE criteria identify indications for which select drug(s) may be appropriate for a given disease state. For example, the use of selected antibiotics for community acquired pneumonia. Use of other antibiotics would fall outside the approved list and require follow-up.

Prescriber-related DUE criteria identify specific physicians whom the P&T committee has determined may use certain drugs. For example, selected antibiotics may be limited to infectious disease specialists or drotrecogin alfa may be limited to critical care specialists.

Drug-specific DUE criteria focus on specific aspects of a select drug such as the dose or dosing frequency. For example, the dosage regimen of a low molecular weight heparin might be reviewed. Dosage regimens outside the criteria would require action.

Pharmacists, working with key physicians, develop criteria for drug use evaluation. The criteria should be focused and limited. Select three to five criteria to evaluate that are meaningful and simple to collect. If possible, data should be collected during the patient visit (concurrent) rather than retrospectively (chart review). Concurrent review often is more complete. It allows the pharmacist to obtain information from the prescriber that may not have been clear in the medical record. It also provides timely information to act on. Because medical information is dynamic, the most meaningful drug use evaluations should reflect current practice patterns rather than those of 6–18 months ago. The criteria should also include a number of patients to be reviewed and the time period. For example, "20 patients each month" receiving the drug are reviewed. The drug use evalu-

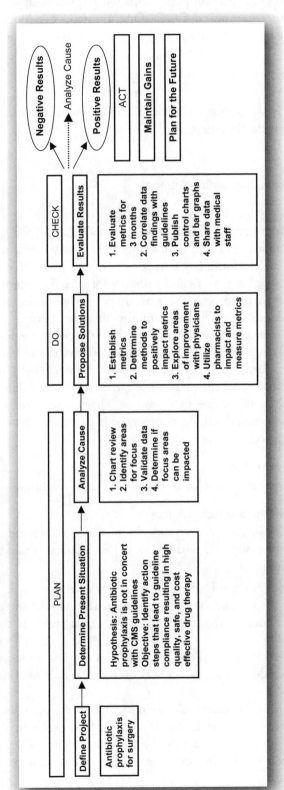

Figure 4-2. PDCA Model: Antibiotic prophylaxis for surgery patients.

ation criteria are presented to the P&T committee for their review and endorsement prior to commencing data collection.

Technology may be used to collect or screen data. Use of information systems to identify patients for review and collate the data will facilitate the process. Hand-held computers or personal data assistants (PDAs) may be useful in the data collection process.

Once the data has been collected, it should be compiled for review. The use of trend graphs or control charts are helpful in identifying opportunities for improvement. The result of a drug use evaluation may be validation that drug use is appropriate and safe. However, it may also indicate an opportunity for improving the way a drug is used. Once the data is collated, it may be beneficial to form a task force to develop an action plan. This task force should include key physicians, nurses, pharmacists, and other health care professional appropriate to the drug therapy under review. The task force should develop an action plan and criteria for ongoing monitoring. The action plan may include development of drug use guidelines, preprinted orders, medication order entry *rules,* professional staff education, formulary changes, or a combination of these actions. The drug use evaluation results and action plan are presented to the P&T committee for consideration. The committee will review and endorse and/or modify the plan for implementation and follow-up. A single drug use evaluation should not continue indefinitely. Once the desired endpoint has been achieved, an ongoing review may be discontinued or conducted less frequently (e.g., once or twice a year).

Medication Use Policies

Medication use policies are critical in the management of medications in the health care settings. Such policies should include the following:

- Formulary management
- P&T committee
- Medication prescribing, dispensing, and administration

Formulary Management

Formulary policies should include information on who may use a specific agent (formulary restrictions), how a drug is added or deleted from the formulary, how a drug is stocked, and which drugs are stocked. The formulary restriction policy should specifically define how items are selected for formulary restriction, rationale for selecting approved prescribers, and a method for managing the process. A formulary policy should describe the method for drug addition and deletion as well as nonformulary drug use. A policy should describe how an agent is added to the pharmacy stock once it is added to the formulary and who gets to decide. For example, the P&T committee approves the addition of a chemical entity added and the pharmacy manager selects dosage forms, strengths, et cetera, or the P&T committee determines the chemical entity and dosage form(s) and the pharmacy manager selects the strengths or sizes to be stocked. The basic policies and procedures governing the formulary system should be incorporated in the medical staff bylaws or in the medical staff rules and regulations.

Pharmacy and Therapeutics Committee

The policy should address the committee membership, operation, and responsibilities.

Medication Prescribing, Dispensing, and Administration

Organizational policies on the prescribing, dispensing, and administration of pharmaceuticals are required and necessary to ensure safe medication use. Such policies should address all aspects of the medication process.

- *writing medication orders or prescriptions*—Defines practitioners that may write medication orders or prescriptions in concert with state and federal regulations. This or related policies may also include the format for order writing and unacceptable abbreviations.
- *verbal orders*—Defines who may accept a verbal order and the transcription process of such an order. This policy should address the reading back of the order to confirm its accuracy.
- *stop orders*—Defines the orders that are automatically terminated, how the prescriber is notified, if appropriate, and the method for their reinstatement. Stop orders are often established for medications that require additional evaluation after a specific time. Examples of stop orders are antibiotic therapy stopped after 7 days and nesiritide therapy stopped after 24 hours.

- *investigational drug orders*—Defines how investigational drugs are managed in the health care system. This policy should include the review process as well as the method for prescribing, dispensing, administering, and monitoring investigational agents.
- *controlled substances*—Defines the flow of controlled substances through the health care system. This policy should include approved prescribers, the ordering process from the pharmacy and the vendor, the distribution and tracking of use, discrepancy tracking and follow-up, and management of diversion.
- *generic and therapeutic substitution*—Defines how a drug is selected for generic substitution and therapeutic equivalents approved by the P&T committee. It should describe how an alternative agent may be prescribed if deemed medically necessary.
- *self-administration of medications*—Defines the conditions and process for the administration of medication by the patient in the hospital setting.
- *medication samples*—Defines the conditions and process for the use of medication samples in the hospital or clinic setting.
- *floor stock*—Defines the criteria for selecting agents for floor stock, process for modifying the stock, and the regular review of the stock by the P&T committee.
- *definition of order interpretation*—Defines the meaning of specific types of orders including sliding scale orders, range orders, as needed orders, tapering orders, and titrating orders.
- *medication administration times*—Defines specific medication administration times and rules for interpretation. This may include the definition of *stat* and related terminology.
- *adverse drug reactions*—Defines an adverse drug reaction, the reporting process, and monitoring methods.
- *medication errors*—Defines a medication error, the reporting process, and monitoring methods.
- *others*—Other topics for policy consideration include pharmaceutical representatives, pharmacy hours of service, emergency medications, and medication delivery devices.

> **Key Point . . .**
>
> Organizational policies on the prescribing, dispensing, and administration of pharmaceuticals are required and necessary to ensure safe medication use.
>
> **. . . So what?**
>
> Policies are developed for common, well understood problems seen in the mediation use process. They are designed to ensure that the produces and services provided by a pharmacy are of consistent high quality. Rather than re-inventing the wheel each time a problem occurs, clear directions are given delineating responsibilities and actions. Policies are not meant to replace professional judgment of pharmacists (e.g., I know it is a bad idea. I am just following our policy). They are meant to supplement and guide pharmacist decision making.

Published Formulary

The published formulary should provide information on the medications approved for use, basic therapeutic information about each item, information on medication use policies and procedures, and special information about medications such as dosing guidelines, etc.

Medication List

The key element of the published formulary is the list of medications approved for use. This section includes both entries for each medication and indexes to facilitate use.

Medication entries may be arranged alphabetically by generic name and trade (synonym) name, therapeutic class, or a combination. At a minimum, each drug entry should include the following:

- *generic name of primary active ingredient*—Combination products may be listed by generic ingredients or trade name.
- *trade or synonym name that is commonly used*—A disclaimer in the introduction to the formulary should explain that the presence or absence of a trade name does not imply that it is or is not the agent stocked by the pharmacy.
- *dosage form, strength, and size stocked by the pharmacy*
- *active ingredients (formulation) for combination products*

Additional information that may be added:

- *DEA schedule (C-II through C-V)*
- *special precautions*—Such as for im use only and protect from light.
- *pediatric or adult dosage ranges*
- *cost information*—Some health-systems have chosen not to publish actual purchase prices for confidentiality reasons but rather to list a cost scale to allow for price comparisons. Cost information is most useful when drugs are arranged within a therapeutic group or class to allow for easy comparison.

The medication list should include one or more indexes. The index should assist the user in locating the medication entry by generic name. The index should include both generic and trade name entries. The trade name entry may state "see generic name, page 123." Such an index may be incorporated into the formulary itself. If that is done, then the formulary listing should be alphabetical and include both generic and trade names. A second index type is the therapeutic index. This index arranges drugs generically by therapeutic or pharmacologic class. It is particularly useful for the prescriber that is not familiar with the formulary of a health-system and desires to prescribe a certain type of drug (i.e., ACE inhibitor).

Medication Use Policy and Procedures

Inclusion of information on the prescribing, dispensing, and administration of medications in the published formulary provides a quick reference for health care providers. Either selected policies may be published or key information summarized in an abbreviated format. Policies for inclusion are the formulary policy, P&T committee policy, and organizational regulations regarding medication use. Information on pharmacy operating procedures may be beneficial. These would include hours of services, prescription policies, medication distribution procedures, contact information and other pharmacy services such as anticoagulation monitoring or pharmacy newsletters.

Medication Use Guidelines

This section should detail guidelines for medication use, which are approved or endorsed by the P&T committee. Such guidelines may include preprinted orders and clinical pathways that have been developed. Examples of medication use guidelines are provided below.

- Antibiotic use guidelines
- Antibiotic use in surgical prophylaxis
- Community acquired pneumonia clinical pathway
- Weight-based heparin orders
- Potassium replacement orders
- ICU sedation guidelines
- Thrombolytic therapy guidelines for stroke
- Alcohol detoxification orders

Special Information

The information in this section is health-system specific. It should be tailored to the needs of the professional and medical staff based on the services provided by the health-system and the pharmacy. Examples of topics to include are below.

- Nutritional products approved for use
- Equivalent dosage tables (e.g., pain medications, corticosteroids)
- Parenteral nutrition formulas
- Pediatric dosages
- Potassium content of drugs or foods
- Antidote list
- Advanced Cardiac Life Support (ACLS) or emergency medication list and dosages
- Metric conversion table
- Serum drug levels
- Standard concentrations of drugs in IV solutions
- Common equations used (e.g., ideal body weight, estimated creatinine clearance, anion gap)
- Antibiograms
- Drug dosing in renal or hepatic dysfunction
- Examples of forms that are routinely used such as nonformulary drug requests, adverse drug reaction reports

Publishing the Formulary

The formulary must be published regularly. The medication list should be readily available to all personnel involved in the medication process. Electronic versions of the formulary may be preferable. Copies of the formulary should be made available where medications are prescribed, administered, and dispensed. Printed formularies are often revised and printed annually. A method should be established for updating the formulary between editions.

Summary

The pharmacist plays a critical role in the management of medication use in the health-system. As the drug expert, the pharmacist can assure safe, efficacious, and cost effective drug use through the formulary system. Ongoing formulary maintenance and routine drug use evaluations are key elements in this process. Focused consideration of medication safety in all medication related discussions optimizes formulary system management.

References

1. Foulke GE, Siepler J. Antiulcer Therapy: An Exercise in Formulary Management. *J Clin Gastroenterol.* 1990;12(suppl 2):S64-8.

2. Kozma CM, Reeder CE, Lingle EW. Expanding Medicaid drug formulary coverage. Effects on utilization of related services. *Med Care.* 1990 Oct;28(10):963-977.

3. Posey LM. Formularies and quality of care: Pharmacoeconomics drives revisionist thinking. *The Consultant Pharmacist.*1996 May;11(5).

4. Blumenthal D, Herdman R, eds. *Description and Analysis of the VA National Formulary.* VA Pharmacy Formulary Analysis Committee, Division of Health Care Services, Institute of Medicine; 2000.

5. Formulary Management. The Academy of Managed Care Pharmacy's concepts in managed care pharmacy. Academy of Managed Care Pharmacy. Available at: http://www.amcp.org/amcp.ark?p=AAAC630C. Accessed June 20, 2010.

6. Tanielian T, Harris K, Suárez A, et al. *Impact of a Uniform Formulary on Military Health-system Prescribers: Baseline Survey Results.* National Defense Research Institute and Rand Health; 2003.

7. White paper: formulary development at express scripts. Available at: http://www.express-scripts.org/research/formularyinformation/development/formularyDevelopment.pdf. Accessed June 20,2010.

8. American Society of Health-System Pharmacists. *ASHP Statement on Medication Use Policy Development.* Bethesda, MD: American Society of Health-System Pharmacists; draft.

9. Pedersen CA, Schneider PJ, Scheckelhoff DJ. ASHP national survey of pharmacy practice in hospital settings: prescribing and transcribing 2007. *Am J Health-Syst Pharm.* 2008. 65: 827-843.

10. American Society of Health-System Pharmacists. ASHP guidelines on the pharmacy and therapeutics committee and the formulary system. *Am J Health-Syst Pharm.* 2008; 65:1272-1283.

11. American Society of Health-System Pharmacists. Principles of a sound formulary system. Bethesda, MD: American Society of Health-System Pharmacists; 2000, 2006.

12. American Society of Health-System Pharmacists. ASHP statement on the pharmacy and therapeutics committee and the formulary system. Bethesda, MD: American Society of Health-System Pharmacists; 2008.

Chapter Review Questions

1. **The following elements of the formulary system are used to manage drug costs (select all applicable).**
    a. Therapeutic interchange
    b. Nonformulary drug use
    c. Generic substitution
    d. Drug Therapy guidelines

    Answer: a, c, d. Nonformulary drug use often drives up drug costs in a health-system.

2. **Once the formulary has been established, no further action is required except to add new pharmaceutical entities as they become available.**
    a. True
    b. False

    Answer: b. False. The formulary must continually be evaluated for additions and deletions.

3. **P&T committees may have subcommittees to facilitate specific objectives. Examples of subcommittees include (select all applicable)**
    a. Medication Safety
    b. Antibiotic/Infectious Disease
    c. Laboratory Testing

    Answer: a, b. Laboratory testing is not under the purview of the P&T committee; but rather the pathology committee of the medical staff or health-system.

4. **When selecting a drug for formulary addition, which of the following should be considered? (select applicable)**
   a. Does it come in unit dose packaging?
   b. Is it a duplication of an existing formulary agent?
   c. How should it be used?
   d. Is it safer than similar agents already on formulary?
   e. Will the vendor give the health-system free samples?

   Answer: b, c, d.

5. **The _____ is responsible for oversight of all medication use in the hospital.**

   Answer: Pharmacy and therapeutics (P&T) committee.

6. **Therapeutic interchange is the**
   a. Interchange of generic equivalents
   b. Interchange of chemically different drugs within the same pharmacologic or therapeutic class
   c. Interchange of chemically different drugs within the same pharmacologic or therapeutic class in accordance with approved written guidelines

   Answer: c. Therapeutic interchange must be approved prior to implementation.

7. **Medication use evaluation is a systematic approach to monitoring drug therapy and associated outcomes. The optimal data collection period is**

   _____

   Answer: Concurrent or during the patient visit.

8. **The Pharmacy and Therapeutics Committee is a multi-disciplinary committee including physicians, pharmacists, and nurses.**
   a. True
   b. False

   Answer: a. True. While pharmacists and nurses may not be permitted to vote, they are important members of the committee.

9. **The rationale for completing a drug use evaluation is to**
   a. Validate drug use is safe and appropriate.
   b. Determine the most common prescribers of a specific drug.
   c. Educate the nursing staff on appropriate medication administration.

   Answer: a. DUE monitoring criteria often include indication for use and adverse events as well as other criteria such as dose, frequency, route of administration, etc.

10. **The pharmacist is *not* responsible for assuring the following**
   a. Quality, quantity and source of all medications in the health-system.
   b. All medications in the health-system meet FDA and USP standards.
   c. All brands of formulary agents are available for use in the health-system.

   Answer: c. Formulary systems seek to reduce the number of brands of medication because offering all brands is inefficient and costly.

Chapter Discussion Questions

1. How do formularies influence medication use within institutions?
2. How can pharmacists take a leadership role in the formulary management?
3. What are key elements in successful and efficient operation of a Pharmacy and Therapeutics Committee?
4. How are Drug Use Guidelines incorporated into the formulary management process?

CHAPTER 5

Clinical Pharmacy

John E. Murphy

Learning Objectives

After completing this chapter, readers should be able to:

1. Discuss different perspectives on the activities and practice of "clinical pharmacy."
2. Contrast clinical pharmacy services with distributive pharmacy services.
3. Identify common clinical pharmacy services offered in hospitals and health-systems.
4. Identify the five clinical pharmacy services that are most closely associated with reduced mortality, decreased drug and total cost of care, and reductions in length of stay and medication errors in hospitals.
5. Advocate for the value of clinical pharmacy services.

Key Terms and Definitions

- **Board certification:** The process by which a clinician specialist may be recognized as possessing a high level of knowledge about the specialty. The initial recognition is by examination after a period of time practicing or doing a residency in the specialty area. Maintenance of specialty recognition may be done by specific education over time or re-examination. Current specialties include: nuclear pharmacy, nutrition support pharmacy, oncology pharmacy, pharmacotherapy, and psychiatric pharmacy. In 2009 the Board of Pharmaceutical Specialties recognized ambulatory care as a pharmacy specialty. The first exam for this specialty is scheduled for 2011.
- **Board of Pharmacy Specialties (BPS):** The board that recognizes, sets standards for, and provides board certification in specific clinical specialties. It oversees the development of specialties and the examinations and continuing education programs for the specialties (http://www.bpsweb.org/).
- **Clinical pharmacist:** An individual in any practice setting who provides a substantial amount of direct patient-oriented care with an emphasis on the science and practice of rational drug use.
- **Clinical pharmacy:** The area of pharmacy concerned with the science and practice of rational medication use. It is patient-directed, evidence-based, and

designed to promote health, wellness, and disease prevention in order to improve the quality of life of patients.

■ **Credentials:** Documented evidence of professional qualifications. For pharmacists, examples of credentials include academic degrees, state licensure, residency program certificate of completion, and board certification in a pharmacy specialty.

■ **Evidence-based:** Refers to health care decisions that incorporate the best evidence currently available in the scientific literature and systematic study of what works best in patient populations.

■ **Fellowship:** A 1- to 3-year research-related experience (usually clinical research) that may contain a small portion of associated clinical practice skill development.

■ **PGY1:** Postgraduate year 1 residency. These residencies are general in nature and designed to expose the resident to a variety of practice areas. PGY1 residents grow beyond entry-level competence in direct patient care and in pharmacy operational services. They also develop leadership skills to apply to any position in any setting. Instructional emphasis in the residency is on the progressive development of clinical judgment under the guidance of model practitioners. Residents acquire competencies in "managing and improving the medication-use process; providing evidence-based, patient-centered medication therapy management with interprofessional teams; exercising leadership and practice management; demonstrating project management skills; providing medication and practice-related education/training; and utilizing medical informatics."[3]

■ **PGY2:** Postgraduate year 2 residency. These residencies are more specialized in nature and prepare the resident to manage the medication therapy of specialty patients. "They are designed to develop accountability; practice patterns; habits; and expert knowledge, skills, attitudes, and abilities in the respective advanced area of pharmacy practice."[3] Completion of a PGY2 program should help prepare the resident for board certification in the specialty practice area, when board certification for the area exists.

■ **Residency:** An organized and directed postgraduate training experience of 1–2 years duration that serves as a bridge between education and practice. The resident is exposed to key areas of practice where they will increasingly take responsibility for the care of patients. They also will focus on learning about the medication use system at the residency site.

■ ■ ■

Introduction

The pharmacy profession has long been evolving its various roles of delivering care to patients. Throughout history the profession has been associated with the delivery of medications as one of its primary values for patients in need of these therapies. As the preparation of medications moved from individual pharmacists to the pharmaceutical industry, and dispensing processes became functions that could be well handled by pharmacy technicians and technology, pharmacists have continually evaluated their purpose and evolved in their optimal roles in patient care.

As early as the 1950s, health-system pharmacy pioneers were advocating that pharmacists go to patient care areas and create a clinical role, including rounding with physicians.[1] These individual pioneers of clinical pharmacy were driven to encourage and enable pharmacists to use their drug knowledge in the clinical care of patients.[2] By the 1970s and 1980s, pharmacists in health-system settings were creating many new clinical roles. Pharmacy organizations began creating policies and activities to enhance the clinical skills of their members and also encouraged the colleges and schools of pharmacy to train their students to become clinicians, something many resisted adopting or even fought against. Thus, creating cross-cutting change required the development of consensus. As momentum built for change, various organizations sought ways to coordinate thought about the new directions. For example, the American Society of Health-System Pharmacists (ASHP; then the American Society of Hospital Pharmacists) held a conference called "Directions for Clinical Practice in Pharmacy" in 1985 on Hilton Head Island in South Carolina that helped galvanize thinking about the clinical future of the profession.

Key Point . . .

The move toward training all pharmacists to take on clinical roles is something that was opposed by many individuals inside and outside of the profession.

. . . So what?

It is easy to take for granted today the opportunities available for pharmacists in clinical practice. However, many pharmacists and others fought for years against the move toward a clinical practice model. Indeed, there are still pharmacists today who resist accepting substantial clinical roles.

What is Clinical Pharmacy?

"It's the Patient, Stupid"

When former U.S. president Bill Clinton was first running for office it was reported that he kept a sign prominently placed in his campaign headquarters stating "It's the economy, stupid!" to keep him focused on the most important issue to the American people at the time. When it is time to consider what clinical pharmacy is or isn't, staying laser-focused on why pharmacy and the health professions exist can be simply stated, "It's the patient." We exist to serve them well. **Clinical pharmacy** has been defined by many over the years, including the American College of Clinical Pharmacy (ACCP), which has done so in simple abridged fashion as "the area of pharmacy concerned with the science and practice of rational medication use."[4] Others have called it "the concept of a patient-oriented rather than a drug product-oriented pharmacy practitioner..."[5] ACCP further states that **clinical pharmacists** "provide patient care that optimizes medication therapy and promotes health, wellness, and disease prevention."[4] They also provide a more detailed unabridged definition that focuses on 1) the discipline of clinical pharmacy, 2) the clinical pharmacist, and 3) the roles of the clinical pharmacist. These three areas will be discussed in greater detail in this chapter.

ACCP and ASHP have developed many documents describing the competencies and training necessary to provide clinical pharmacy services (direct patient care), including the necessity for residency training and the vision that pharmacists will increasingly become board certified if they provide direct patient care in specialty areas.[6-10]

The Joint Commission of Pharmacy Practitioners (JCPP), a forum for the chief executive and chief elected officers of the 11 premier national pharmacy organizations, has published its vision for what pharmacy practice will look like in 2015.[11] Their vision is that "Pharmacists will be the health care professionals responsible for providing patient care that ensures optimal medication therapy outcomes," and that this will occur because pharmacists "will have the authority and autonomy to manage medication therapy and will be accountable for patients' therapeutic outcomes." These are clearly clinical pharmacy functions that are unrelated to dispensing.

The ultimate goal of clinical pharmacy should be that "every patient who needs the clinical drug knowledge and skill of the pharmacist does in fact receive the services."[2] This isn't the case in most practice settings, and though progress has surely been made, there have been suggestions that little real change has occurred in the profession over the last 15 years despite the great need that exists.[12] Because medication therapy has become an extremely important part of healthcare, the need for medication therapy experts is critical. ASHP stated in their long-range vision for the pharmacy work force document that "Medication use in hospitals and health-systems is a prominent therapy for virtually all patients, and it is inherently complex and dangerous."[10] Clearly this is also the case for many patients on multiple medications who are virtually on their own when it comes to understanding their drug therapy. Clinical pharmacists have the education and training to help these patients when given the opportunity.

As clinical pharmacy developed over the years, some pharmacy leaders began to suggest that it was "a reactive service supplied on the request of physicians for physicians," rather than direct care for the patient themselves.[13] This, in part, led to the redefining concept of pharmaceutical care, which may be considered "Responsible provision of drug therapy for the purpose of achieving definite outcomes that improve a patient's quality of life."[14] "Pharmaceutical care" later transformed to "pharmacy care" in the lexicon of several pharmacy organizations. "Pharmacy care" is essentially a rebranding of the pharmaceutical care concepts to focus on pharma-

Key Point . . .

Clinical pharmacy is patient-oriented rather than drug product–oriented.

. . . So what?

The pharmacy profession has attempted to move from an orientation toward a thing (i.e., drug) to a focus on a person (i.e., the patient). This reorientation has been slow for a number of reasons. One, pharmacists are the only professionals uniquely associated with medications and the effective distribution of drugs is sufficiently large without taking on other responsibilities. Two, payment for pharmacist services revolves around the dispensing of drugs— not managing the impact of those drugs on patient health outcomes. Thus, that which gets paid for gets accomplished. Three, barriers in health care still exist toward pharmacists having greater patient-orientation: antiquated laws, perceptions of the public, inadequate technology, and the structure and financing of the health care system.

cy rather than pharmaceuticals, since the proponents of "pharmaceutical care" indicated that the services could be provided by many health care providers.[15] In truth, all of these terms and the functions describe the role of pharmacists in ensuring optimal outcomes for patients through rational drug therapy, which is the ideal of clinical pharmacy practice.[13]

The Discipline and the Process

As members of a health science discipline, clinical pharmacists optimize medication therapy and promote health, wellness, and disease prevention. Further, the discipline embraces pharmaceutical care by blending "a caring orientation with specialized therapeutic knowledge, experience, and judgment for the purpose of ensuring optimal patient outcomes."[2]

An Evidence-Based Process

Determining the best use of medications for individuals and populations must be **evidence-based** because such guidelines for performance improvement have been shown to improve patient care outcomes.[16] Clinical pharmacists have long provided valuable services to health care teams through analysis of the literature and development of treatment guidelines and a number of pharmacy organizations have created policies promoting the pharmacists' role in these processes. An example of this comes from the American Pharmacists Association (APhA). APhA states that pharmacists should be directly involved in developing, evaluating, and implementing clinical guidelines for diseases. They further suggest that guidelines can promote interprofessional team approaches to patient care where pharmacists' expertise in optimizing patient outcomes can be used. APhA also believes that clinical guidelines should be developed using interprofessional approaches and be built on the best scientific data that is evaluated regularly to ensure the guidelines reflect current practice standards.[17] The latter is an important consideration since new knowledge can, on occasion, substantially change the thinking on how patients should be treated for a given disease. Thus, clinical pharmacists must commit to lifelong learning and frequent assessment of the literature to ensure that treatment approaches are the best possible for patients.

Another example of an organization promoting the value and role of pharmacists in developing and applying evidence-based approaches is ASHP's 2015 Initiative, which states that by 2015 pharmacists in 90% of hospitals "will be actively involved in providing care to individual patients that is based on evidence, such as the use of quality drug information resources, published clinical studies or guidelines, and expert consensus advice."[18] They further propose that pharmacists will be active participants in developing and implementing drug therapy protocols and/or order sets that are evidence-based.[18] Development of evidence-based guidelines and ensuring their use provides outstanding opportunities for clinical pharmacists to impact large numbers of patients in a variety of healthcare delivery settings.

Therapeutic Problem Solving Processes

Clinicians generally follow fairly standard processes to evaluate patients, determine appropriate treatments, and document the findings in patient charts. Common approaches in pharmacy are SOAP and FARM notes. SOAP stands for *S*ubjective findings, *O*bjective findings, *A*ssessment, and *P*lan. FARM stands for *F*indings, *A*ssessment, *R*ecommendations, and *M*onitoring. Other approaches have also been suggested for pharmacists to organize their evaluation of patients. For example, the Clinical Pharmacist Recommendation (CPR) Taxonomy was developed for clinical use by pharmacists and also to be able to compare clinical pharmacy intervention trials.[19] Another, the Pharmacists' Management of Drug-Related Problems (PMDRP), was designed to reduce variation in monitoring forms and to focus more specifically on the identification and management of drug-related problems.[20] All of these methods serve to consistently organize a clinician's evaluation of a patient and each allows for similar information to be incorporated, though under slightly different headings. No matter which rubrics are used, there is value in consistency of approaches to evaluating patients.

The Clinical Pharmacist

Competencies

The clinical pharmacist is a highly educated and well-trained individual, with specialized knowledge and experience, who contributes to the outcomes of patients by using this knowledge to enhance drug therapy. In addition to the development of specific competencies, clinical pharmacists must be dedicated to life-long learning to ensure their value to the interprofessional health care team. Specific competencies and roles of the clinical pharmacist have been outlined in a number of publications and in policies and guidelines of various pharmacy organizations. For example, the ACCP created a task force to outline the competencies they considered of greatest importance for clinical pharmacists.[6] An extensive list was developed, a summary of which is shown in Table 5-1.

Education, Training, and Credentials

Many early clinical pharmacists honed their skills with on-the-job training and just getting involved; they may or may not have had an advanced degree or residency training prior to beginning their participation. Though this pathway clearly remains possible today, the academic and training environment has changed. On the education side, all pharmacists in the U.S. graduate with a Doctor of Pharmacy degree that provides more clinical education than ever before. But, medication therapy is becoming increasingly complex as well, particularly in the health-system setting.

After graduation from pharmacy school, opportunities to advance skills and knowledge exist through continuing professional development programs, postgraduate training (e.g., **residencies** and **fellowships**), and graduate school. Organizations like ACCP and ASHP have gone on record stating that all pharmacy students planning on providing *direct patient care clinical services* should be adding **PGY1 (post-**

Key Point . . .

Attaining advanced degrees or residency training are well-recognized and accepted paths to becoming a clinical pharmacist, although rigorous on-the-job training is still a challenging and possible option.

. . . So what?

The automatic answer that many educators and clinical pharmacists provide to students seeking a clinical career is, "Do a residency." However, this traditional path toward becoming a clinical pharmacist is not the only one. Many clinical pharmacists learned on-the-job: a path requiring exceptional and highly motivated individuals for success.

Table 5-1.
Clinical Pharmacist Competencies[6]

I.   Clinical problem solving, judgment, and decision making

   A.   Monitor patients in the health care setting.
   B.   Assess patient-specific medical problems.
   C.   Evaluate patient-specific drug therapy and therapeutic problems.
   D.   Design a comprehensive drug therapy plan for patient-specific problems.
   E.   Collaborate with patients, caregivers, and other health care professionals.

II. Communication and education

   A.   Educate patients.
   B.   Educate other health care professionals.
   C.   Communicate effectively.
   D.   Document interventions in the patient medical record.

III. Medical information evaluation and management

   A.   Demonstrate the motivation and commitment to become a lifelong learner.
   B.   Retrieve biomedical literature using appropriate search strategies.
   C.   Interpret biomedical literature with regard to study design, methodology, statistical analysis, significance of reported data, and conclusions.
   D.   Integrate data obtained from multiple sources to derive an overall conclusion or answer.

IV. Management of patient populations

   A.   Patient safety and drug therapy evaluation.
   B.   Critical pathways.

V.   Therapeutic knowledge areas

   A.   Apply disease-oriented knowledge of the following areas (various areas provided in document—some examples include anatomy, epidemiology, prognosis, interpretation of laboratory tests).
   B.   Demonstrate competence in the pharmacotherapy of the following medical problems (various areas provided in document—example categories include bone and joint, cardiovascular, dermatologic, endocrine, infectious diseases, etc. There are also subcategories under each of these).
   C.   Apply the following principles in the setting of each disease state, patient population, and/or therapeutic category (examples of included items are: pharmacokinetics, pharmacogenomics, health screening, drug interactions, immunizations, considerations for geriatrics and pediatrics, etc.).
     1.   Additional details of competencies are provided under each subcategory

graduate year one) **residency training** to their credentials by the year 2020, with the assumption that the percent of graduates will continually increase up to that point.[8,21] The organizations realized that some graduates would pursue other opportunities that would not require the extensive clinical education and training provided by a residency, such as graduate school in a basic science discipline, and law school. ACCP also suggested that most clinical faculty should have a **PGY2 (post-graduate year two) specialty residency** as might clinicians practicing in specialty areas of the health-system. Some clinical pharmacists will also desire to advance their research skills and may pursue graduate degrees or fellowships, particularly if they are interested in an academic or industry position with research as an important component.

In addition to the education and training credentials available to individuals, increasing numbers of specialist pharmacists seek to demonstrate their knowledge through board certification. These **credentials** can enhance an individual's ability to gain clinical privileges to provide patient care services. In addition, **board certification** will increasingly be recognized by purchasers of clinical pharmacy services. The issues of credentialing and privileging for pharmacists have been well articulated in two papers that are worth reading by anyone interested in the processes and terminology.[22,23] Both ACCP and ASHP have stated that most clinical pharmacists providing direct patient care in specialty areas will be board certified in the future.[9,10] Pharmacy students should learn about the **Board of Pharmaceutical Specialties** and the processes for attaining specialty certification in order to determine the value that such certification might provide for them (see http://www.bpsweb.org/).

Key Point . . .

Both ACCP and ASHP have stated that most clinical pharmacists providing direct patient care in specialty areas will be board certified in the future.

. . . So what?

As the profession evolves, requirements for practice will evolve too. The trend in clinical practice is an expectation that clinical specialists become board certified. New pharmacists should consider board certification as a possible way of differentiating themselves for future clinical positions.

Roles of the Clinical Pharmacist

There are a wide variety of activities associated with clinical pharmacy practice. Bond and Raehl evaluated associations of clinical pharmacy services and level of pharmacy staffing with reductions in hospital mortality rates.[24,25] The services evaluated and the percent of responding hospitals offering the services at the time included: drug use evaluation (94.5%), pharmacokinetic consultations (80.3%), adverse drug reaction management (70.4%), drug protocol management (69.6%), in-service education (65.5%), drug therapy monitoring (53.5%), drug therapy counseling (46.3%), TPN team participation (43.6%), participation on cardiopulmonary resuscitation team (31.8%), drug information services (25.7%), participation on medical rounds (22.9%), poison information (15.5%), clinical research (11.8%), and the taking of admission drug histories (4.2%).[24]

Pharmacokinetic consultations can be used as an example of growth and evolution of a clinical service over time as well as an indicator of the types of medications for which pharmacists are providing consultations, since pharmacists have been active in providing pharmacokinetic consultations for a long time. In the early days of these services, hospitals may have had specific dosing services with pharmacokinetics specialists, but now most of the consults are provided by the clinical pharmacy staff in the institutions.[26] These pharmacy directed services were provided in 86.8% of hospitals responding to a 2006 survey, a 117.5% increase from an earlier survey in 1989.[27] The 2006 survey determined that more than 60% of the institutions provide drug therapy consultations and therapeutic monitoring for the aminoglycosides and vancomycin while 20% to 40% provided these services for warfarin, low-molecular-weight and unfractionated heparins, fluoroquinolones, antiparkinsonian drugs, proton pump inhibitors, HIV drugs, and cephalosporins.[27]

When Bond and Raehl combined all of their previous study data they found five key clinical pharmacist services that were associated with reductions in patient mortality, decreased drug and total cost of care, and reductions in length of stay and medication errors.[27] The authors suggested that the profession must agree to consistently provide these services in order to increase the potential for recognition as healthcare providers. The five services were:

1. Drug information
2. Adverse drug reaction management
3. Drug protocol management
4. Participating in medical rounds
5. Admission drug histories

In their earlier work, Bond and Raehl found that the number of clinical pharmacists and pharmacy administrators/100 occupied beds was also associated with reduced mortality rates.[24] This is an indicator of the value of managing and providing clinical services.

Other Clinical Pharmacy Services

Pharmacists have been involved in many innovative clinical services over time. In April of 2009, a PubMed literature search of publications over the last 5 years using the term "role of the pharmacist" yielded over 3,000 references to publications containing this phrase. This is an indicator of efforts by pharmacists to create new, primarily clinical roles. Some of the roles described in the literature include caring for diabetic patients, patients with chronic renal failure, patients in prisons, medication therapy management services, patients with hypertension and hyperlipidemia, and migraine. Other important clinical services include the following:

- Medication reconciliation—Medication reconciliation is a relatively new service provided by pharmacists in response to the understanding that medication errors occur too frequently when patients are transferred from one setting to another and medications are added or deleted without determining whether they are needed or not. The Joint Commission established medication reconciliation as an important quality service for hospitals and pharmacists increasingly provide these reviews.
- Education—Though education, per se, is not a solely a clinical service, institutions associated with educating pharmacy students generally provide more clinical pharmacy services than institutions that do not.[28]
- Collaborative practice—Laws and regulations permitting collaborative practice arrangements between pharmacists and prescribers have been enacted in over 40 states in the US. These arrangements allow pharmacists to control the medication therapy of specified patients and sometimes specified diseases in collaboration with one or more prescribers.
- Immunizations—The physical aspect of administering an injection should not be considered a clinical pharmacy service. Conversely, determining a patient's need for an immunization and setting up a tracking and reminder program to ensure that patients are immunized would be a clinical service.
- Primary care—Pharmacists have opportunities to participate in providing primary care services for patients. These are most often done as part of a collaborative practice in setting where access to patient data is easiest. As electronic medical records are more readily available, access may become more virtual (i.e., electronically) than site-dependent, creating new opportunities for collaboration of pharmacists and primary care providers.

- Identifying and resolving drug related problems in population based care—Clinical pharmacists provide valuable population based care through the development and enforcement of guidelines in managed care settings. Medication therapy management programs provided to large groups of patients also provide these opportunities.
- Designing systems that prevent drug related problems at the individual and population level—Many pharmacists are involved as medication safety officers in hospital settings, developing programs designed to identify and prevent drug problems for both individual patients and for groups of patients.

Contrasting Clinical and Distributional Activities

Clinical and drug distribution services are distinct but complementary activities in ensuring safe medication use. Medication distribution to patient attempts to ensure that the correct physical product gets to the patient. However, important clinical opportunities exist at the point of patient medication distribution to reduce medication problems and enhance the potential for the medications to be beneficial. These include, among other possibilities, determining that the medication is appropriate for the patient (e.g., avoidance of serious drug-drug interactions or allergies, correct dose) and ensuring that the instructions for safe and effective use of the medication are understood by the patient or their caregiver. The actual technical functions that make up the distribution process such as determining the medication ordered and instructions for use, creating a label, and preparing the medication in an appropriate container, are activities that do not require the clinical skills and knowledge of a pharmacist. While it is abundantly clear that distribution systems must be safe so that patients do not get the wrong medications or incorrect doses of medication, and that pharmacists should ensure that these processes work correctly, pharmacists should have limited involvement with these technical aspects of the process as they can be appropriately done by well-trained technicians and by technology.

A review of controlled studies that included evaluation of comprehensive patient counseling services by pharmacists at discharge or at the time of dispensing demonstrated that these services led to improved patient outcomes.[29] Unfortunately, such comprehensive services or even cursory instructions for use are not consistently provided to patients who may need them. In community settings, research by Elizabeth Flynn and colleagues showed that less than a third of patients were automatically counseled by pharmacists when receiving new prescriptions for medications whose misuse could lead to

Key Point . . .

Clinical and drug distribution services are distinct but complementary activities in ensuring safe medication use.

. . . So what?

The patient-centered integrated model of practice described in Chapter 1 of this text recognizes the responsibility of pharmacists for both clinical and distributional roles because of the realization that both are essential for managing the medication use process. Clinical practice relies on an efficient, well-run distribution system, while getting the right drug in the right dose to the right patient at the right time via the right route of administration relies on good clinical services.

harm.[30] Of interest in this study, pharmacist counseling was unrelated to the busyness of the store.

This highlights a problem with the current dispensing processes—pharmacists are not providing even minimal discussions that patients may need about medications. Indeed, this problem has existed for decades. Over 28 years ago, Russell Miller said that dispensing-oriented practices led to the "frustration of many pharmacists who had completed five or more years of difficult studies only to enter a rather undemanding, unprofessional practice."[5] Unfortunately, the same can be said today for much of the dispensing-oriented practices in too many pharmacy settings. Even worse, another year of training is now associated with getting a pharmacy degree. It is clear that pharmacy must make the full transition to clinical practice. Graduating pharmacy students are too highly trained to be limited to only dispensing medications, and it is hard to justify to employers the high salaries of pharmacists, if they are underemployed in routine dispensing tasks.

One of the most important areas for clinical pharmacy service provision lies in identifying and resolving drug related problems in direct patient care. Research has shown the unfortunately extensive incidence of drug related problems that can lead to morbidity and mortality as well as huge economic burden.[31-33] Since many studies have demonstrated that pharmacists providing clinical services directly to patients can decrease these problems, it is unfortunate that such services are not consistently provided while routine technical functions continue to dominate the practice of many pharmacists.[24-27,34]

Payment for clinical services is an important criterion for the advancement of clinical pharmacy. When (or if) payment for clinical pharmacy services (either directly for the service or in the hiring of pharmacists to provide them consistently) becomes the norm in all settings, there will be better justification for pharmacists to move from the tasks of medication dispensing to the provision of clinical pharmacy services. When this occurs, patients and payers will be far better served.

Evidence of the Value of Clinical Pharmacy

Numerous studies have been conducted and published examining the outcomes of clinical pharmacy services, though the majority were not designed in a manner that could yield convincing results. However, several reviews have evaluated studies that were appropriately designed that documented both the economic and patient care outcome value of clinical pharmacist services.[35-39] One group of researchers evaluated two decades of evidence establishing the association between clinical services in hospital settings with important patient outcomes.[24,25,27,40,41] Their work showed that core services not only save money, but enhance patient outcomes. The task that remains for the profession is to

> **Key Point...**
>
> Change in pharmacy practice will only occur when pharmacists actively lobby stakeholders about the benefits of the medication therapy expertise of clinical pharmacists.
>
> **...So what?**
>
> Currently, many pharmacists do not advocate for change in pharmacy practice. However, the collective effort of the more than 200,000 practicing pharmacists in the U.S. could make things happen.

convince key stakeholders (e.g., hospital administrators, insurers, and other payers) that clinical services should be provided in all hospitals.[42] This will only occur when pharmacists actively lobby stakeholders about the benefits of the medication therapy expertise of clinical pharmacists.

Summary

Clinical pharmacy is a patient-oriented, evidence-based practice that uses the medication-related expertise of pharmacists to enhance patient outcomes and improve quality of life. Hallmarks of a patient-oriented clinical pharmacy practice include focus on the patient, taking responsibility for medication therapy outcomes, and identifying and preventing medication errors and preventable adverse drug events. Although important, services related to the product-oriented dispensing process such as determining the drug name, correct directions for use, and placing the medication in an appropriate container for use cannot be classified as clinical pharmacy services. Neither is determining formulary status of the medication in order to ensure reimbursement and providing simple directions on use (e.g., take twice daily until gone and refrigerate).

Clinical pharmacists provide patient care that optimizes medication therapy and promotes health, wellness, and disease prevention to improve the lives of patients. Five clinical pharmacy services have been shown to be associated with reductions in patient mortality, decreased drug and total cost of care, and reductions in length of stay and medication errors; drug information, adverse drug reaction management, drug protocol management, participating in medical rounds, and admission drug histories.

The value of certain clinical pharmacy services has been demonstrated in a number of studies and patients deserve to have the expertise of clinical pharmacists as participants in their treatment. To accomplish this pharmacists need to move their focus away from dispensing-related activities that can be managed by technology and well-trained technicians. Direct payment for clinical services or the hiring of pharmacists to provide these patient-oriented services is necessary to accomplish this goal and the profession must continue to advocate for these changes to optimally benefit the patients it serves.

Suggested Reading

American College of Clinical Pharmacy. The definition of clinical pharmacy. *Pharmacotherapy.* 2008;28(6):816-817.

Bertin RJ. Credentialing in pharmacy. *J Manag Care Pharm.* 2001;7:22-31.

Bond CA, Raehl CL. Clinical pharmacy services, pharmacy staffing, and hospital mortality rates. *Pharmacotherapy.* 2007;27:481-493.

Elenbaas RM, Worthen DB. *Clinical Pharmacy in the United States: Transformation of a Profession.* Lenexa, KS: American College of Clinical Pharmacy; 2009.

Murphy JE, Nappi JM, Bosso JA, et al. American College of Clinical Pharmacy's vision of the future: Postgraduate pharmacy residency training as a prerequisite for direct patient care practice. *Pharmacotherapy.* 2006:26(5):722-733. (See also the editorials accompanying this paper.)

Galt KA. Credentialing and privileging for pharmacists. *Am J Health-Syst Pharm.* 2004;61:661-670.

Joint Commission of Pharmacy Practitioners. Vision statement for pharmacy practice in 2015. http://www.accp.com/docs/positions/misc/JCPPVisionStatement.pdf Accessed May 26, 2009.

References

1. Elenbaas RM, Worthen DB. Clinical Pharmacy in the United States: Transformation of a Profession. Lenexa, KS: American College of Clinical Pharmacy; 2009.

2. Smith WE. Clinical pharmacy: Reflections and forecasts. *Ann Pharmacother.* 2007;41:325-328.

3. ASHP. Residency accreditation frequently asked questions. Available at: http://www.ashp.org/Import/ACCREDITATION/ResidentInfo/FAQs.aspx. Accessed May 30, 2009.

4. American College of Clinical Pharmacy. The definition of clinical pharmacy. *Pharmacotherapy.* 2008;28(6):816-817.

5. Miller RR. History of clinical pharmacy and clinical pharmacology. *J Clin Pharmacol.* 1981;21:195-197.

6. Burke JM, Miller WA, Spencer AP, et al. Clinical pharmacist competencies. *Pharmacotherapy.* 2008;28(6):806-815.

7. ASHP Policy Statements: Medication therapy and patient care. Available at: http://www.ashp.org/Import/PRACTICEANDPOLICY/PolicyPositionsGuidelinesBestPractices/BrowsebyTopic/MedicationTherapyandPatientCare.aspx. Accessed May 30, 2009.

8. Murphy JE, Nappi JM, Bosso JA, et al. American College of Clinical Pharmacy's Vision of the future: Postgraduate pharmacy residency training as a prerequisite for direct patient care practice. *Pharmacotherapy.* 2006:26(5):722-733.

9. Saseen JJ, Grady SE, Hansen LB, et al. Future clinical pharmacy practitioners should be board-certified specialists. *Pharmacotherapy.* 2006;26(12):1816-1825.

10. ASHP. ASHP long-range vision for the pharmacy work force in hospitals and health-systems. *Am J Health-Syst Pharm.* 2007;64:1320-1330.

11. Joint Commission of Pharmacy Practitioners. Vision statement for pharmacy practice in 2015. Available at: http://www.accp.com/docs/positions/misc/JCPPVisionStatement.pdf Accessed May 26, 2009.

12. Tse CST. Clinical pharmacy practice 30 years later. *Ann Pharmacother.* 2007;41:116-118.

13. Bosso JA. Clinical pharmacy and pharmaceutical care. *Pharmacotherapy.* 2004;24:1499-1500.

14. Hepler CD, Strand LM. Opportunities and responsibilities in pharmaceutical care. *Am J Pharm Educ.* 1989;53(suppl):S7-15.

15. Hepler CD. Clinical pharmacy, pharmaceutical care, and the quality of drug therapy. *Pharmacotherapy.* 2004;24:1491-1498.

16. Fonarow GC, Abraham WT, Albert NM, et al. Influence of a performance-improvement initiative on quality of care or patients hospitalized with heart failure. *Arch Int Med.* 2007;167:1493-1502.

17. APhA. 1995 Pharmacists' role in the development and implementation of disease-based clinical guidelines. *Am Pharm.* 1995;NS35(6):37.

18. ASHP. 2015 Health-System Pharmacy Initiative. Available at: http://www.ashp.org/s_ashp/docs/files/2015_Goals_Objectives_0508.pdf. Accessed June 5, 2009.

19. Hoth AG, Carter BL, Ness J, Bhattacharyya A, Shorr RI, Rosenthal GE, Kaboli PJ. Development and reliability testing of the clinical pharmacist recommendation taxonomy. *Pharmacotherapy.* 2007;27:639-646.

20. Winslade NE, Bajcar JM, Bombassaro AM, Caravaggio CD, Strong DK, Yamashita SK. Pharmacist's management of drug-related problems: A tool for teaching and providing pharmaceutical care. *Pharmacotherapy.* 1997;17:801-809.

21. ASHP House of Delegates Policy Statement 0701: Requirement for residency. Available at: http://www.ashp.org/DocLibrary/BestPractices/EducationandTrainingPositions.aspx. Accessed June 1, 2009.

22. Bertin RJ. Credentialing in pharmacy. *J Manag Care Pharm.* 2001;7:22-31.

23. Galt KA. Credentialing and privileging for pharmacists. *Am J Health-Syst Pharm.* 2004;61:661-670.

24. Bond CA, Raehl CL. Clinical pharmacy services, pharmacy staffing, and hospital mortality rates. *Pharmacotherapy.* 2007;27:481-493.

25. Bond CA, Raehl CL, Franke T. Clinical pharmacy services and hospital mortality rates. *Pharmacotherapy.* 1999;19:556-564.

26. Murphy JE, Slack MK, Campbell S. National survey of hospital-based pharmacokinetic services. *Am J Health-Syst Pharm.* 1996;53:2840-2847.

27. Bond CA, Raehl CL. 2006 national clinical pharmacy services survey: Clinical pharmacy services, collaborative drug management, medication errors, and pharmacy technology. *Pharmacotherapy.* 2008;28:1-13.

28. Raehl CL, Bond CA, Pitterle ME. Clinical pharmacy services in hospitals educating pharmacy students. *Pharmacotherapy.* 1998;18:1093-1102.

29. Morrison A, Wertheimer AI. Evaluation of studies investigating the effectiveness of pharmacists' clinical services. *Am J Health-Syst Pharm.* 2001;58:569-577.

30. Flynn EA, Barker KN, Berger BA, Braxton Lloyd K, Brackett PD. Dispensing errors and counseling quality in 100 pharmacies. *J Am Pharm Assoc.* 2009;49:171-180.

31. Johnson JA, Bootman JL. Drug-related morbidity and mortality: a cost-of-illness model. *Arch Int Med.* 1995;155:1949-1956.

32. Ernst FR, Grizzle AJ. Drug-related morbidity and mortality: updating the cost-of-illness model. *J Am Pharm Assoc.* 2001;41:192-199.

33. Institute of Medicine. Preventing medication errors: Quality chasm series. Institute of Medicine, 2007. Available at: http://www.nap.edu/catalog.php?record_id=11623#toc.

34. Johnson JA, Bootman JL. Drug-related morbidity and mortality and the economic impact of pharmaceutical care. *Am J Health Syst Pharm.* 1997;54:554-558.

35. Hatoum HT, Catizone C, Hutchinson RA, Purohit A. An eleven-year review of the pharmacy literature: documentation of the value and acceptance of clinical pharmacy. *Drug Intell Clin Pharm.* 1986;20:33-41.

36. Schumock GT, Meek PD, Ploetz PA, Vermeulen LC. Economic evaluations of clinical pharmacy services: 1988-1995. *Pharmacotherapy.* 2009;Jan 29(1):1-2.

37. Schumock GT, Butler MG, Meek PD, Vermeulen LC, Arondekar BV, Bauman JL. Evidence of the economic benefit of clinical pharmacy services: 1996-2000. *Pharmacotherapy.* 2003;23:113-132.

38. Perez A, Doloresco F, Hoffman JM, Meek PD, Touchette DR, Vermeulen LC, Schumock GT. Economic evaluations of clinical pharmacy services: 2001-2005. *Pharmacotherapy.* 2008;28:285e-323e.

39. De Rijdt T, Willems L, Simoens S. Economic effects of clinical pharmacy interventions: A literature review. *Am J Health-Syst Pharm.* 2008;65:1161-1172.

40. Bond CA, Raehl CL, Franke T. Interrelationships among mortality rates, drug costs, total cost of care, and length of stay in United States hospitals: Summary and recommendations for clinical pharmacy services and staffing. *Pharmacotherapy.* 2001;21:129-141.

41. Bond CA, Raehl CL, Patry R. Evidence-based core clinical pharmacy services in United States hospitals in 2020: Services and staffing. *Pharmacotherapy.* 2004;24:427-440.

42. Schumock GT. We've been shown the money, and we now know how to spend it. *Pharmacotherapy.* 1999;19:1349-1351.

Chapter Review Questions

1. **Which of the following pharmacist-provided services are not associated with reduced patient mortality in the hospital setting?**
   a. Pharmacokinetic consultation
   b. Adverse drug reaction management
   c. Drug protocol management
   d. TPN team participation
   e. Medical rounds participation

   Answer: a and d. A study by Bond and Raehl was unable to find an association between reduced mortality and pharmacokinetic consults or participation on Total Parenteral Nutrition teams.

2. **What is the approximate percentage of patients receiving an offer to counsel on new prescriptions in community pharmacies?**
    a. 67%
    b. 50%
    c. 40%
    d. 33%

    Answer: d. A study by Flynn and colleagues found that less than one third of patients with a new prescription received on offer to counsel.

3. **The likelihood of a patient receiving an offer to counsel on a new prescription is associated with the busyness of the pharmacy.**
    a. True
    b. False

    Answer: b. False. According to the study by Flynn and colleagues, an offer to counsel on new prescriptions was unrelated to how busy was the pharmacy.

4. **Clinical pharmacy and pharmaceutical care practice approaches have opposing goals.**
    a. True
    b. False

    Answer: b. False. Though some individuals consider clinical pharmacy to be focused more on providing services to physicians, the reality is that both services are defined as focusing on the patient's medication therapy for optimal outcomes that improve the patients' lives. Some would suggest that pharmaceutical care can be provided by other healthcare professionals though, while clinical pharmacy is usually defined as a service provided by a clinical pharmacist.

5. **ACCP and ASHP have stated that all pharmacy graduates should undertake a PGY1 residency.**
    a. True
    b. False

    Answer: b. False. Both organizations have said that all pharmacy graduates who intend to provide direct patient care (clinical) services should plan on a residency. Both organizations realized that graduates often have plans that could include graduate school for an MS, PhD, MBA, JD, etc. Further, both targeted 2020 as the time when this should have been completed in order to give time for more evolution of the profession and development of more residency programs and positions.

6. **Specialty board certification can be achieved by:**
    a. Attending specific continuing education programs focused on the specialty topics
    b. Passing a specialty examination after graduation and passing the NAPLEX exam.
    c. Passing a specialty examination after practicing in the specialty for a specific time period
    d. a or c

    Answer: c. All of the specialties require time in practice in the specialty before taking the exam. This can be achieved in a residency or specialty practice.

7. **Which of the following is least likely to be offered by pharmacists in U.S. hospitals?**
   a. Pharmacokinetic consultations
   b. Drug use evaluation
   c. Participation on medical rounds
   d. Adverse drug reaction management
   e. In-service education

   Answer: c. Participation on medical rounds. Although rounding with physicians is common in teaching hospitals where students receive clinical training, it is less common in non-teaching institutions. A study in 2007 by Bond and Raehl found services being offered by the following percent of hospitals: drug use evaluation (94.5%), pharmacokinetic consultations (80.3%), adverse drug reaction management (70.4%), in-service education (65.5%), and participation on medical rounds (22.9%).

8. **The evidence showing the impact of clinical pharmacy services on economic and clinical outcomes is overwhelming.**
   a. True
   b. False.

   Answer. a or b depending on the level of evidence one needs to declare something "overwhelming." There are many well-designed trials that provide definitive conclusions demonstrating the value of pharmacist services. However, the majority of outcomes research on the impact of pharmacist services have study design limitations that preclude definitive decisions about the value of the services.

9. **Which of the following healthcare professionals are NOT recognized as patient care providers by the Federal government (for service payment)?**
   a. Pharmacists
   b. Podiatrists
   c. Nurses
   d. Physicians
   e. All of the above are recognized

   Answer: a. Pharmacists. Though some pharmacists are recognized by certain payers and are paid directly for their services, this is not routine. The federal government does not recognize pharmacists as providers.

10. **In what year was the following quote made about dispensing-oriented pharmacy practice? It has lead to "frustration of many pharmacists who had completed five or more years of difficult studies only to enter a rather undemanding, unprofessional practice."**
    a. Last year
    b. Ten years ago
    c. Twenty years ago
    d. Thirty years ago

    Answer: d. Thirty years ago. However, this quote could have been made almost any time in the last 40 years because it is still true for many pharmacy practice settings.

Chapter Discussion Questions

1. What are the differences between providing basic information about a medication to a patient at the time of dispensing and true counseling of a patient to enhance medication outcomes?
2. If a number of clinical pharmacy services have been shown to improve patient care, why hasn't there been development of structures to pay pharmacists for these services or to have sufficient numbers of pharmacists to provide the services in all settings?
3. What do you think needs to happen within and outside of the profession for it to move toward a greater role in clinical practice?

CHAPTER 6

Medication Safety

David A. Holdford

■ ■ ■
Learning Objectives

After completing this chapter, readers should be able to:

1. Describe the extent of medical errors in the U.S. health care system.
2. Define key terms in medication safety.
3. Describe and classify various medication errors.
4. Identify potential causes for medication errors.
5. List strategies for improving medication safety in health-system pharmacy practice.

Key Terms and Definitions

■ **Administration error:** An incorrect medication administration that includes the wrong dose, omitted dose, additional dose, wrong administration time, incorrect handling of drugs during administration, and wrong infusion rate.

■ **Adverse drug event (ADE):** An ADE is an injury, large or small, preventable or unpreventable, that may be caused by the use or lack of intended use of a drug.

■ **Adverse drug reaction (ADR):** An ADR is a drug related problem that consists of an unexpected, unintended, undesired, or excessive response to a drug that requires some type of medical response (e.g., discontinuing the drug, changing therapy, making major dose modifications) or results in a negative outcome (e.g., hospital admission, prolonged treatment, harm, disability, death). It may or may not be the result of a medication error.

■ **Allergic drug reactions:** An allergic drug reaction is a type of ADR resulting from immunologic hypersensitivities to drugs.

■ **Dispensing error:** A mistake during the dispensing process where a patient receives the wrong drug, the correct drug for the wrong patient, wrong galenic form (e.g., tablet for patient who is NPO) or wrong dose.

■ **Drug misadventure:** An iatrogenic hazard or incident associated with indicated drug therapy resulting in patient harm that can be attributable to error, immunologic response, or idiosyncratic response—consisting of the sum of medication errors, ADRs, and ADEs.

- **Drug-related morbidity:** The failure of a drug to achieve its intended health outcome due to unresolved drug-related problems. It is a negative outcome associated with an error.

- **Drug-related problems (DRPs):** DRPs are events associated with drug therapies that can or do hamper optimal patient health outcomes.

- **Error of commission:** An error that results when the patient receives the correct drug in a way that does not result in optimal patient outcomes or an incorrect drug which puts the patient at risk of negative outcomes.

- **Error of omission:** An error that results in a patient failing to receive a beneficial drug.

- **Idiosyncratic reaction:** A type of ADR resulting from abnormal responses to drugs that are peculiar to individuals.

- **Latent injury:** A propensity or predisposition for harm during the process of care that actually does not result in patient injury.

- **Medication error:** Any error in the medication process (prescribing, dispensing, administering of drugs), whether there are adverse consequences or not.

- **Medication reconciliation:** The process of resolving discrepancies as patients transition across departments (e.g., a medical ICU to a step down unit), locations (e.g., inpatient to outpatient), or other places.

- **Monitoring error:** The failure to review a prescribed regimen for appropriateness and detection of problems, or failure to use appropriate clinical or laboratory data for adequate assessment of patient response to prescribed therapy.

- **Outcome:** The end result attributable to health care products or services

such as mortality, infection, myocardial infarction, and pain.

- **Potential adverse drug event:** A mistake in prescribing, dispensing, or medication administration that has the potential to cause an ADE but did not, either by luck or because it was intercepted.

- **Prescribing error:** An incorrect drug, dose, dosage form, quantity, route, concentration, rate of administration, or instructions for use that has been ordered or authorized by a prescriber. It includes illegible prescriptions or medication orders that lead to errors that reach the patient.

- **Process:** These are actions associated with quality such as reviewing patient orders prior to dispensing, conducting drug use evaluation, and counseling patient prior to discharge.

- **Sentinel event:** An unexpected occurrence involving actual or potential death or serious injury. These events signal the need for immediate investigation and response.

- **Side effect:** An expected, well-known reaction resulting in little or no change in patient management (e.g., drowsiness or dry mouth associated with certain antihistamines).

- **Structure:** The presence of something that is reasonably associated with quality such as a pharmacy, a pharmacist, available references, 24-hour pharmacy services, a formulary, and a computerized prescriber order entry system.

- **Transcription and/or interpretation error:** An error in transcribing or interpreting prescriptions due to causes including misinterpretation of abbreviations, illegible hand-written prescriptions, or misinterpretation of spoken prescriptions.

- **Trigger event:** An event occurring during patient treatment that causes a latent injury that may become an actual discernible injury.

Introduction

Medication safety has been a priority of health-system pharmacy practice in recent years. Driven by landmark publications including the Institute of Medicine's (IOM) report, *To Err Is Human: Building a Safer Health System*,[1] pharmacists have been attempting to reduce medication risks in institutions. The report highlighted the pervasive nature of injuries associated with both appropriate and inappropriate use of medications—reframing medical error as a chronic threat to public health.[2] Some of the following findings were revealed in the report[1]:

- Medical errors are common—one medication error per patient per day.
- Medical errors are tragic—over 7,000 preventable deaths occur each year due to medication errors.
- Medical errors are expensive—resulting in annual costs of $17 billion to $37 billion in the United States due to lost income, disability, and health care expenditures.
- Medical errors are preventable—at least 400,000 adverse drug events (ADEs) in hospitals are preventable.
- Medical errors are not fully appreciated—they cause more deaths each year than breast cancer, motor vehicle accidents, and AIDS.

In a follow-up report, the IOM committee published *Crossing the Quality Chasm: A New Health System for the Twenty-first Century*,[3] which highlighted the causes of medical error and called for fundamental changes to improve the quality of health care. This chapter deals with many of the issues identified by the IOM and discusses their impact in institutional pharmacy settings.

> **Key Point . . .**
>
> The IOM concluded that medical errors are common, tragic, expensive, preventable, and not fully appreciated.
>
> **. . . So what?**
>
> It is shocking that medical errors are still so common more than a decade after *To Err Is Human*. The public would allow no other industry to put so many people at risks that are so easily preventable.

Definitions

The terminology of medication safety can be confusing because of the variety of ways of defining and classifying medication errors. This section of the chapter defines key terms and describes various classification systems in order to give a foundation for subsequent sections on preventing, reporting, and managing medication errors.

Drug-related problems (DRPs) are events associated with drug therapies that can or do hamper optimal patient health outcomes[4,5] (Figure 6-1). DRPs include medication errors, adverse drug reactions, adverse drug events, and side effects. A term very similar to DRPs commonly used in institutional safety studies is medication misadventures. **Medication misadventures** are iatrogenic hazards or incidents associated with indicated drug therapy resulting in patient harm that can be attributable to error, immunologic response, or idiosyncratic response.[4,6,7] Medication misadventures cover the sum of medication errors and adverse drug events,[8] as do DRPs, so the two terms will be considered synonymous in this text.

Figure 6-1. Various types of drug-related problems.

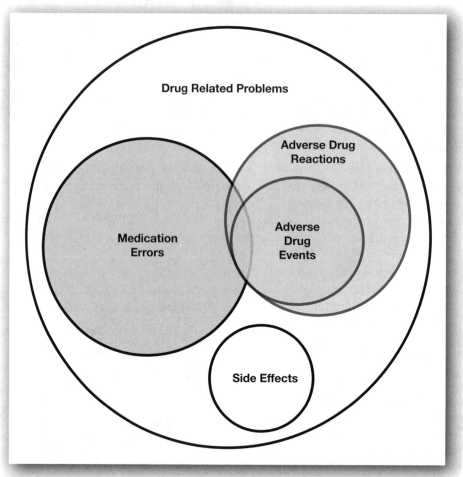

Medication errors are errors or mistakes in the medication use process (prescribing, dispensing, administering of drugs) that may result in negative outcomes. [9] Not all DRPs are medication errors because problems in medication use can occur even when best medication practices are applied. For example, side effects are DRPs that occur through no one's mistake—indeed, they are expected, unavoidable reactions of the appropriate use of many drugs (e.g., potential upset stomach associated with nonsteroidal anti-inflammatory drugs). In addition, medication errors may or may not cause adverse consequences, because some mistakes have no negative clinical effects (e.g., a missed dose of blood pressure medicine may not cause any change in blood pressure). In these situations, errors are said to only increase the *risk* of adverse consequence.

Medication errors can be classified in a variety of ways. One way is to classify them by their impact on patients such as that seen in Figure 6-2. This figure shows errors that range from Category A where circumstances have no capacity for harm to Category I where circumstances result in patient death.

Another way is to classify medication errors according to where they exist within the medication use system (Figure 6-3).[10] **Administration errors** occur when patients are administered something other than that prescribed for the patient—the wrong dose,

Figure 6-2. The National Coordinating Council for Medication Error Reporting and Prevention (NCC MERP) Index for Categorizing Medication Errors.[20]

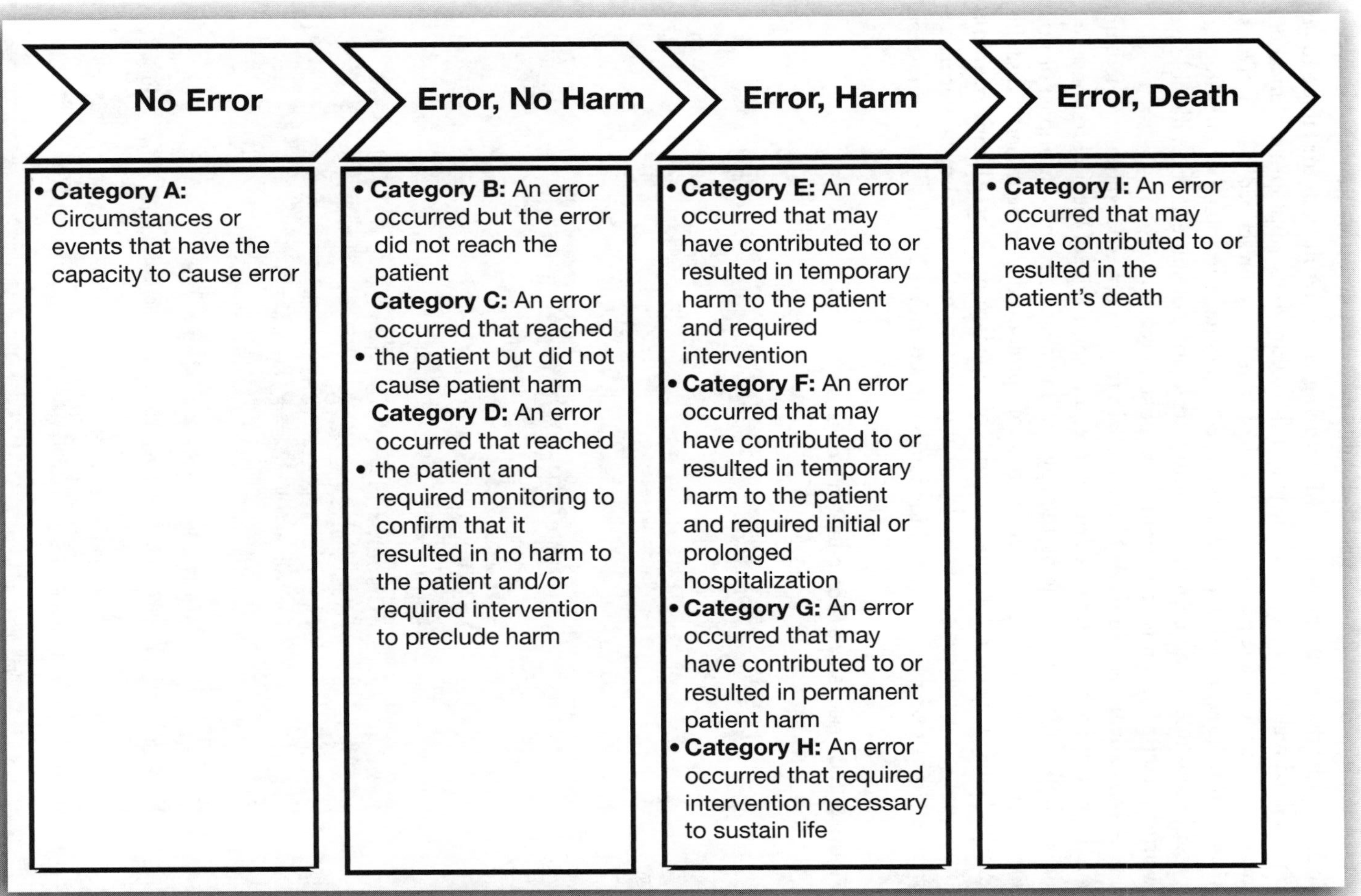

No Error	Error, No Harm	Error, Harm	Error, Death
• **Category A:** Circumstances or events that have the capacity to cause error	• **Category B:** An error occurred but the error did not reach the patient • **Category C:** An error occurred that reached the patient but did not cause patient harm • **Category D:** An error occurred that reached the patient and required monitoring to confirm that it resulted in no harm to the patient and/or required intervention to preclude harm	• **Category E:** An error occurred that may have contributed to or resulted in temporary harm to the patient and required intervention • **Category F:** An error occurred that may have contributed to or resulted in temporary harm to the patient and required initial or prolonged hospitalization • **Category G:** An error occurred that may have contributed to or resulted in permanent patient harm • **Category H:** An error occurred that required intervention necessary to sustain life	• **Category I:** An error occurred that may have contributed to or resulted in the patient's death

omitted dose, additional dose, wrong administration time, incorrect handling of drugs during administration, or wrong infusion rate. **Dispensing errors** are mistakes made during the dispensing process where a patient receives the wrong drug, the correct drug for the wrong patient, wrong galenic form (e.g., tablet for patient who is NPO) or wrong dose. **Prescribing errors** occur when prescriptions have an incorrect drug selection, dose, dosage form, quantity, route, concentration, rate of administration, or instructions for use of a drug product. These include illegible prescriptions or medication orders that lead to errors that reach the patient. **Monitoring errors** result from the failure to review a prescribed regimen for appropriateness or the failure to use appropriate clinical or laboratory data for adequate assessment of patient response to prescribed therapy. **Transcription and/or interpretation errors** are made during the transcribing or interpreting of prescriptions due to causes including misinterpretation of abbreviations, illegible handwritten prescriptions, misinterpretation of spoken prescriptions.

Adverse drug reactions (ADRs) are DRPs that are unexpected, unintended, undesired, or excessive responses to a drug that require some type of medical response (e.g., discontinuing the drug, changing therapy, making major dose modifications) or resulting in a negative outcome (e.g., hospital admission, prolonged treatment, harm, disability, death).[11] They may or may not be the result of a medication error. **Allergic reactions** (immunologic hypersensitivities to drugs) and **idiosyncratic reactions** (abnormal responses drugs that are peculiar to individuals) are considered ADRs.[11] In contrast, **side**

Figure 6-3. Consequences of drug-related problems.

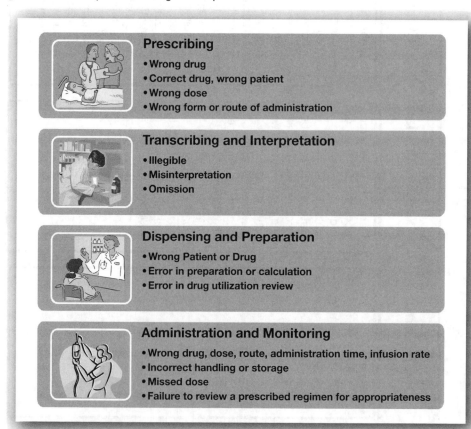

effects (expected, well-known reactions that require little or no change in patient management) are *not* ADRs.[11] Neither are other expected, well-known responses such as drug withdrawal symptoms, drug-abuse syndromes, accidental poisonings, and drug-overdose complications.[11] **Adverse drug events (ADEs)** are ADRs that result in an injury—large or small—preventable or unpreventable—due to the use or lack of intended use of a drug.[4,10] Expected, well-know reactions to medications that are severe enough to require extensive medication management are *not* side effects—they are ADEs.

DRPs associated with errors can have negative outcomes or no negative outcomes (Figure 6-4). Any error in the medication use process can lead to actual or potentially negative health outcomes. Negative outcomes associated with medical errors are called drug-related morbidity. **Drug-related morbidity** is defined as the failure of a drug to achieve its intended health outcome due to unresolved DRPs.[4,5] **Sentinel Events** are unexpected incidents resulting in death or the potential for serious physical or psychological injury. These events are labeled "sentinel" because they signal the need for immediate investigation and response.

In truth, most medication errors do not lead to negative health outcomes. Rather, they elevate the potential for injury associated with drugs. These types of errors are called either latent or potential injuries. **Latent injuries** are defined as a propensity or predisposition for harm during the process of care that actually does not result in patient injury.[4] **Potential injuries** are mistakes in prescribing, dispensing, or medication administration that have the potential to cause an injury but did not, either by luck or because they were intercepted.[4,12]

Errors that lead to DRPs typically result because of something that an individual did (i.e., an error of commission) or didn't do (i.e., an error of omission) (Figure 6-5). **Errors of commission** can occur when the patient receives either a correct drug or an incorrect drug. DRPs associated with receiving the correct drug occur when the patient

Figure 6-4. Various drug-related problems associated with errors.

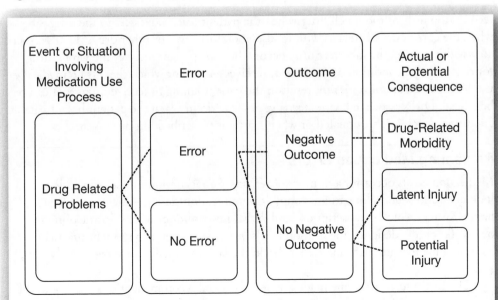

Figure 6-5. Types of medication errors.

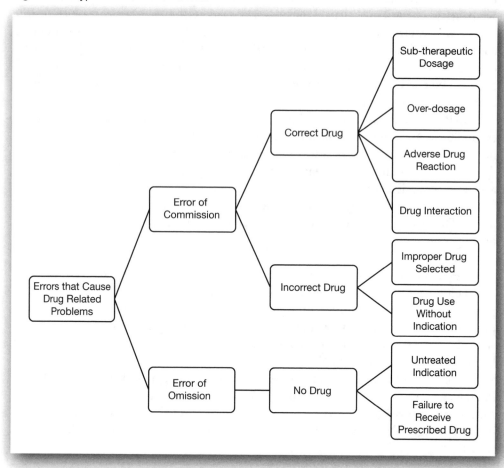

receives too little or too much drug, when the patient reacts adversely to the drug, or when the correct drug interacts with foods, laboratory tests, or other drugs. DRPs associated with receiving the incorrect drug occur when the patient receives the wrong drug for that patient's condition or the patient receives a drug for which there is no medically valid reason. **Errors of omission** result in the patient failing to receive drugs that can be beneficial. DRPs associated with receiving no drug occur when the patient has a treatable condition which is left untreated or when a drug is prescribed but not taken.

Preventing Medication Errors

Medication errors occur for a number of reasons. Some common reasons include look-alike and sound-alike drugs; sloppy communication practices including illegible handwriting, incorrect transcription, and verbal miscommunications; distractions and overwork; poorly designed medication labels; poor personnel management practices including inadequate performance feedback; the lack of a quality improvement system; and equipment failures.[12]

The Institute of Medicine made a series of general recommendations relating to the prevention of medication errors.[13]

- Involve the patient in the medication use process. This includes formalizing the rights of patients, educating them, and consulting with them.
- Consumer-oriented medication resources should be made available to support patient self-management of their medication use.
- Health care providers should have access to patient information and decision-support tools and technologies to enable them to be more active in monitoring and intervening.
- Medication labeling needs to be improved along with methods for communicating medication information to consumers.
- Health information technology must be improved to support the medication use process.
- Congressional funding should be increased to study safe and appropriate medication use and error prevention.
- Health care payers and oversight organizations should be more active in promoting good medication use practices.

Recommendations specific to pharmacies and pharmacists suggest a more active role in ensuring safe medication use.[14] None of these recommendations are surprising except in the fact that they are not being followed in many pharmacy settings.

- Pharmacists must keep up with the medication literature for drug error information and take action for prevention.
- Pharmacists should verify the accuracy of new prescription data, monitor for errors and near misses, make corrections as needed, and report errors to external reporting programs.
- Patient identities should be verified using bar codes.
- Patients should be educated about ways to prevent medication errors.
- Patients should be engaged in managing their own medication regimens.
- Electronic prescribing should be used.
- Trivial warnings to prescribers and pharmacists should be avoided in medication decision-support systems.
- Prescription filling technology needs to be assessed and improved.
- Pharmacists should monitor patients for high risk side effects.
- Pharmacists should routinely review patient medication records especially when transitioning between types of care (e.g., hospital to community).

Culture of Safety

One major reason medication safety problems have remained persistent in health care is providers and professionals do not have a culture of safety. Clearly, no one wants errors to happen and professionals make efforts to avoid errors, but a culture of safety is more than just having people who make efforts to avoid medical errors. A **culture of safety** exists where safety is a key element of everyone's job—from the leadership to the technicians and unit secretaries. In a culture of safety, leaders encourage workers to seek out and implement new ways of ensuring the safety of patients. This is done through actions (e.g., developing systems that promote safety) and words (e.g., asking people what the leader can do to help them ensure patient safety). In a culture of safety, people are obligated to take responsibility for protecting the well being of patients. Inaction is frowned upon by everyone—pressure to solve medication problems comes from technicians, pharmacists, and supervisors. Information is shared in a culture of safety because reducing patient risk is more important than concerns about disclosure.

However, sharing information about patient safety is easier said than done. In many pharmacies, the reporting of medication errors is discouraged by attempts to find someone to blame and punish for the error. In a culture of blame, adverse events and errors are rarely identified because the risk of reprisal discourages anyone from reporting them. Ignorance about the existence of medication errors means that they will continue to occur. A culture of safety tries to avoid blaming individuals, and instead focuses on identifying errors in the system that lead to errors. Thus, ensuring patient safety requires a change in the culture of work, medicine, medication use systems, and human interactions.

■ ■ ■

Key Point . . .

A culture of safety exists where safety is a key element of everyone's job—from the leadership to the technicians and unit secretaries.

. . . So what?

The steps in a safe medication use system are like the links of a chain. The system is only as good as the weakest link in the chain. Any individual involved in the medication use process can influence patient safety for the good or bad—from the housekeeper to the chief executive officer. A culture is needed to promote the importance of everyone in ensuring patient safety.

Models of Quality Improvement

Organizations that seek to improve medication safety apply common models of quality improvement. A variety of models are available such as total quality management, continuous quality improvement, six-sigma, LEAN, or others. All share the following principles:

- The status quo is unacceptable. According to the IOM and almost every other health care leader, the status quo harms patients and wastes money. [1] Therefore, change must occur, and it must be continuous. What was acceptable yesterday is no longer acceptable today. What is satisfactory now may be intolerable tomorrow.
- Safety can be enhanced by improving the core processes of the medication use system. This means that safety will increase by identifying essential elements of the medication use process and improving the process by eliminating duplication, avoiding unnecessary steps, decreasing process time, reducing errors, and simplifying the overall process.
- Safety efforts must be patient-centered. Unlike in the past—where practice revolved around the needs of the health care workers—the patient is now the emphasis. Solutions should then seek to serve the patient.
- Quality must be measured. Identifying problems with core processes requires establishing key measures of the process and monitoring them. For example, the quality of compounded IVs might be assessed by periodically culturing laminar flow hoods or systematically observing the process used by technicians in compounding. Unless quality is measured, it is not a priority, and there will be no way to identify whether it is improving, worsening, or staying the same.
- Solutions to safety problems should address the system, not individuals. Most DRPs are built into the system by design. Handwritten orders, use of abbreviations, tran-

scribing orders by hand, paper-based charts, and numerous other quality deficiencies increase the likelihood that errors will occur and ADEs will take place. Attempts to blame single individuals or departments do not get at problems within the system. Indeed, errors in the system can strike anyone—pharmacist, technician, physician, or nurse—no matter how conscientious and competent. Poorly designed systems set up individuals to fail. Therefore, solutions to safety problems must address the overall system and cross organizational and professional lines.

PDSA Cycle of Safety Improvement

A well-recognized process for improving the safety of medication use systems consists of four steps—Plan, Do, Study, and Act—called the PDSA cycle (Figure 6-6). The PDSA cycle starts by first asking the following questions:

1. What do we want to accomplish?
2. How will we know when we are successful?
3. What changes will result in success?

■ ■ ■

Key Point . . .

Unless quality is measured, it is not important.

. . . So what?

There is no way of telling if an institution provides high quality health care if it is not measured. Saying "We're the best!" is a hollow boast without providing evidence to back it up. Quality must be measured because individuals can be held accountable for things that are measurable (e.g., number of consultations provided, frequency of reported errors). In addition, quality measures can be used in performance evaluations and affect compensation. Unless quality is measured, there is no accountability.

Figure 6-6. Plan-Do-Study-Act (PDSA) cycle of quality improvement.

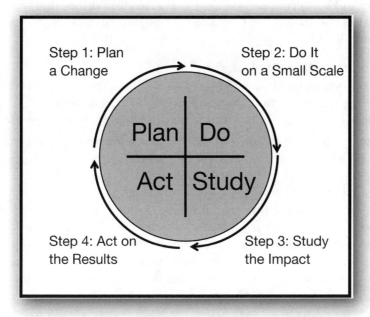

Step 1: Plan a Change

Step 2: Do It on a Small Scale

Plan | Do
Act | Study

Step 4: Act on the Results

Step 3: Study the Impact

Then the following steps are conducted:

PLAN. This step attempts to clarify the purpose of the quality improvement effort. In this step, a bottom-up approach is typically preferred where everyone potentially involved in the process is consulted and engaged in the change—especially frontline health care workers. This is because frontline workers are more likely to understand the problems and ways to fix them. Within the medication use system, technicians, pharmacists, nurses, unit secretaries, managers, and physicians might be consulted. Based upon that input, a clear description of the problem is developed. An example problem statement might be, "The average time from prescription to patient receiving a medication is 4 hours. This delay in therapy results in unnecessary longer lengths of stay for patients."

The next part of the plan stage is to clarify the expected actions. Details need to be made clear including what actions will be taken, when and where, who will do them and the specific responsibilities of those involved. This process can be made clear by mapping out the medication use process with flow charts, root cause analyses, failure mode effects analyses, or other tools. For details about the many tools used in improving medication use, visit the American Society of Health-Systems Pharmacists (ASHP) and Institute for Healthcare Improvement (IHI) websites.

DO. Once a plan has been established, it needs to be implemented. Implementation is typically done on a small scale to allow adjustments to the plan as experience with the problem is gained. Questions of interest include the degree to which the plan is implemented as designed and anything unexpected that occurs during the implementation.

STUDY. This step (also called "CHECK" by some) studies the effect of the change on the safety measure. Collected data are analyzed to determine if the change has been successful and if any unintentional consequences (good or bad) have resulted due to the change. Questions of interest during this stage are the degree to which the desired results are achieved, what new knowledge is gained, and what adjustments might need to be made to improve the results.

ACT. In this step, the small scale change is implemented on a larger level, and the entire process of monitoring and assessment starts over again. Changes from the small scale study might be warranted requiring further PDSA cycles. The key is that once a desired safety goal is achieved, a new goal is established that further improves the safety of patients within the medication use process. The status quo is never acceptable, and change is continuous.

Measures of Heath Care Quality

Health care quality can be measured in many ways. One of the frameworks most widely used is one suggested by Donabedian—Structure, Process, and Outcome.[15] Donabedian stated that quality measures can be divided into the following three categories:

- **Structures**—These are measures of the presence of something that is reasonably associated with quality. One might expect the presence of a pharmacist and electronic medical records to be associated with safer use of medications. Structures are desirable for assessing the quality of health care because they are easy to measure—the number of pharmacists can be counted and the presence or absence of electronic medical records can be easily established. Table 6-1 provides a list of structures associated with patient medication safety. The problem with structures is that their relationship with quality and patient safety is not always clear or established. Just because a pharmacist is there, for instance, does not mean that the pharmacist is doing the right things to ensure patient safety.

Table 6-1.
Structures That Should Be Present for Ensuring Safe Medication Use

STRUCTURES

▨ A *formulary system*, governed by a multidisciplinary pharmacy and therapeutics committee (or its equivalent) should have responsibility for formulating policies regarding the evaluation, selection, and therapeutic use of drugs.

▨ Effective *human resources management* must be present to effectively hire, manage, and train personnel involved in medication ordering, preparation, dispensing, administration, and patient education.

▨ *Adequate staffing* must be available to perform tasks effectively and ensure reasonable employee workloads and working hours.

▨ *Suitable work environments* should exist that minimize interruptions and distractions that might cause errors.

▨ *Lines of authority* and *areas of responsibility* within the medication use process should be clearly defined for all individuals involved.

▨ An ongoing, systematic program of *quality improvement* and *peer review* relating to the safe use of medications should be present.

▨ *Clinical information about patients* (including medications, allergies, and hypersensitivity profiles; diagnoses; pregnancy status; and laboratory values) needs to be available to pharmacists and others responsible for processing drug orders.

▨ *Patient medication profiles* should be maintained for all patients. Profiles should include information that allows monitoring of medication histories, allergies, diagnoses, potential drug interactions and ADRs, duplicate drug therapies, pertinent laboratory data, and other information.

▨ *The pharmacy department must be responsible* for the procurement, distribution, and control of all drugs used within the organization.

▨ *Computerized pharmacy systems* should be in place to automate the drug use process and provide better management of information.

▨ *Unit dose systems* are strongly recommended as the preferred method of drug distribution.

▨ Pharmacists should have access to *electronic health records*.

▨ *Computerized prescriber order entry* is the preferred method for prescribing medication orders.

▨ *Medication references* should be available to all health care providers.

▨ *Standard drug administration times* should be established to ensure consistency in when patients receive drugs.

▨ *Standard abbreviations* should be established for medication ordering.

▨ A *review mechanism* must be in place to conduct retrospective reviews of drug-related problems.

▨ *Educational programs* should be in place to discuss medication errors, their causes, and methods to prevent their occurrence.

Source: Adapted from reference 12.

▨ **Processes**—These are actions reasonably associated with quality such as the checking of patient medication profiles prior to dispensing, double checking technician work, and electronic prescribing. Table 6-2 provides a list of processes associated with patient medication safety. Although assessing the quality of processes is better than simply measuring the presence of structures, it is still possible that widely accepted practices are not always associated with positive patient health consequences. For example, many common preventive health care practices such as annual breast cancer screenings for women do not necessarily lead to positive patient health outcomes.

■ **Outcome**—Ultimately, the quality of safety systems needs to be assessed by their impact on patient health outcomes—dissatisfaction, discomfort, disability, disease, and death. Achieving positive health outcomes is the real purpose of having quality structures and processes. At the same time, they are the hardest to link to safety efforts.

Table 6-2.

Processes Associated with Safe Medication Use

PROCESSES

■ *All drugs should be dispensed from the pharmacy department* except in emergency situations.

■ *Storage of nonemergency floor stock medications* on the nursing units or in patient-care areas should be minimized.

■ *Routine inspections* should be conducted of all drug storage areas.

■ *Use of a patient's own or "home" medications* should be discouraged.

■ All *discontinued* or *unused drugs should be returned* to the pharmacy immediately after discontinuation or at patient discharge.

■ *Discharge counseling* of patients about their medication should be conducted.

■ When in doubt, *pharmacists should clarify any prescription*.

■ *Manual transcription* of physician orders should be minimized.

■ *Pharmacists should collaborate with the prescriber* in developing, implementing, and monitoring a therapeutic plan to produce defined therapeutic outcomes for the patient.

■ *Pharmacists should participate in drug therapy monitoring* including assessing therapeutic appropriateness, possible duplication, potential interactions, and clinical data.

■ *Pharmacists should make themselves available* to prescribers and nurses to offer information and advice about therapeutic drug regimens and the correct use of medications.

■ *Use of technology and support personnel* in the medication use process should be encouraged.

■ *Checks should be conducted on all work* performed by support personnel or automated devices.

■ *For high risk drug products*, additional checks should be conducted when possible.

■ *Ready-to-administer medication dosage forms* should be used whenever possible.

■ *Manipulation of drugs by nurses* (e.g., measure, repackage, and calculate) prior to administration should be minimized.

■ *Timely delivery of medications* to nursing units should occur.

■ *Monitoring of actual administration* should be conducted periodically to ensure safe administration by nurses.

■ *Pharmacists should collaborate with nurses* to ensure safe administration of medications.

■ *Medications returned to the pharmacy should be reviewed* for potential system breakdowns or medication errors (e.g., omitted doses and unauthorized drugs).

Source: Adapted from reference 12.

Thus, Donabedian suggested that a mix of structure, process, and outcome measures be collected to gain a true understanding of the quality of health care.[15]

Monitoring, Reporting, and Communicating

ADR-Monitoring and Reporting Programs

All institutions should have a comprehensive ADR-monitoring and reporting program.[11] Any surveillance program should be conducted both concurrently and prospectively. One form of concurrent (during drug therapy) surveillance system is based on reports of suspected ADRs by pharmacists, physicians, nurses, or patients. Another form of concurrent surveillance monitors for "alerting orders." **Alerting orders** are prescriptions which alert pharmacists that an ADR may have occurred and that an investigation needs to be conducted.[11] Several types of alerting orders occur. One is for "tracer" drugs commonly used to treat ADRs (e.g., orders for immediate doses of antihistamines, epinephrine, and corticosteroids). When tracer drugs are used, an ADR may have occurred. Another form of an alerting order is any abrupt discontinuation or decrease in dosage of a drug—the assumption being that the discontinuation occurred because of a negative reaction to the medication. The last type of alerting order concerns stat orders for laboratory assessments of therapeutic drug levels. This type of order alerts the pharmacist that some concern exists in the mind of the prescriber that too much or too little drug is in the patient's system.

Key Point . . .

Alerting orders warn pharmacists that a potential ADR has occurred and an investigation needs to be conducted.

. . . So what?

Alerting orders are identified by understanding the best medical evidence and using the experience of pharmacists and other health care professionals. Alerting orders are based upon the Pareto Principle—that 80% of all drug related problems are associated with 20% of the orders. Knowing which orders are associated with the most problems allows pharmacists to give them more attention and develop specific strategies to deal with them (e.g., provide computer-generated warnings).

One type of prospective (before drug therapy) surveillance system focuses on monitoring high-risk drugs or patients with a high risk for ADRs.[11] High-risk drugs include the following[16]:

- Adrenergic agonists (IV) (e.g., epinephrine)
- Adrenergic antagonists (IV) (e.g., propranolol, metoprolol)
- Anesthetics (e.g., ketamine)
- Antithrombotics (e.g., warfarin, low molecular weight heparin)
- Cardioplegic solutions
- Chemotherapeutic agents
- Hypertonic dextrose
- Dialysis solutions
- Epidural and intrathecal medications
- Hypoglycemic agents (P.O.)

- Inotropic agents (e.g., digoxin, milrinone)
- Insulin
- Methotrexate for non-oncologic use)
- Sedatives (e.g., midazolam)
- Narcotics/opiates
- Neuromuscular blocking agents (e.g., succinylcholine)
- Nitroprusside
- Oxytocin (IV)
- Potassium chloride and sodium chloride for injection
- Promethazine (IV)
- Radiocontrast agents
- Total parenteral nutrition

Populations at greatest risk for ADRs are those with the most trouble adjusting to the negative consequences.[17] Pediatric patients are at greater risk because drug responses are less predictable than with adults due to pharmacokinetic variations. This problem is aggravated because of the lack of clinical trials conducted in pediatric populations. On the other end of the age spectrum, the elderly are at greater risk due to issues of polypharmacy, multiple prescribers, adherence problems (due to memory or vision problems), changes in renal function and metabolism, and greater sensitivity to medications. Oncology patients commonly suffer ADRs because they are exposed to highly toxic therapeutic regimens and often are immunocompromised. Therefore, greater attention should be given to surveillance programs in these populations.

When suspected ADRs occur, several actions should occur.[11] First, prescribers, nurses, and pharmacists should be notified. Notification should also be made to the pharmacy surveillance program for recording and analysis. Attempts should be made to determine the cause or causes of each suspected ADR using the patient's medical and medication history, the circumstances of the adverse event, and what might be found in any literature review. Ideally, a systematic method for assigning the probability of the reported or suspected ADR (e.g., confirmed or definite, likely, possible, and unlikely) should be used to categorize each ADR. Serious or unexpected ADRs should be reported to the Food and Drug Administration (FDA) or the drug's manufacturer (or both).

Medication Reconciliation

In health care systems, confusion can occur about patient medication regimens as they transition throughout the system. Medication reconciliation is promoted as a solution. **Medication reconciliation** is the process of resolving discrepancies with what a patient has been taking in the past with what the patient should be taking at the moment. Medication reconciliation is an opportunity for pharmacists to use their knowledge and skills to enhance patient safety by identifying and resolving drug-related problems as patients transition throughout the health care system.

Reconciliation attempts to correct problems such as omissions in therapy, medication duplications, errors in dosing, and potential drug interactions. Medication reconciliation is meant to be conducted each time a patient transitions across departments (e.g., a medical ICU to a step down unit), locations (e.g., inpatient to outpatient), or other location.

The medication reconciliation process consists of the following steps.[18]

1. Verification. The most up-to-date list of medications currently being taken by the patient within the hospital or other institution is developed by using one or more sources of

information—pharmacy profile, medical records, patient or caregiver interview, and patient medications brought to the institution.

2. Clarification. The medication and dosages are checked for appropriateness.
3. Reconciliation. Clinical decisions are then made based upon a comparison of newly prescribed medications against what was prescribed previously. This might include discontinuing unnecessary medications and reordering medications placed on hold or temporarily discontinued. Changes to pharmacotherapy are documented in all relevant records.
4. Transmission. Therapy changes are communicated to those people who need to know about the changes including providers on both ends of the transition (e.g., hospital pharmacist and community pharmacist, surgeon and internist), caregivers, and the patient. This step typically includes providing the patient or caregiver with a copy of the final medication list with administration instructions.

Key Point . . .

Medication reconciliation requires pharmacists to take responsibility for patient medication safety as they transition to different parts of the health care system.

. . . So what?

In the past, what happened to patients after they left a pharmacy or institution was not a major role for pharmacists. Accreditation organizations have now started to require institutions to conduct medication reconciliation. This is a key opportunity for pharmacists.

National Quality Organizations

Numerous national organizations exist to promote health care quality and patient safety. Key organizations are listed below.[19]

- The Institute of Medicine (IOM)—The IOM is a component of the National Academy of Sciences. Its mission is to "serve as adviser to the nation to improve health." It has published a series of reports focusing on assessing and improving the nation's quality of care including "Crossing the Quality Chasm," "To Err is Human," and "Preventing Medication Errors."
- IHI Institute for Healthcare Improvement—IHI is a not-for-profit organization with a goal of improving health care throughout the world. One major initiative of IHI was its 100,000 Lives Campaign that had a purpose of introducing proven best practices to extend or save as many as 100,000 lives. Its 5 Million Lives Campaign seeks to "prevent 5 million incidents of medical incidents over a two year period."
- NQF National Quality Forum—The NQF's primary role is in improving health care quality measurement and reporting. It endorses consensus-based national standards for measurement and public reporting of health care performance data that provide meaningful information about whether care is safe, timely, beneficial, patient-centered, equitable, and efficient. It has endorsed more than 300 measures, indicators, events, practices, and other products to help assess quality.
- The Leapfrog Group—The Leapfrog Group is a voluntary program of employers who use employer purchasing power to encourage the health industry to make big leaps in health care safety, quality, and customer value. It conducts the Hospital Quality and Safety Survey which asks hospitals to rate themselves on four "leaps" of quality and

safety practices. It also conducts the Hospital Rewards Program which measures performance in five areas for effectiveness and affordability and rewards excellent hospitals.

- Joint Commission—Joint commission assesses and accredits the quality of health systems. See Chapter Three: Key legal and regulatory issues in Health-System Pharmacy Practice for more information about Joint Commission.
- CMS Centers for Medicare and Medicaid Services—CMS manages Medicare and Medicaid programs which contracts with a private Quality Improvement Organization (QIO) in each state to monitor care to Medicare beneficiaries. It sets quality standards that must be met to be able to serve CMS patients.
- AHRQ Agency for Healthcare Research and Quality—AHRQ conducts and supports research for the U.S. Department of Health and Human Services (HHS) in the areas of quality improvement and patient safety, outcomes and effectiveness of care, clinical practice and technology assessment, and health care organization and delivery systems. It sponsors the National Quality Measures Clearinghouse (NQMC)—a public repository for evidence-based quality measures and measure sets.
- NCQA National Committee for Quality Assurance—NCQA manages the Health Plan Employer Data and Information Set (HEDIS). HEDIS measures are used to provide purchasers and consumers with information about the quality of healthcare plans.
- ASHP American Society of Health-System Pharmacists—ASHP supports health systems pharmacists in quality and safety through publishing (e.g., books, American Journal of Health-System Pharmacy), education (e.g., professional meeting CEs, ASHP website), advocacy, and guidance documents (e.g., ASHP guidelines on adverse drug reaction monitoring and reporting).
- PQA Pharmacy Quality Alliance—PQA is a consortium of pharmacy organizations that brings key stakeholders together to agree on strategies for measuring performance at the pharmacy and pharmacist-levels; collecting data in the least burdensome way; and reporting meaningful information to consumers, pharmacists, employers, health insurance plans, and other healthcare decision-makers to help make informed choices, improve outcomes and stimulate the development of new payment models.

Summary

Medication safety is a fundamental responsibility of all pharmacists who work in institutional practice, and it is part of their core mission. The complexity of the medication use process requires pharmacists to have knowledge about types of safety problems, the causes of errors and drug-related morbidity, and practices that can reduce them. The inter-connections between various components of the medication-use process require pharmacists to take responsibility for the entire process—not only what goes on in the pharmacy. The problems of medication safety are complex, and therefore, quick fixes and simplistic solutions will not resolve them. Commonly recommended solutions like the use of technologies such as bar code monitoring, computerized prescriber order entry systems, and electronic medical records are not panaceas. They are only part of the solution. Other parts may incorporate training, improved workflow, and good leadership.

Suggested Reading

ASHP guidelines on preventing medication errors in hospitals. *Am J Health Syst Pharm.* 1993;50:305-314.

ASHP statement on reporting medical errors. *Am J Health Syst Pharm.* 2000;57:1531-1532.

Bates DW. Preventing medication errors: A summary. *Am J Health Syst Pharm.* 2007;64:S3-S9.

Berwick DM. Improving patient care. My right knee. *Ann Intern Med.* 2005;142:121-125.

Chassin MR. Assessing strategies for quality improvement. *Health Aff (Millwood).* 1997;16:151-161.

Cohen MR. *Medication Errors.* 2nd ed. Washington, DC: American Pharmacists Association; 2009.

Flynn EA, Barker KN. Medication Errors Research: Medication Errors: Causes, Prevention, and Risk Management. Sudbury, MA: Jones and Bartlett, Publishers; 2000.

Frank, JR, Brien S, and editors on behalf of the Safety Competencies Steering Committee. The Safety Competencies: Enhancing Patient Safety Across the Health Professions. Safety Competencies Steering Committee. 2008. Ottawa, Ontario, Canadian Patient Safety Institute.

Holdford DA. Recognizing and defining quality problems. In: Warholak TL, Nau D, eds. *Pharmacy Quality: Improving the Safety and Effectiveness of Pharmacy Services.* New York: McGraw Hill; 2009.

Institute of Medicine. *Crossing the Quality Chasm: A New Health System for the Twenty-first Century.* Institute of Medicine. Washington, DC: National Academy Press; 2001.

Institute of Medicine. *Health Professions Education: A Bridge to Quality.* Washington, DC: National Academies Press; 2003.

Institute of Medicine. *Preventing Medication Errors: Quality Chasm Series.* Washington, DC: National Academy Press; 2001.

McCarthy ID, Cohen MR, Kateiva J, McAllister JC, Ploetz PA. What should a pharmacy manager do when a serious medication error occurs? A panel discussion. *Am J Health Syst Pharm.* 1992;49:1405-1412.

Schmidek JM, Weeks WB. What do we know about financial returns on investments in patient safety? A literature review. *Jt Comm J Qual Patient Saf.* 2005;31:690-699.

Senge PM. *The Fifth Discipline. The Art and Practice of the Learning Organization.* New York: Currency Doubleday; 1990.

Taylor-Adams S, Brodie A, Vincent C. Safety skills for clinicians: An essential component of patient safety. *J Patient Saf.* 2008;4:141-147.

Walton M. *The Deming Management Method.* New York: Perigree Books; 1986.

Warholak TL, Nau D, eds. *Pharmacy Quality: Improving the Safety and Effectiveness of Pharmacy Services.* New York: McGraw Hill; 2010.

References

1. Kohn, LT, Corrigan, JM, Donaldson, MS. "To err is human: building a safer health system." Committee on Quality and Health Care in America. Institute of Medicine. Washington, DC: National Academy Press; 1999.

2. Berwick DM. A user's manual for the IOM's 'Quality Chasm' report. *Health Aff (Millwood).* 2002;21:80-90.

3. Institute of Medicine. *Crossing the Quality Chasm: A New Health System for the Twenty-first Century.* Washington, DC: National Academy Press; 2001.

4. Ackroyd-Stolarz S, Hartnell N, MacKinnon NJ. Demystifying medication safety: Making sense of the terminology. *Research in Social and Administrative Pharmacy.* 2006;2:280-289.

5. Hepler CD, Strand LM. Opportunities and responsibilities in pharmaceutical care. *Am J Hosp Pharm.* 1990;47:533-543.

6. Manasse HR, Jr. Medication use in an imperfect world: drug misadventuring as an issue of public policy, Part 2. *Am J Health Syst Pharm.* 1989;46:1141-1152.

7. Manasse HR, Jr. Medication use in an imperfect world: drug misadventuring as an issue of public policy, part 1. *Am J Health Syst Pharm.* 1989;46:929-944.

8. Suggested definitions and relationships among medication misadventures, medication errors, adverse drug events, and adverse drug reactions. *Am J Health Syst Pharm.* 1998;55:165-166.

9. Leape LL. Preventing adverse drug events. *Am J Health Syst Pharm.* 1995;52:379-382.

10. Krahenbuhl-Melcher A, Schlienger R, Lampert M, Haschke M, Drewe J, Krahenbuhl S. Drug-related problems in hospitals: A review of the recent literature. *Drug Safety.* 2000;30:379-407.

11. American Society of Health-Systems Pharmacists. ASHP guidelines on adverse drug reaction monitoring and reporting. *Am J Health Syst Pharm.* 1995;52:417-419.

12. ASHP guidelines on preventing medication errors in hospitals. *Am J Health Syst Pharm.* 1993;50:305-314.

13. Institute of Medicine. *Preventing Medication Errors: Quality Chasm Series. Institute of Medicine.* Washington, DC: National Academy Press; 2001.

14. Bates DW. Preventing medication errors: A summary. *Am J Health Syst Pharm.* 2007;64:S3-S9.

15. Donabedian A. The seven pillars of quality. *Archives of Pathology and Laboratory Medicine.* 1990;114:1115-1118.

16. Institute of Safe Medication Practices. List of high-alert medications. http://www.ismp.org/Tools/high alertmedications.pdf Accessed March 31, 2010.

17. Hartman, C. Medication Safety and Quality. Part 3: Managing High-Alert Medications. *Pharmacy Practice News.* April 11, 2009. American Society of Health-System Pharmacists.

18. Karapinar-Carkit F, Borgsteede SD, Zoer J, Smit HJ, Egberts A, van den Bernt P. Effect of medication reconciliation with and without patient counseling on the number of pharmaceutical interventions among patient discharged from the hospital. *Ann Pharmacother.* 2009;43:1001-1010.

19. American Society of Health-System Pharmacists. The Pharmacist's Role in Quality Improvement. 9-11. 2007.

20. Error Taxonomy. The National Coordinating Council for Medication Error Reporting and Prevention. 2009. 11-3-2009.

Chapter Review Questions

1. **Drug-related problems include medication errors, adverse drug reactions, medication side effects, and adverse drug events.**
   a. True
   b. False

   Answer: a. True. They are all drug-related problems because they are events associated with drug therapies that can or do hamper optimal patient health outcomes.

2. **Which of the following is never caused by a medication error?**
   a. Side effect
   b. Adverse drug event
   c. Adverse drug reaction
   d. Allergic reaction

Answer: a. Medication errors are errors or mistakes in the medication process (prescribing, dispensing, administering of drugs) that may result in negative outcomes. Side effects are well known reactions that are expected and not due to error. Adverse drug reactions and adverse drug events are unexpected, undesired, and often result from error. Allergic reactions are types of adverse drug reactions that can be caused by errors.

3. **Which of the following sometimes directly results in drug-related morbidity?**
    a. A latent injury
    b. A potential injury
    c. An adverse drug event
    d. An allergic reaction
    e. An adverse drug reaction

    Answer: c, d, and e. Negative health outcomes associated with medical errors are called drug-related morbidity. Latent injuries and potential injuries do not actually result in patient injury—they are only a propensity or predisposition for harm. Adverse drug events and adverse drug reactions such as an allergic reaction may result in harm and may be due to error.

4. **Pharmacists in health-system practice are responsible for errors in dispensing.**
    a. True
    b. False

    Answer: a or b depending on how the question is interpreted. If the statement is interpreted as "only responsible for errors in dispensing," then the answer is false, because pharmacists are responsible for all parts of the drug use process including prescribing, administration, and monitoring. If the question is interpreted as this being one responsibility in the drug use process, then the answer is true.

5. **Latent injuries are not important because they do not result in actual injury.**
    a. True
    b. False

    Answer: b. False. Latent injuries indicate problems in the medication use process. They may not result in injury but they do warn pharmacists of issues that might eventually hurt patients.

6. **Which of the following is NOT an important principle of quality improvement?**
    a. The status quo is unacceptable.
    b. People are the reason for poor patient safety.
    c. Safety can be enhanced by improving the core processes of the medication use system.
    d. Safety efforts must be patient-centered.
    e. Quality must be measured.

    Answer: b. People may make errors and do less they are capable of doing in health care but quality improvement works under the assumption that the system is the problem. Individuals make mistakes because of flaws in the system, whether those flaws are due to poor human resources management, work flow problems, lack of necessary tools and technology, and the like.

7. **In which step of the PDSA cycle is a quality problem statement developed?**
    a. Plan
    b. Do
    c. Study
    d. Act

    Answer: a. In this stage, the problem is defined and a plan is developed. The plan is implemented on a small scale in the Do stage. The results are assessed in the Study stage. An finally, the plan is implemented on a larger scale in the Act stage based upon lessons learned in the other stages.

8. **The best indicator of health care quality is positive patient health outcomes.**
    a. True
    b. False

    Answer: a. True. Ultimately, positive patient health outcomes are what is sought by health care. Structures (e.g., a clinical pharmacist) and processes (e.g., providing clinical therapy) are means to achieve an end—positive health outcomes. However, an argument can be made that the answer is False because the best indication of quality really depends on the circumstances. Depending on the situation, structures, processes, or outcomes could be superior indicators.

9. **Which of the following is classified as a STRUCTURE according to Donabedian?**
    a. Health related quality of life
    b. Medication reconciliation
    c. A unit dose system
    d. Mortality
    e. Collaborating with nurses

    Answer: c. A unit dose system is classified as a structure because its presence is associated with quality health care. Health related quality of life and mortality are outcomes of health care. Medication reconciliation and collaborating with nurses are processes.

10. **Which of the following organizations conducts and supports research for the U.S. Department of Health and Human Services (HHS) in the areas of quality improvement and patient safety, outcomes and effectiveness of care, clinical practice and technology assessment, and health care organization and delivery systems?**
    a. Leapfrog group
    b. IHI
    c. NQF
    d. NCQA
    e. AHRQ

    Answer: e. Agency for Healthcare Research and Quality is the health services research arm of the U.S. Department of Health and Human Services (HHS). IHI Institute for Healthcare Improvement is a not-for-profit organization that promotes healthcare quality improvement including its 100,000 Lives Campaign. The NQF National Quality Forum endorses consensus-based national standards for measurement and public reporting of healthcare performance data. The Leapfrog Group is a voluntary program of employers who seek to recognize and reward excellent health care organizations. NCQA National Committee for Quality Assurance manages the Health Plan Employer Data and Information Set (HEDIS) which are used to provide purchasers and consumers with the information about the quality of healthcare plans.

Chapter Discussion Questions

1. Which types of errors are easier to detect, errors of omission or errors of commission?
2. What features might you expect to see in a pharmacy that has a culture of safety?
3. What is a pharmacist's responsibility within the medication use system? What is not the pharmacist's responsibility?
4. What do you think are the biggest barriers to a safe medication use process?
5. What do you think are the biggest barriers to pharmacist involvement in the medication use process (other than time).

CHAPTER 7

Medication Distribution Systems

Stephen F. Eckel and Fred M. Eckel

■ ■ ■

Learning Objectives

After completing this chapter, readers should be able to:

1. Describe the advantages and disadvantages of floor stock, patient prescription, and unit dose medication distribution systems.
2. Contrast the advantages and disadvantages of centralized and decentralized models of distribution.
3. Discuss the evolution of medication distribution over time and its impact on the professional role of pharmacists.
4. Identify technologies used in managing medication distribution.
5. List the attributes of a good medication distribution system.
6. Define key terminology associated with medication distribution systems.

Key Terms and Definitions

■ **Automated dispensing cabinets (ADCs):** ADCs are point-of-use medication storage devices located in patient care areas designed to allow nurses to have quick but accountable access to medications. Most systems have some form of user identifier or password that restricts access to the medications. More advanced systems are linked to pharmacy electronic medication profiles.

■ **Centralized pharmacy services:** This model distributes medications from a centralized pharmacy location.

■ **Decentralized pharmacy services:** This model distributes medications from a decentralized satellite pharmacy located in or near a patient care area.

■ **Floor stock system:** A system of distribution that consists of an individual storage area on each nursing unit where drugs are stored prior to preparation and administration by the nurse. The medications are usually unsecured in this system and the role of pharmacy is primarily distributional.

■ **Medication administration record (MAR):** An MAR is a record of all current medications prescribed for each patient. The records contain information on the drugs, administration times, and directions for use. MARs are used by the nurse to know what medication each patient should receive at what time and how. They are also used to document that the drug was given by whom and at what time.

- **Medication profile:** The medication profile is the primary record used by pharmacists to document patient medications.
- **Patient prescription system:** An antiquated system of medication distribution that consists of patient-specific containers with 2-day to 5-day supply of drugs delivered to and stored on nursing units. Within this system, drug orders are transcribed by the nurse and reviewed by a pharmacist although no patient information is available to the pharmacist.
- **Unit dose system:** A system of distribution coordinated by the pharmacy that dispenses medication orders to be administered, not prepared, by the nurse. This system is characterized by medications contained in unit dose packages, dispensed in ready-to-administer form, and no more than a 24-hour supply being delivered or available on the patient care unit at any time. Pharmacists monitor and coordinate unit dose systems by reviewing all medication prescriptions against patient medication profiles and managing the distribution and storage process.
- **Unit of use package:** A container with the exact dose needed for patients in a ready-to-administer form, not requiring any preparation or selection by the nurse.

Introduction

The role of the pharmacist has always been to ensure that patients receive the appropriate medication in an acceptable dosage form that facilitates safe administration and improved outcomes. At different times in pharmacy's evolving responsibilities, some aspects of this role seemed to receive more attention. In the early days of institutional pharmacy, the pharmacist's role was distributional—developing systems of drug delivery that reduced waste and medication errors. As time has progressed, pharmacists have become more and more involved in clinical responsibilities. Despite the expanding clinical role of pharmacists, distribution of drug products will continue to be an important responsibility of pharmacists in health care institutions.

The evolution of institutional pharmacy practice was transformed by the unit dose system.[1] The system changed the hospital pharmacist into an integral member of the health care team by requiring that pharmacists receive individual patient medication orders. The pharmacist would review those orders against patient medication records prior to preparing and dispensing patient-specific doses in a ready-to-administer form. This allowed the hospital pharmacist to assume responsibility for a patient's drug therapy. Over the past 40 years, there have been many improvements to the unit dose system, mostly through advancements in technology.

This chapter provides a brief overview of the history of the medication distribution system leading to unit dose, a discussion of the unit dose system, an analysis of different technologies that assist drug distribution today, and thoughts on the future of medication distribution.

History of Medication Distribution Systems Leading to the Unit Dose Concept

The role of the hospital pharmacist 50 years ago was primarily confined to the basement.[2] The space was small and the personnel involved in drug distribution were few.

The pharmacist's primary role was to purchase and prepare medications to be used on the nursing unit. The physician would prescribe the medication and the nurse would administer it to the patient. The pharmacist was rarely involved in assessing the appropriateness of therapy. They simply made sure that the nurse had a supply of medication for the patient. If repackaging or compounding of the medication was required, the pharmacist accepted responsibility for this function with the exception being IV admixtures, which were usually prepared by the nurse on the nursing unit.

There were at least two distinct distribution methods the pharmacist would utilize for the nurse to obtain the medications for patient use.[2] The first was referred to as the floor stock system and the second was the patient prescription system.

Floor Stock System

The **floor stock system** consisted of an individual storage area on each nursing unit where medications were kept prior to the nurse preparing them to administer to patients. The medications were largely unsecured. The pharmacist was responsible for stocking the nursing unit storage area. The pharmacist would place bulk containers of medications in the unit storage area, often called the drug room. There were multiple doses in each bottle to supply all patients receiving that drug on the nursing unit. The nurse was the professional responsible for preparing the patient-specific medications for both oral and intravenous use. The nurse would read the physician order, go into the drug room to select the drug and prepare it, and then administer it to the patient. In this selection process, the nurse could choose from many different medications. If a medication needed to be refilled or a patient was started on a different drug, the nurse would request the new medication to be stocked on the nursing unit. The pharmacist would likely never see the physician order and would stock the medication on the floor solely from the nursing request. This system was utilized because it required minimal pharmacy resources, and it was assumed that this distribution system was safe. Patients were only charged for the drugs administered to them or were billed a daily fee, also termed per diem, for the drugs.

Patient Prescription System

In contrast, the **patient prescription system** involved the pharmacist to a greater extent than the floor stock system by requiring a review of the patient order. After the physician wrote the order, the nurse would transcribe the medication order and send it to pharmacy for preparation. The pharmacist would prepare a 2- to 5-day supply of medications for the patient and charge the patient for the medications dispensed. The nurse would store the medication on the nursing unit. This system still required the nurse to prepare the individual dose for the patient. When the drug needed to be refilled, the nurse would con-

Key Point . . .

In the floor stock system, the nurse was the professional responsible for preparing the patient-specific medications for both oral and intravenous use.

. . . So what?

Nurses receive only a fraction of the training pharmacists get in the preparation and handling of medications. In addition, nurses have numerous responsibilities that can force them to give medication preparation less attention than desirable. Distribution systems have evolved to allow pharmacists to take much of the burden of medication preparation from nurses.

tact the pharmacist who would prepare it and send it to the floor for continued use. When the drug was discontinued or the patient was discharged, the prescription containers were returned to the pharmacy and the unused drugs were credited to the patient's account. Even though the pharmacist had the opportunity to review the patient order, the pharmacist would place only limited judgment on whether it was correct or appropriate for the patient. This was because the pharmacist did not have access to pertinent patient information and it was not expected of them.

Unit Dose System

The move from floor stock and patient prescription systems to unit dose was driven by several studies that found the floor stock and individual prescription system to be error-prone.[3-5] Based upon these studies, a few hospitals began experimenting with the unit dose system which seemed to be safer and was believed to offer more opportunities for pharmacists to help improve the medication use cycle.[4,6] This move to unit dose placed the pharmacist in a position to begin affecting a patient's medication therapy.

The **unit dose system** is defined as a pharmacy-coordinated method of dispensing and controlling medications in health care institutions.[7] This system is characterized by medications contained in unit dose packages, dispensed in ready-to-administer form, and not more than 24-hour supply being delivered or available on the patient care unit at any time. The pharmacist dispenses patient-specific medications to be administered, not prepared, by the nurse. Figure 7-1 compares the unit dose process with features of floor stock and patient prescription systems.

The U.S. General Accounting Office concluded in 1971 that the unit dose system was the most cost-effective of any distribution system—especially when the entire medication use cycle is considered.[2] Studies have shown the reduction of medication errors when transitioning from the floor stock system to the unit dose system to be 2% to 11% of all orders studied.[3-5] Advantages of the unit dose system are listed in Table 7-1. Unit dose distribution has been adopted by almost all hospital pharmacies in the U.S.[8,9]

Figure 7-1. Comparing key features of medication distribution systems. *Source:* David Holdford.

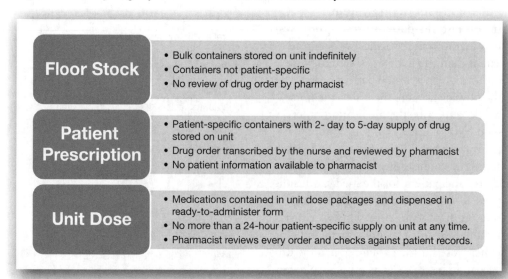

Role of Unit Dose on Drug Use Control

Implementation of unit dose systems in institutions had a critical role with involving pharmacists in the process of medication prescribing, distribution, and administration. Unit dose placed pharmacists front and center in the medication use cycle. It required pharmacists to review every medication order prior to dispensing. Duplicate carbon copies of the original orders were provided to pharmacists to prevent transcription errors seen in systems that had nurses or unit secretaries hand copy the originals for pharmacists. Seeing prescription orders prior to dispensing let pharmacists intervene if needed prior to the first dose of any order being made available to the patient. This important step provided a new role for pharmacists that made much better use of their knowledge and training.

Another important advance for pharmacists provided by the unit dose system was that it required the pharmacy to have and maintain a **patient medication profile**.[10] This allowed pharmacists to gain access to patient-specific information including the following[10]:

Table 7-1.

Advantages of the Unit Dose Distribution Method[7]

Reduction in medication errors
Decrease in total cost of medication-related activities
More efficient use of pharmacy and nursing personnel
Improved drug control and drug use monitoring
More accurate patient billing for medications
Minimization of credits for drugs
Greater control by pharmacist over work patterns and scheduling
Reduction of inventories maintained on nursing units

- Patient's name and location
- Generic name of medication
- Dosage in metric system, where feasible
- Frequency of administration
- Route of administration
- Signature of the physician
- Date and hour the order was written

The enhanced role of pharmacists helped propel clinical pharmacy services. Instead of being focused solely on getting the correct drug to the nursing unit (for nurse selection and administration), pharmacists also began evaluating whether the drugs sent were appropriate for the patient.

Efficient distribution systems are essential for developing the credibility to provide clinical pharmacy services. If pharmacists cannot ensure that they can provide reliable and responsive distribution of medications for patients, it will be difficult for them to convince physicians and nurses that pharmacists can be relied

Key Point . . .

An efficient and well-run distribution system lends essential credibility to the pharmacy department and facilitates the ability of pharmacists to provide more clinical services.

. . . So what?

A pharmacist's ability to influence others involved in the medication use process is based in large part on the pharmacist's reputation. That reputation can be damaged by a poorly run distribution system. Indeed, the best clinical pharmacy services can be undercut by a distribution system that is inept and wasteful.

upon to provide clinical services. Hence, clinical services can only be built upon the foundation of excellent medication distribution systems.

The Unit Dose Process

The process of unit dose varies with each institution. Therefore, the following description of unit dose systems in this section may not be completely illustrative of that seen in many institutions. Nevertheless, this section provides a general description of key steps in the unit dose order fulfillment process (Figure 7-2).

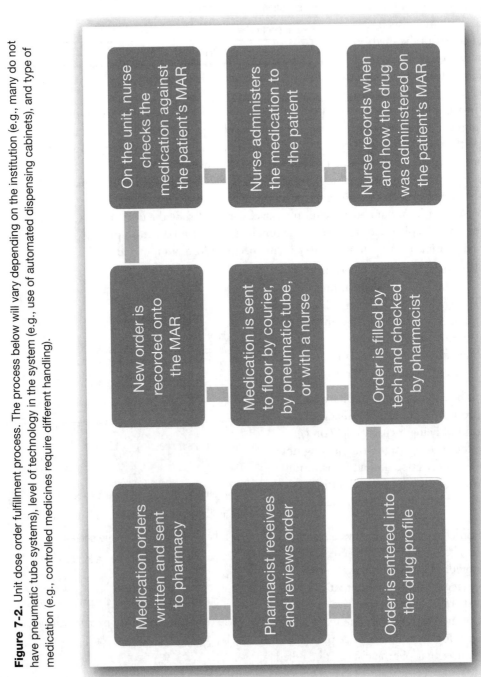

Figure 7-2. Unit dose order fulfillment process. The process below will vary depending on the institution (e.g., many do not have pneumatic tube systems), level of technology in the system (e.g., use of automated dispensing cabinets), and type of medication (e.g., controlled medicines require different handling).

Orders are written on the patient care area and sent to the pharmacy through various methods. Some hospitals have couriers that routinely go to nursing units to collect orders and deliver medications. Others rely on pneumatic tube systems (i.e., pressurized tubes that move small containers throughout institutions) for order delivery or facsimile devices for order transmission. Some orders are delivered to decentralized pharmacy satellites located near or within nursing units. Increasingly, physician orders are being sent to the pharmacist through computerized physician order entry (CPOE). With CPOE, pharmacists can review orders any place they have computer access to patient specific information. As computer systems evolve, CPOE will likely become the primary form of order delivery.

After receiving the medication order, the pharmacist clarifies any discrepancies with the prescriber. After the order is reviewed and deemed appropriate for the patient, the medication is entered into a medication profile in the pharmacy information system. The medication profile is the primary record used by pharmacists to document patient medications.

A label is usually generated and filled by the technician for enough doses until the next cart fill. If automated dispensing cabinets are not used, institutions typically utilize a 24-hour cart-fill, whereby a 24-hour supply of drug is sent to the floor at a specified time period each day. From the label entered into the computer system, the technician fills the medication and sends it to the unit after the pharmacist has checked it for accuracy and appropriateness.

After each physician order, the nurse's **medication administration record (MAR)** is updated on the nursing unit. The MAR is a record located on nursing units of all the medications that are prescribed for the patient, including administration times. Figure 7-3 shows a copy of an electronic MAR. Prior to giving the new medication to the patient, the nurse double-checks the MAR against the patient order to ensure that it is appropriate. After patient administration, the nurse initials the MAR to denote that the drug was given and at what time.

Pharmacy medication profiles and the nursing MARs are linked within each institution's computerized medication system. In completely computerized record keeping systems, the MAR is electronic and is updated instantaneously with each new order entered in the pharmacy medication profile. For some systems, however, a hard copy of each MAR is printed every 24 hours from the pharmacy's computerized patient profile and delivered to the nursing unit. Any changes in the patient medications are updated manually on the nursing unit until the next computerized MAR is delivered.

One goal of unit dose systems is to reduce the cognitive burden on nurses in the administration process. One way of accomplishing this is the **unit of use** package.[2] Unit of use packages (also known as unit dose packages) contain the correct dose for the patient in a ready-to-administer form and do not require any preparation by the nurse. The medication will have a label that bears the name of the medication, the corresponding strength, expiration date, and bar code identifier. The nurse should be able to check the MAR, find the exact unit of use package in an individual patient's medication bin, and give it to the patient with minimal effort beyond double checking the MAR and directions for administration. The majority of drugs in institutions can be purchased from manufacturers in unit dose packaging. Medications from bulk bottles can also be repackaged into unit of use packages in the pharmacy.

On the nursing unit, medications are typically stored in either automated dispensing cabinets or locked medication carts. Medication carts have two major sections. One is a common area of the cart where bulk medications and floor stock can be stored. The other section contains individual patient medication bins. Each patient bed has a

Figure 7-3. Copy of a Medication Administration Record (MAR). MARs vary according to the software system used. *Source:* Available at: http://www.medical.siemens.com/siemens/en_US/rg_marcom_FBAs/images/presskits/HIMSS_2008/Siemens_Medication_Administration_Check_screenshot.jpg

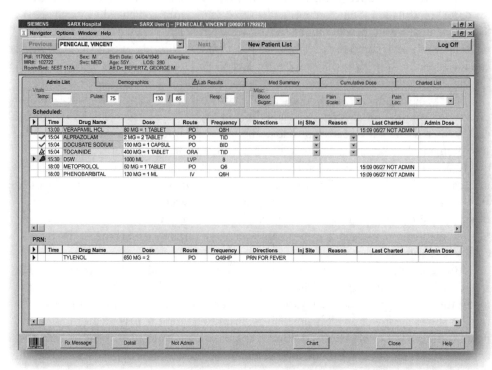

separate compartment (i.e., bin) where an individual patient's unit of use medications are stored. These patient medication bins are filled by the pharmacy and can only be accessed by a nurse or other appropriate representative. Carts have wheels but are usually kept stationary. Carts also have a flat surface for the nurse to use for preparation prior to administering the dose and for documentation needs.

Each day, the medications in this cart are exchanged with new ones for the day. The previous day's medications are returned to the pharmacy and medications that have not been given are evaluated as to why they were not given (e.g., Was an error made?). The unused medications are also credited to the patient, since many systems charge upon dispensing. Following this, the cart replenishment process starts again, where medications are placed

■ ■ ■

Key Point . . .

One goal of unit dose systems is to reduce the cognitive burden on nurses in the administration process.

. . . So what?

Spend some time on the nursing unit and watch the numerous tasks nurses have to perform. Research studies in the social sciences have concluded that multi-tasking by anyone, including nurses, increases the chances for error due to inattention and distraction. Unit dose systems seek to reduce the cognitive burden and errors associated with multitasking.

in the cart for the next day. The carts are filled by the pharmacy technician and checked by a pharmacist before being exchanged. If done properly, this cart replenishment can be completed in a short period of time.[11] In some states, technicians can substitute for pharmacists in double checking the accuracy of filling the unit dose cart.

If the pharmacy receives a new medication order for a patient or a dose request from the nurse, the pharmacist provides the medication to the floor before the next cart exchange. The number of items sent for a new order will provide enough doses until the next cart exchange. Drugs can be delivered to the floor either through a courier or pneumatic tube system.

Although unit dose systems rely on cart delivery for many drugs, some medications have unique handling and delivery instructions. Therefore, unit dose systems exist alongside floor stock and other distribution systems. Table 7-2 lists a sample of the different delivery methods and doses needed for a typical patient care unit at a tertiary care hospital.

Narcotics, PRN (as needed) medications, and emergency drugs follow a different process than the classic unit dose system. Schedule II narcotics, because of Drug Enforcement Agency requirements, cannot be stored in the individual patient bins in a medication cart because they do not provide sufficient security. Instead, they are usually stored in a locked cabinet with access limited to a few individuals (e.g., nurse-in-charge). Prior to giving controlled medication doses, the nurse takes an inventory of the medication and documents the doses removed. Discrepancies are reported immediately. Nursing also takes an inventory at each shift change to reconcile the number of orders against the number of medications given to minimize the chance of diversion. Periodically, pharmacy personnel take inventory of the controlled medications on the nursing unit to verify records and ensure that no diversion has taken place. Although time intensive, this process effectively reduces diversion.[12,13] Another more commonly used option is an automated dispensing cabinet (described later in the chapter).

Table 7-2.

Medication Delivery from Pharmacy to Patient Care Unit[2]

Medication Category	Delivery/Storage Method
1. Stable scheduled medications	A 24-hr supply is kept in a patient-specific bin on the medication cart in the unit
2. Unstable scheduled medications	Automatic delivery of medications to the unit 1 hr before administration time
3. Scheduled IV/TPN solutions	Automatic delivery of medications to the unit before administration time
4. PRN medications	A limited supply is kept in a patient-specific bin on the medication cart. Some PRN medications are kept in a limited floor stock supply and delivered by the pharmacy in response to request by the unit
5. Controlled medications	A limited patient-specific supply is secured in an automated dispensing cabinet or in a medication cart
6. STAT medications	Delivered by the pharmacy in response to a request from the unit
7. Emergency medications	Emergency drug kits are located on units and replaced by the pharmacy in response to a request from the unit
8. Investigational medications	Per investigational drug protocol

As needed (PRN) medications are handled according to different institution-specific methods. One method is to keep them in the pharmacy and dispense upon request. This system provides the most control over medication distribution, but it is rarely used because of the time burden on nurses and pharmacists and resulting delays in dispensing and administration. Another method is to send up a small amount of PRN medications for each patient in their medication drawer. If the patient requests a dose, the nurse retrieves the medication from the medication cart. The downside to this process is that many doses are sent daily to the nursing unit and returned unused. This is inefficient because it adds time to the cart replenishment process and reduces inventory turnover.[14,15] Most hospitals now use a limited floor stock system where medications with low potential for misuse and patient harm (laxatives, antacids) are stored in small quantities in the medication cart. If the patient requests a dose, the nurse removes the medication from the drawer, administers the dose, and records its use on the MAR. Medications with greater risk potential may be kept in individual patient bins or locked in automated dispensing cabinets (described later in this chapter).

Distribution of emergency medications is another area for pharmacy oversight. Emergency medications are a select number of drugs needed to be kept on-site to respond immediately to patients who deteriorate quickly due to failure of major organ systems. Emergency medications must be available instantly because any delay can be catastrophic for the patient. These medications are made available throughout the hospital in tamper-evident boxes or carts (sometimes called "crash or code carts"). An example of a cart is shown in Figure 7-4. Carts typically contain nondrug items (e.g., defibrilla-

Figure 7-4. Picture of an emergency crash cart. Emergency medications are stored in the tamper-evident red drawers. *Source:* Available at: http://www.ucdmc.ucdavis.edu/cne/resources/clinical_skills_refresher/crash_cart/

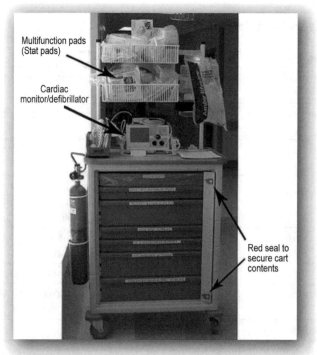

tor, medical supplies), intravenous solutions, and medications (e.g., epinephrine). Medications are in ready-to-administer form and located on nursing units or any other location an emergency may occur in an institution. Carts are checked periodically by pharmacy personnel to ensure that they have not been tampered with and to replace expired medications. In many institutions, pharmacists respond to medical codes and assist in the drug selection, preparation, and administration.[16, 17]

Models of Unit Dose Delivery

There are two main models used to structure unit dose services: centralized and decentralized models. A **centralized model** emanates from the main pharmacy (a centralized location). Medication orders are received in the central pharmacy, and all of the processing for patients occurs there: order processing, drug packaging, cart fill, and medication dispensing. The advantages of this model are that all resources can be localized into one area and drug inventory can be minimized. The biggest disadvantage is that the pharmacist is not able to directly interact with the physician and nurse. Clinical services are limited since the pharmacy is not closely located to patient care areas.

The **decentralized model** is characterized by having pharmacy satellites located throughout the institution.[18] A physician order is routed to a designated satellite where the pharmacist there processes the order and dispenses the first dose of the medication directly to the nursing station. Since pharmacists are closely located to patient care areas, it is very easy for physicians and nurses to stop by to ask a question. The pharmacist can also go into the patient care areas to speak with a patient or provide clinical services. The pharmacy satellite still needs to be supported by a centralized pharmacy which provides cart fill and serves the decentralized satellites. The centralized pharmacy is also needed to provide services to the hospital after the satellites close. Pharmacy satellites can provide specialized services in pediatrics, oncology, critical care, the emergency room, and the operating room.[19–23] The advantages with a decentralized model compared to a centralized model include faster order filling, increased physician and nursing satisfaction, better professional relationships between pharmacy and other departments, expansion of clinical services, fewer dispensing errors, and decreased need for floor stock medications.[24]

> **Key Point . . .**
>
> In many institutions, pharmacists respond to medical codes and assist in the drug selection, preparation, and administration.
>
> **. . . So what?**
>
> The public perception of pharmacists is of an individual working in an out-of-the-way, calm, and quiet area. Many people would be surprised to see pharmacists responding to medical codes in nursing units and advising physicians and nurses on appropriate use of emergency medications.

Rise of Technology to Assist Drug Distribution

As medication options continue to expand, the personnel demands of maintaining the unit dose method also increase. Computers and other technology have helped pharmacists respond to this demand.

One technological advance is the use of robots to fill medication carts. These robots are centralized automated dispensing devices that typically contain a medication selection station, a bar-code reader, and packaging and bar-coding equipment. Through the use of bar-code scanning, the robot selects the appropriate medication and number of doses for a medication drawer.[25] Robotic fill technology supports a centralized model of drug distribution, where carts are filled in a single location. The computerized information from the pharmacy patient profile system is transferred to the robotic dispensing system before filling. Once started, a bar-code label for each patient is generated and placed on a medication bin. These bins are placed on a conveyor belt, and the patient label is read by a scanner. The robotic filling device immediately recognizes the specific patient's medication needs, picks those medications, and places them in the bin. Once completed, the conveyor belt starts and advances the next bin. The process starts all over again, continuing until all medication carts are filled.

The benefit of the robotic fill system is that it replaces the tedious manual cart fill. Another benefit is its accuracy, since the use of bar-codes removes confusion over sound-alike drug names, skipped medications, or errors in choosing the wrong strength. It also frees up technician and pharmacist time and overall inventory costs are reduced, because medications are stored in the central pharmacy and not throughout the institution.[26]

The downside is that special preparation is needed before medications can be loaded into robotic filling systems. All medications need to be placed in unit dose packages that can be read and handled by the robot. This can take significant money and effort on the part of the pharmacy. In addition, robotic breakdowns or routine maintenance require pharmacy staff to return to filling medication carts by hand.

For that reason and others, **automated dispensing cabinets (ADCs)** are used frequently in medication distribution. An ADC is a point-of-use medication storage device located on patient care areas designed to replace traditional floor stock systems and unit dose cart exchange systems (Figure 7-5). They allow nurses to have quick drug access to medications but provide accountability by having an audit trail for all medications

Figure 7-5. Picture of an automated dispensing cabinet. This automated dispensing cabinet has a computer monitor for access to patient records and locked medication drawers, one of which is open. *Source:* Available at: http://www.webmm.ahrq.gov/media/cases/images/case36_fig1.jpg

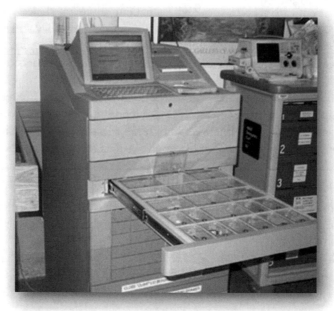

removed. Most systems have some form of user identifier or password to restrict access to the cart. More advanced systems are linked to pharmacy electronic medication profiles, not allowing a nurse to remove a medication prior to the pharmacist reviewing the order.

The advantage of ADCs is that they permit quick order filling while still maintaining control of the medication use system. When linked to the pharmacy drug profile, pharmacists can control access to first doses of new drug orders. Another advantage is that waste is reduced with ADCs because the nurse only needs to remove a dose from the cabinet if it is needed. This provides more accurate patient charges and minimizes the number of credits processed, since doses are administered upon removal.

The major disadvantage of the ADC system is that it is similar to the floor stock system, a system that reduced pharmacy oversight of medication use. This could increase medication errors compared to the unit dose system although the evidence of this is not clear. Another disadvantage is that it increases drug inventory on patient care areas and it places some of the burden of medication use back on the nurse.

Key Point . . .

A major disadvantage of the ADC system is that it increases drug inventory on nursing units and it places some of the burden of medication use back on the nurse.

. . . So what?

It is important for pharmacists not to forget the evolution of medication use systems. Pharmacists became involved because control over medication use was inadequate, errors were made, nurses were overburdened, and a lot of waste occurred. When adopting and using medication dispensing technology, policies and procedures must seek pharmacy oversight on medication use and reduce cognitive burden on nurses.

Some of these disadvantages have been minimized however by linking ADC systems with pharmacy information systems. ADCs on the floor can now be controlled by pharmacists at computer terminals working from up-to-date patient specific profiles. Nurses can only gain access to medications when they log into the system with a unique password or by using bio-ID scanning of fingerprints. Nurses are guided by a computer screen on the ADC system that matches the patient of interest with medications contained in the cabinet. Once the nurse removes a drug and closes the cabinet drawer, the patient is automatically charged for the dose and the inventory is decremented by what was removed. This allows for accurate patient billing and the maintenance of a perpetual drug inventory.

ADCs can be very useful in controlling narcotic use. The ADC can provide tracking required by the DEA and can store the narcotics in a safeguarded location where distribution is limited. In configuring these machines, different drawer types can be configured to manage access ranging from very restrictive (only housing the medication of interest) to less restrictive (gaining access to all of the medications in this drawer, trusting the nurse to choose the correct medication).

Future of the Medication Use System

As technology progresses, it will continue to take over the many manual tasks involved with the medication distribution system. Although it still takes time to fill the medication cart (if it is done manually), replenish the robotic dispensing device, or refill the ADC, automation will further decrease the number of people involved with the dispensing of medications.

In the future, drugs may be provided to nursing units from the pharmacy within the institution or it can be outsourced to wholesalers or other providers (Figure 7-6). Most pharmacies will likely maintain a mix of centralized, decentralized, and automated dispensing managed by the pharmacy. However, outsourcing of medication distribution to wholesalers may also become more widespread; dramatically changing medication distribution systems. Presently, wholesaler outsourcing may be limited to delivering totes specific for an ADC. Depending on various state laws, outsourcing can expand where wholesalers go to nursing units and replenish the ADCs, reducing the amount of time that a pharmacy department needs to be involved. The wholesaler may even own the inventory and charge for it when the patient uses it.

Bar-code technology will continue to be important in medication distribution. Bar codes help pharmacists track medication use and ensure that patients receive the correct medication. Bar codes also help robots and other technology read package labels.

Figure 7-6. Sources of Medications for Nursing Units. Nursing units in U.S. hospitals receive medications from a variety of sources—both within and outside of the hospital. Within the hospital (i.e., insourcing) medications can be dispensed from the centralized pharmacy, decentralized satellite, or automated dispensing cabinet. Outside of the hospital (i.e., outsourcing) medications may be directly delivered to the nursing unit from a wholesaler or other supplier.

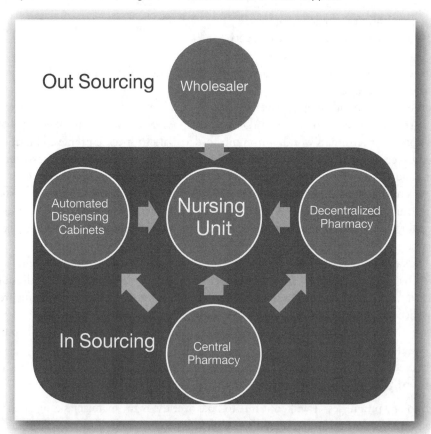

Technicians will also continue to play a large role in the medication distribution system. Studies have demonstrated that a tech-check-tech system for checking unit dose carts is as good as, if not better than, pharmacist checking a technician.[27,28] The pharmacist's value lies in using professional judgment in the profiling of medication orders, monitoring the medication use process, taking medication histories, conducting discharge counseling and the like. The technician's value lies in the distribution process.

Requirements of Any Good Medication Distribution System

As pharmacy medication distribution systems evolve, several requirements must be demanded by pharmacists of all new systems. The first is that pharmacists must always maintain quality control over drug use in institutions where patients are assured of receiving the right drug at the right time in the right way. This means that pharmacists need to be involved in efforts to prevent the diversion of drugs, reduce medication errors and waste, minimize adverse drug events, and ensure that drugs maintain potency through proper storage and handling.

Another requirement is that any system must be efficient in how it achieves drug use control. Thus, trade-offs may need to be made in some traditional practices that may not be cost effective. For instance, many distribution activities traditionally done by pharmacists, such as checking medication carts, might better be delegated to pharmacy technicians.

Finally, current and future medication distribution systems must always attend to the needs of those served by these systems—patients, physicians, and nurses. Therefore, the systems need to reduce the effort and inconvenience associated with the medication use process and enhance patient outcomes.

Key Point . . .

Studies have demonstrated that a tech-check-tech system for checking unit dose carts is as good as, if not better than, pharmacist checking a technician.

. . . So what?

There is still resistance by some pharmacists to the idea of systems that allow technicians to check the work of technicians. One concern is that technicians lack the professional training and experience to adequately monitor the quality of the dispensing process. Studies have shown that this is not the case in some situations. Indeed, pharmacists may be overqualified for this task and better used elsewhere for improving the medication use process.

Summary

The unit dose system and the development of automation for drug distribution have had a profound impact on elevating the practice of hospital pharmacy. The unit dose system reduces medication errors and supports the concept of clinical pharmacy. Technology has further enhanced the distribution of medications, allowing pharmacists to become more involved with patient care. The use of technology should further improve medication use by helping maintain pharmacist oversight of the process and allow the pharmacist to better care for patients' medication needs.

Suggested Reading

American Society of Hospital Pharmacists (ASHP). ASHP technical assistance bulletin on single unit and unit dose packages of drugs. *Am J Hosp Pharm.* 1985;42:378-379.

American Society of Health-System Pharmacists (ASHP). ASHP guidelines on the safe use of automated medication storage and distribution devices. *Am J Health-Syst Pharm.* 1998;55:1403-1407.

ASHP statement on the pharmacist's responsibility for distribution and control of drug products. In: Deffenbaugh JH, ed. *Practice Standards of ASHP 1996–97.* Bethesda, MD: American Society of Health-System Pharmacists; 1996.

Barker KN. Ensuring safety in the use of automated medication dispensing machines. *Am J Health-Syst Pharm.* 1995;52:2445-2447.

Borel JM, Rascati KL. Effect of an automated, nursing unit-based drug-dispensing device on medication errors. *Am J Health-Syst Pharm.* 1995;52:1875-1879.

Botwin KJ, Chan J, Jacobs R, et al. Restricted access to automated dispensing machines for surgical antimicrobial prophylaxis. *Am J Health-Syst Pharm.* 2001;58:797-799.

Cina JL, Gandhi TK, Churchill W, Fanikos J, McCrea M, Mitton P, et al. How many hospital pharmacy medication dispensing errors go undetected? *Jt Comm J Qual Patient Saf.* 2006 Feb;32(2):73-80.

Guerrero RM, Nickman NA, Jorgenson JA. Work activities before and after implementation of an automated dispensing system. *Am J Health-Syst Pharm.* 1996;53:548-554.

Klibanov OM, Eckel SF. Effects of automated dispensing on inventory control, billing, workload, and potential for medication errors. *Am J Health-Syst Pharm.* 2003;60:569-572.

Lee LW, Wellman GS, Birdwell SW, et al. Use of an automated medication storage and distribution system. *Am J Hosp Pharm.* 1992;49:851-855.

Max BE, Itokazu G, Danzinger LH, et al. Assessing unit dose system discrepancies. *Am J Health-Syst Pharm.* 2002;59:856-858.

Oren E, Griffiths LP, Guglielmo BJ. Characteristics of antimicrobial overrides associated with automated dispensing machines. *Am J Health-Syst Pharm.* 2002;59:1445-1448.

Pedersen CA, Gumpper KF. ASHP national survey on informatics: Assessment of the adoption and use of pharmacy informatics in U.S. hospitals—2007. *Am J Health-Syst Pharm.* 2008 Dec 1;65(23):2244-2264.

Pedersen CA, Schneider PJ, Scheckelhoff DJ. ASHP national survey of pharmacy practice in hospital settings: Dispensing and administration—2005. *Am J Health-Syst Pharm.* 2006 Feb 15;63(4):327-345.

Pedersen CA, Schneider PJ, Scheckelhoff DJ. ASHP national survey of pharmacy practice in hospital settings: Prescribing and transcribing—2007. *Am J Health-Syst Pharm.* 2008 May 1;65(9):827-843.

Pedersen CA, Schneider PJ, Scheckelhoff DJ. ASHP national survey of pharmacy practice in hospital settings: Monitoring and patient education—2006. *Am J Health-Syst Pharm.* 2007 Mar 1;64(5):507-520.

Schwarz HO, Brodowy BA. Implementation and evaluation of an automated dispensing system. *Am J Health-Syst Pharm.* 1995;52:823-828.

Shirley KL. Effect of an automated dispensing system on medication administration time. *Am J Health-Syst Pharm.* 1999;56:1542-1545.

Sutter TL, Wellman GS, Mott DA, et al. Discrepancies with automated drug storage and distribution cabinets. *Am J Health-Syst Pharm.* 1998;55:1924-1926.

References

1. Black HJ. Unit dose drug distribution: A 20-year perspective. *Am J Hosp Pharm.* 1984;41:2086-2088.

2. Black HJ, Nelson SP. Medication Distribution Systems. In: Brown TR. *Handbook of Institutional Pharmacy Practice.* 3rd ed. Bethesda, MD: American Society of Hospital Pharmacists; 1992:165-174.

3. Shultz SM, White SJ, Latiolais CJ. Medications Errors Reduced by Unit-Dose. Hospitals. *JAHA.* 47, March 16, 1973:106-112.

4. Barker KN, Heller WM. The development of a centralized unit-dose dispensing system for UAMC—part VI: the pilot study—medication errors and drug losses. *Am J Hosp Pharm.* 1964;21:609-625.

5. Hynniman CE, Conrad WF, Urch WA, et al. A comparison of medication errors under the University of Kentucky unit dose system. *Am J Hosp Pharm.* 1970;27:802-814.

6. Black HJ, Tester WW. Decentralized pharmacy operations utilizing the unit dose concept. *Am J Hosp Pharm.* 1964;21:344-350.

7. American Society of Hospital Pharmacists (ASHP). ASHP Statement on Unit Dose Drug Distribution. *Am J Hosp Pharm.* 1975;32:835.

8. Pedersen CA. Schneider PJ. Schecklehoff DJ. ASHP national survey of pharmacy practice in hospital settings: Prescribing and transcribing-2007. *Am J Health-Syst Pharm.* 2008;65:827-843.

9. Pedersen CA. Schneider PJ. Schecklehoff DJ. ASHP national survey of pharmacy practice in hospital settings: Dispensing and administration—2005. *Am J Health-Syst Pharm.* 2006;63:327-345.

10. American Society of Hospital Pharmacists(ASHP) ASHP technical assistance bulletin on hospital drug distribution and control. *Am J Hosp Pharm.* 1980;37:1097-1103.

11. McGovern D. Print, prepare, check, and deliver a 24-hour supply of unit dose medication for 600 patients in one hour. *Hosp Pharm.* 1981;16:193-206.

12. Woller TW, Roberts MJ, Ploetz PA. Recording schedule II drug use in a decentralized drug distribution system. *Am J Hosp Pharm.* 1987;44:349-353.

13. Norvell MJ, McAllister JC, Bailey E. Cost analysis of drug distribution for controlled substances. *Am J Hosp Pharm.* 1983;40:801-807.

14. Baker GE. Reducing the handling of prn doses in a unit dose drug distribution system. *Am J Hosp Pharm.* 1987;44:2255-2256.

15. Woller TW, Kreling DH, Ploetz PA. Quantifying unused orders for as-needed medications. *Am J Hosp Pharm.* 1987;44:1347-1352.

16. Shimp LA, Mason NA, Toedter NM, et al. Pharmacist participation in cardiopulmonary resuscitation. *Am J Health-Syst Pharm.* 1995;52:980-984.

17. Gonzalez ER, Ornato JP. Cardiopulmonary resuscitation documentation: a survey of 135 medical centers. *Drug Intell Clin Pharm.* 1988;22:559-562.

18. Kelly WN, Meyer JD, Flatley CJ. Cost analysis of a satellite pharmacy. *Am J Hosp Pharm.* 1986;43:1927-1930.

19. Tisdale JE. Justifying a pediatric critical-care satellite pharmacy by medication-error reporting. *Am J Hosp Pharm.* 1986;43:368-371.

20. Sauer KA, Nowak MM, Coons SJ, et al. Justification and implementation of a cancer center satellite pharmacy. *Am J Hosp Pharm.* 1989;46:1389-1392.

21. Caldwell RD, Tuck BA. Justification and operation of a critical-care satellite pharmacy. *Am J Hosp Pharm.* 1983;40:2141-2145.

22. Powell MF, Solomon DK, McEachen RA. Twenty-four hour emergency pharmaceutical services. *Am J Hosp Pharm.* 1985;42:831-835.

23. Vogel DP, Barone J, Penn F. Ideas for action: the operating room pharmacy satellite. *Top Hosp Pharm Mgt.* 1986;6(2);63-81.

24. Rascati KL. Brief review of the literature on decentralized drug distribution in hospitals. *Am J Hosp Pharm.* 1988;45;639-641.

25. Crawford SY, Grussing PG, Clark TG, et al. Staff attitudes about the use of robots in pharmacy before implementation of a robotic dispensing system. *Am J Hosp Pharm.* 1998;55:1907-1914.

26. Perini VJ, Vermeulen LC. Comparison of automated medication-management systems. *Am J Hosp Pharm.* 1994;51:1883-1891.

27. Ness JE, Sullivan SD, Stergachis A. Accuracy of technicians and pharmacists in identifying dispensing errors. *Am J Hosp Pharm.* 1994;51:354-357.

28. Andersen SR, St. Peter JV, Macres MG, et al. Accuracy of technicians versus pharmacists in checking syringes prepared for a dialysis program. *Am J Health-Syst Pharm.* 1997;54:1611-1613.

Chapter Review Questions

1.   Floor stock systems are no longer used in institutional pharmacy practice.
   a. True
   b. False

Answer: b. False. Floor stock systems are common for low risk medications used for PRN use, controlled medicines locked on nursing units, emergency medications, and other medications. Medication dispensed from automated dispensing cabinets may be considered to be part of a form of floor stock system. Floor stock systems exist alongside of unit dose and other types of distribution systems.

2.   Under what circumstances should pharmacists give up their responsibility to control drug distribution in health care institutions?
   a. Whenever medications can be delivered cheaper and faster than from a pharma-
       cist controlled system.
   b. As soon as possible because the future of pharmacy practice is clinical pharmacy.
   c. Never. Distribution is a fundamental responsibility of pharmacists.

Answer: c. The role of pharmacists is drug use control. Giving up control of the distribution process would be counter to the profession's mission. Drug use control is more than getting medications to the patients fast and cheap and clinical pharmacy is complemented by the distribution process.

3.   Decentralized pharmacy services are better than centralized pharmacy services.
   a. True
   b. False

Answer: b. False. Neither centralized nor decentralized models of mediation distribution have been shown to be clearly superior according to all the requirements of a good medication system. In general, centralized models offer efficiencies in the preparation and management of medications. Decentralized models better allow pharmacists to be part of the clinical team of physicians, nurses, and other health care professionals.

4.   Improvements in drug distribution have led the way for clinical pharmacy services.
   a. True
   b. False

Answer: a. True. When pharmacists accepted responsibility for and improved the distribution of drugs in health systems, they were able to establish credibility as experts in drug use control. Clinical pharmacy services were built upon that credibility.

5. **A centralized pharmacy is no longer needed if satellite pharmacy services are provided throughout the hospital.**
    a. True
    b. False

    Answer: b. False. Satellite services must still be supported by centralized services. Centralized pharmacies are typically provide preparation of refill medications, inventory control, managerial support, and other services that satellites cannot easily and efficiently provide.

6. **Institutional pharmacy services can be outsourced to wholesalers.**
    a. True
    b. False

    Answer: a. True. There is no reason why pharmacy services must be provided inhouse if superior services can be provided by wholesalers or other suppliers. Therefore, institutional pharmacist must make a case that in-house pharmacy services run by pharmacists can be more cost-effective than outsourcing competitors.

7. **Emergency medications are made available throughout the hospital in tamperevident containers called _____.**
    a. Lock boxes
    b. Crash carts
    c. Tackle boxes

    Answer: b. Also known as code carts, these containers are distributed throughout the hospital to have critical medications and supplies available to respond to emergencies. They are tamper evident to reduce the temptation for health care personnel to borrow medicines from the cart for non-emergency situations. If tampered with, the cart must be immediately replaced with another cart that is fully stocked with supplies and medicines.

8. **Who is responsible for maintaining MARs?**
    a. Nurses
    b. Pharmacists
    c. Physicians

    Answer: a. Nurses maintain MARs on nursing units to record information on the drugs, administration times, and directions for use.

9. **It is not clear how ADC systems affect the medication administration error rate in institutions.**
    a. True
    b. False

    Answer: a. True. Surprisingly, ADC systems have been adopted without much study of their impact on medication administration errors.

10. **Some type of electronic identification system like bar codes is needed on all unit-of-use packages with robotic fill technology.**

a. True
b. False

Answer: a. True. Robots need bar codes to identify medications. If unit of packages with bar codes are not available from the manufacturer, they must be packaged in the pharmacy from bulk medicine containers.

Chapter Discussion Questions

1. Compare the advantages and disadvantages of floor stock, patient prescription, and unit dose systems from the pharmacist's perspective.
2. Compare the advantages and disadvantages of floor stock, patient prescription, and unit dose systems from the nurse's perspective.
3. Clinical pharmacy in institutions did not blossom until pharmacists started taking greater responsibility for drug use. What lessons does this have for pharmacists practicing in community pharmacy settings?
4. Compare the advantages and disadvantages of centralized versus decentralized pharmacy services on service to nurses, speed of filling orders, cost of medication distribution, pharmacist and technician satisfaction, and demands on pharmacy managers.

CHAPTER 8

Controlled Substances Management

George J. Dydek and David J. Tomich

■ ■ ■

Learning Objectives

After completing this chapter, readers should be able to:

1. Discuss the federal and state laws governing controlled substances in IPP.
2. Identify organizations involved in regulating and managing controlled substances use.
3. Define key terms associated with controlled substances management.
4. Explain the pharmacist's role in handling, distribution, and control of controlled substances.
5. Describe the handling, distribution, and control of controlled substances in IPP.

Key Terms and Definitions

■ **Code of Federal Regulation (CFR):** A set of general or permanent rules that are published in the Federal Register by the federal government. The regulation is divided into 50 titles encompassing executive departments and agencies covering broad areas subject to federal regulation.

■ **Controlled Substance Act (CSA):** Also known as the Comprehensive drug Abuse Prevention and Control Act of 1970. The CSA is the federal government's drug policy governing the manufacturing, importation, possession, and distribution of certain substances that have been classified into five schedules based on their potential for abuse and accepted medical use in the United States.

■ **Drug Enforcement Administration (DEA):** A law enforcement agency under the Department of Justice that is responsible enforcement of the drug policy of the United States as required under the CSA.

■ **Failure modes and effects analysis:** A systematic approach of examining and analyzing a process to determine potential areas where errors or failures may occur (failure modes) and determine the effects (effects analysis) of those failures on a process so as to identify opportunities for improvements.

The opinions or assertions contained herein are the private views of the authors and are not to be construed as official or reflecting the views of the U.S. Department of Army or the Department of Defense.

- **Institute of Safe Medication Practices (ISMP):** A non-profit organization with the mission of enhancing patient safety through education, collecting and analyzing adverse drug events, disseminating medication safety information, collaborating with healthcare organizations, and conducting research.
- **Medication utilization evaluation (MUE):** An examination of a specific medication; most often within the context of a defined healthcare system. It is a method usually incorporated into an organization's performance improvement program that examines the utilization of a medication and its effects on patient outcomes.
- **Policies and procedures:** A set of written requirements dictated by an organization (polices) that provide the foundation for the written procedural instructions in an organization (procedures).

- **Power of attorney authorizations:** A legal document that allows another person to act on your behalf (i.e., allowing another pharmacist to order or receive controlled substances).
- **Stop order:** An order that automatically discontinues a medication based on pre-established parameters (e.g., time, clinical conditions).
- **Taper order:** An order that changes the dose of a medication; the dose is either progressively decreased or increased based on pre-established parameters (e.g., time, clinical conditions).
- **United States Pharmacopoeia (USP)-ISMP Medication Errors Reporting Program (USP-MEDMARX):** A national program designed for the voluntary reporting, categorizing, and expert data analysis of medication errors and adverse drug reactions.

■ ■ ■

Introduction

This chapter reviews the management of controlled substances within a health-system pharmacy practice. It is not intended to give a detailed description of applicable federal or state laws and regulations regarding the management of control substance medications (subsequently referred to as controlled substances). Rather, this chapter will take a medication-use systems approach in examining the management of controlled substances in the health-system environment. Strategies and resources for pharmacists are offered. The approach is similar to the approach taken in the Joint Commission (formerly known as the Joint Commission on Accreditation of Healthcare Organizations or JCAHO) medication management standards instituted in 2004.[1] It allows for the systematic examination of controlled substances within an organization from selection and procurement through storage, inventory management, dispensing, administration, surveillance, and system evaluation.

Several factors influence the need for health-system pharmacist involvement in controlled substances management. First, pharmacists must ensure that all federal and state laws and regulations are obeyed. Second, pharmacists need to ensure that controlled substances are used safely with minimal medication errors resulting in adverse patient outcomes. Last, pharmacists must ensure that controlled substances are used appropriately to achieve optimal health for patients. Each of these factors will be discussed in the following sections of this chapter.

Federal and State Laws and Regulations

The overriding influence on the management of controlled substances in the health care environment are federal and state laws and regulations. The principal federal law regulating controlled substances is the **Controlled Substance Act (CSA)**, also referred to as Title II of the Federal Comprehensive Drug Abuse Prevention and Control Act of 1970, under Title 21 United States Code, starting at Section 801.[2] The **Drug Enforcement Administration (DEA)** is the federal entity charged with enforcing and implementing the CSA. The main mission of the DEA is to work in concert with state agencies and other federal agencies (e.g., Food and Drug Administration) to prevent the diversion of controlled substances for illicit reasons. The DEA is able to carry out its mission through regulations contained in the **Code of Federal Regulations (CFR)**, Title 21, starting at Part 1300.[3] Additionally, the DEA provides an informative manual targeted for pharmacists that can be readily retrieved from their website.[4]

Controlled substances are classified according to their potential for abuse, accepted medical use, and potential for physical or psychological dependence which places them into different schedules (I–V). A list of these classified medications can be viewed through a hyperlink from the DEA website.[5] State laws and regulations regarding controlled substances for the most part mirror the CSA and may have more stringent requirements, but not less than the federal law required in the CSA. Due to variations in state laws regarding controlled substances, it is beyond the scope of this chapter to detail every state law regarding these medications. Pharmacists can obtain guidance about specific state laws and regulations regarding controlled substances from regulatory agencies in the state where they practice. Another source of information regarding some state and national activities involving controlled substances can be found at a website maintained by the National Association of State Controlled Substance Authorities (NASCSA).[6]

Patient Safety

Patient safety is another concern for pharmacists managing controlled substances. This is evident by measures adopted by both The **Institute of Safe Medication Practices (ISMP)** and the Joint Commission. The ISMP has designated controlled substances, specifically opiates in several dosage forms (intravenous, transdermal, and oral preparations) as *High Alert* medications.[7] Medication errors involving controlled substances have a greater risk of causing negative outcomes for patients. This designation for opiates has resulted from national reported medication errors through the **United States Pharmacopoeia (USP)-ISMP Medication Errors Reporting Program (USP-MEDMARX)**. Data obtained from nationally reported medication errors collected through the USP-MEDMARX program revealed that medication errors involving controlled substances were among the most frequently reported. Morphine was second only to

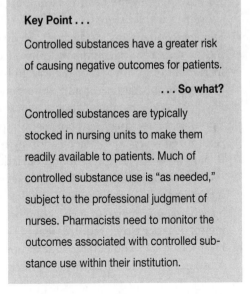

Key Point . . .

Controlled substances have a greater risk of causing negative outcomes for patients.

. . . So what?

Controlled substances are typically stocked in nursing units to make them readily available to patients. Much of controlled substance use is "as needed," subject to the professional judgment of nurses. Pharmacists need to monitor the outcomes associated with controlled substance use within their institution.

insulin in medications associated with errors that cause patient morbidity.[8] The ISMP Medication Safety Alert program for acute care environments recently described problem errors relating to the use of patient-controlled analgesia, specifically, narcotic toxicity due to inappropriate dosing.[9] In addition, the ISMP publishes and readily updates a list of drugs with similar sounding names that can be confused with each other resulting in errors. That list includes several controlled substances.[10]

Complexity of Pharmacotherapy

The complexity of pharmacotherapy and medication delivery systems can lead to negative health outcomes for patients. Many new formulations of older agents, such as morphine in sustained release forms or in novel administration forms (e.g., nasal) can lead to therapeutic problems. Medication complexity has lead to morphine/ hydromorphone mix-ups and morphine concentrate/non-concentrate solution mix-ups.[11] An example in the complexity of medication delivery systems and the effect on different patient populations is in a decision by the Food and Drug Administration in March 2009 to remove from the market an unapproved version of morphine concentrate liquid preparations widely employed in the hospice patient population.[12] The FDA subsequently reversed their decision after widespread outcries from the healthcare community. The health-system practicing pharmacist will continue to be challenged as new controlled and non-controlled agents are developed with novel pharmacologic applications and delivery systems.

Selection of Controlled Substances

Formulary

In most health systems the selection of all medications, including controlled substance medications, is performed by the pharmacy and therapeutics committee. When any controlled substance medication is considered for inclusion onto a formulary, a detailed evaluation of the medication is conducted. Data on the safety, efficacy, toxicity, potential for adverse events and abuse, and the pharmacoeconomics related to the population served by the health system are reviewed. Some of the criteria considered include the following:

- Location within the health system, other than the pharmacy, where the controlled substance will be stored.
- Storage requirements for the controlled substances based on manufacturer requirements, such as refrigeration. As controlled substance inventory increases due to increased utilization and/or increase in formulary additions, the pharmacy needs to consider immediate needs and project ahead for appropriate space.
- Physical security requirements at the location to ensure federal or state standards are met.
- Appropriate stocking levels both within pharmacy and outside in patient care areas.
- Authorized access to the medication by health care staff.
- Requirement for any prescribing restrictions based on providers' scope of practice.
- Incorporation of the controlled substances into to any prescribing or clinical guidelines (i.e., pain guidelines).
- Specific requirements for medication ordering by prescribers (i.e., **stop order requirements** or **taper order requirements**).
- Health care staff and patient education requirements on the use of the controlled substances prior to release into the institution.

- Any new policies and procedures that need to be addressed with the addition of the controlled substances.

Risk Assessment

Use of a **Failure Mode and Effects Analysis (FMEA)** or similar process is useful when evaluating the controlled substances for formulary addition and prior to procurement and distribution within a health system.[13] FMEA examines the potential for failures by identifying, classifying, and assessing the impact of failures on the system. **Failure modes** are any errors or defects in a process, design, or item, especially those that affect the customer, and can be potential or actual. **Effects analysis** refers to studying the consequences of those failures. Pharmacists can use FMEA to identify and examine potential deficiencies in medical processes or oversight of federal and state legal requirements associated with physical security, accountability, documentation, and audit trail. A critical analysis of the processes involved in the medication-use system for controlled substances can identify risk reduction strategies to enhance patient safety.

Key Point . . .

Failure Mode and Effects Analysis (FMEA) or similar process is useful when evaluating the controlled substances for formulary addition and prior to procurement and distribution within a health system.

. . . So what?

FMEA attempts to be proactive in addressing problems with the medication use process. Rather than waiting for a problem to occur, FMEA in control substance systems seeks to identify and address potential problems that might lead to a negative patient health outcome or an investigation by a state or federal agency for inadequate oversight and documentation of controlled substance inventory.

Procurement of Controlled Substances

Federal Registration Requirements

Procurement of controlled substances requires that the health-systems pharmacy be registered with the Drug Enforcement Agency (DEA) by submitting DEA Form 224, Application for New Registrant.[14] The registration is required to be renewed every 3 years with both the initial and renewal involving fees. The procurement of Schedule II's requires the use of DEA Form 222. The pharmacist in charge of the health system pharmacy needs to acquire a complete understanding of federal requirements for procurement and processes within the medication-use system to ensure integrity in accountability and documentation of controlled substances.[4]

Inventory and Storage Management of Controlled Substances

Inventory and Record Requirements

Once the controlled substance has been procured, the pharmacist must assure compliance with regulations pertaining to accountability and documentation. The inventory system must allow for an audit trail of complete and accurate documentation of the controlled substance through the medication-use system from the point of procurement and receipt in the pharmacy, through storage and distribution points within the institution to administration to a patient. Certain records must be maintained for 2 years in paper or electronic format to be readily retrievable on demand by state or federal inspectors. Records for Schedule II substances are segregated from all other records, whereas records for Schedules III–V substances may be either kept separate from other records or mixed with other records if kept in a readily retrievable form. Federal law and regulations require the following records to be maintained:

- Official order forms such as the official record of receipt and sale for Schedule II controlled substances, DEA Form 222.
- **Power of attorney** to sign for DEA order forms.
- Receipts and invoices for Schedule III–V controlled substances.
- Initial inventory taken when a new DEA registration is required. The CFR requires the date and time of the initial inventory be documented; the name of the drug, strength, and dosage form; the number of units or volume and total quantity of the controlled substance.
- Biennial inventory is conducted following the initial inventory, with the same required information as in the initial inventory. An actual count is required for all Schedule II controlled substances. The inventory for Schedule III–V controlled substances allows for an estimated count, unless the container holds more than 1,000 dosage units and has been opened.
- Records of controlled substance distribution and dispensing records (i.e., prescriptions).
- Records, if needed, relating to theft or loss (DEA Form-106).
- Inventory of controlled substances surrendered for disposal (DEA Form-41).
- Records of any transfers of controlled substances between pharmacies.
- DEA registration certificate.

All of the above records must contain the drug name, drug strength, dosage form, number of units or volume, and total quantity of the controlled substances.

Physical Security and Storage

Federal requirements for physical security for controlled substances require that the medications be in a "securely locked, substantially constructed cabinet" to deter theft and diversion. Pharmacies are allowed to place the controlled substances among the non-controlled medications as long as there are barriers to theft of the controlled substances.[2,4] This requirement provides a lot of latitude in where the controlled substances can be stored. Pharmacists need to evaluate the storage location of all controlled substances within their health system to

> **Key Point . . .**
>
> A controlled substance inventory system must allow for an audit trail of complete and accurate documentation of the controlled substance procurement, receipt, storage, distribution, and use.
>
> **. . . So what?**
>
> Imagine that you are a director of pharmacy standing before a representative of the Drug Enforcement Agency (DEA) who has responded to a report that controlled substances have been diverted from your pharmacy's inventory. Now imagine how much worse the situation would be if you could not identify the point where the diversion occurred within the system because the institution's record keeping for controlled substances was inadequate.

consider the level and type of physical security warranted. In some cases a locked cabinet, with minimal stock levels, and limited access to health care staff may be sufficient security. In other cases the requirement for a safe with intrusion detection devices and alarm systems may be warranted. The following are suggested factors to consider in determining the level of security required[15,16]:

- Location of the storage site (pharmacy, inpatient wards, surgical suites, ambulatory clinics).
- Level of activity of the storage site for controlled substances (bulk storage in the pharmacy, hospital ward, or clinic stock).
- Quantity of controlled substances expected to be stored at the site.
- Dosage form of controlled substances handled at the storage site.
- Level of physical security that the container provides that will be utilized for storage of the controlled substances (safe, fixed cabinet, movable cabinet, automated storage and dispensing device).
- Policies and procedures for restricting access to the storage site (authorized personnel, access code management, key control, and safe combination procedures).
- Adequacy of electronic detection and alarm systems.
- Amount of unsupervised access, or potential for unsupervised access and procedures for handling patients and visitors.
- Amount of oversight of health care staff, whether they have immediate access to the controlled substances or not.
- Audit capability and inventory management of controlled substance at storage site.
- Review of applicable state laws and regulations and institutional policies and procedures.

Automated Storage and Distribution Devices

Automated storage and distribution devices greatly enhance the process of controlled medication distribution within health systems in both patient safety and inventory control. The devices permit better inventory control by allowing electronic documentation of all controlled medication use. All access to storage of drugs is limited to those with unique passwords that permit easy identification of individuals. User identification of access to the storage devices provides an audit trail if any discrepancies of records occur. As more health systems adopt bar code technology applications at the point-of-administration, the ability to control controlled drug use will improve. The American Society of Health-System Pharmacists provides an excellent overview of considerations for requirements in automated storage and distribution devices.[17]

Disposal of Controlled Substance Medications

When controlled substances need to be disposed of due to expiration, damage, or for other quality control reasons, they must be segregated and inventoried separately from all other drugs. The CFR requires that the inventory for these medications include the inventory date, drug name, strength, and dosage form, total quantity or total number of units or volume, the reason for the substance being maintained in the disposal inventory, and whether the substance is capable of being used in the manufacturing of other controlled substances. A company that disposes of expired medications (a reverse distributor) may be used for controlled substances, as long as that distributor is registered with the DEA. Pharmacists can contact the local DEA Diversion Field Office to determine which reverse distributor is registered with the DEA. Complete inventory documentation of any transfer of disposed controlled substances need to be retained.

Ordering and Dispensing of Controlled Substances

Medication Orders
The institution pharmacist practices in a different environment with regards to medication orders and dispensing than the pharmacist practicing in the ambulatory (outpatient) environment. Typically, the pharmacists practicing in health systems will find themselves in the position of reviewing medication orders from a provider (prescriber) entering that order into a pharmacy informatics system to be processed and the dispensed directly to the provider, nursing staff, or released from an automated storage device.

The ordering of medications is covered under Title 21 CFR, Section 1300. This section of Title 21 CFR defines a *prescription* as a means of ordering medication intended to be dispensed for a patient who is the ultimate user. The regulation goes on to clearly state that a *prescription* does not cover medication orders that are written for the purpose of being dispensed for immediate administration to a patient in a hospital setting. Pharmacists dispensing a prescription for controlled substances for patients in an ambulatory (outpatient) setting have strict requirements for container labeling. The same requirements for Schedule III–V controlled substances are not required for hospital dispensing from a federal CSA perspective and is covered in Title 21 CFR.[18] Pharmacists should be aware that specific requirements for controlled substances dispensed in institutions may be covered within state law or regulations. Applying Joint Commission requirements for medication orders and labeling of dispensed medications of controlled substances within a hospital will more than adequately cover any federal requirements.

In an institutional practice, individual practitioners (physicians, mid-level practitioners) employed at an institution or hospital may conduct medication related activities such as administering, dispensing, or prescribing controlled substances under the hospital's DEA registration. These activities are allowed as long as the practitioner is engaged in the usual course of professional practice while in the employment of the hospital and allowed by state law and regulations. Pharmacists are advised to seek out state law and regulations regarding mid-level practitioners' prescriptive authority. Additionally, within health systems there may be established formulary prescribing restrictions placed on controlled substances based on clinical practice guidelines or through the hospital's credentialing process of restricting certain prescribing privileges to individual practitioners.

Electronic Prescribing
There is continued movement across the nation to migrate most, if not all, of health care transactions currently being conducted on paper to an electronic format. There is a governmental initiative to migrate health care records to an electronic medical record. Certainly from a patient safety perspective, the migration of medication ordering has been identified as major tool to prevent medication related errors. Facsimile of Schedule II substances prescriptions has been authorized by the DEA since 1994. This authorization is allowed if an original prescription is presented at the time of actual dispensing of the controlled substances. Exceptions to this requirement for an original prescription are for medication orders related to home intravenous infusions for pain therapy, patients in long term care facilities, and patients in hospice care. Facsimile prescriptions for Schedule III-V substances are authorized without the requirement for an original prescription to be presented at the time of dispensing. With the advent of physician computer order-entry and the strong movement within health systems across the nation to adopt this technology, both federal

and state laws and regulations will need to address the electronic transmission of medication orders in the absence of paper. After the DEA conducted pilot projects to examine technology to ensure appropriate security requirements in the electronic transmission of controlled substances prescriptions, revised regulations have been published to allow this process to proceed.

Administration of Controlled Substances

As has been highlighted previously, the three primary factors requiring increased scrutiny of controlled substances are attributable to federal and state laws and regulations, patient safety, and the complexity of pharmacotherapy. Pharmacists must take an active role in working primarily with the nursing staff to reduce the risk of controlled substances diversion and enhancing patient safety at the point of administration. The complexity of pharmacotherapy is certainly contributory to the environment of increasing the potential for medication errors, with multiple medications and dosage forms, medications with look-alike and sound-alike names, and the increased utilization of infusion devices. Risk reduction strategies for minimizing medication errors prior to administration on patient care units include limiting access to the controlled substances; limiting the availability of some products, especially look-alike and sound-alike identified controlled substances; requiring redundancies involving a double check system; educating the health care staff and patients; and monitoring patients.[19]

> **Key Point . . .**
>
> Physician computer order-entry within health systems will require changes in both federal and state laws and regulations.
>
> **. . . So what?**
>
> The electronic transmission of orders for controlled substances offers both opportunities and risks. Electronic order transmission can permit more accurate communication of orders and better record keeping. However, it can also lead to new ways of diverting drugs outside of approved channels. Pharmacists' expertise will be necessary to ensure that the negatives of computerized prescriber order entry do not outweigh the positives.

Evaluation of Controlled Substances

Medication Utilization Evaluation (MUE) Program

A **medication utilization evaluation (MUE) program** can provide pharmacists with a mechanism for examining the utilization of controlled substances within the health system. A MUE is a method usually incorporated into an organization's performance improvement program that examines the utilization of a medication and its effects on patient outcomes.[20] The MUE process can be a tool to study the use of controlled substances throughout the medication-use system or to focus on one particular process of the system. If employed as part of a multidisciplinary program, it can be used to enhance patient safety, ensure compliance with regulation and laws, and most importantly effect on patient outcomes.

Controlled Substances Surveillance Program

Controlled substances by definition are medications that have various potential for abuse and diversion within the medication system. The fact remains that in our society there is the potential for abuse and diversion of controlled substances within the health care system by all professionals. Data from the DEA indicates a 114 percent increase from 2001 to 2005 in unintentional deaths involving prescription opioids, with most of the prescriptions obtained illegally from friends, family, physician shopping, theft or fraud.[21] In concert with a MUE program that is primarily focused on patient outcomes and performance improvement, there needs to be a controlled substances surveillance program that focuses on controlled substances diversion and subsequent abuse. Controlled substances surveillance is a required program that every pharmacist must be actively engaged in. The deployment of automated storage and distribution devices previously noted has enhanced inventory control management of controlled substances. These devices not only serve as excellent inventory management tools for controlled substances but can serve as tools in any surveillance program. There are several commercial vendors on the market that offer storage devices with computer software enhancements, data capture, and report capabilities to allow pharmacists in any health system monitor controlled substances. Wellman et al. describe an efficient computer assisted surveillance program utilizing data capture from automated storage and dispensing devices.[22] Any surveillance system built to monitor controlled substances will invariably have deficiencies. An article by O'Neal describes the inherent flaws in current automated surveillance systems and presents diversion scenarios with some recommendations for resolutions.[23] One recommendation is to ensure that controlled substances surveillance program information is readily available for pharmacy and nursing managers. Any controlled substances surveillance program will not only need to exploit automated data collection and analyses tools but also fully engage staff members within pharmacy and key departments or services outside the pharmacy.

Clinical Practice Guidelines

Pharmacists should not lose sight of the tremendous therapeutic potential that controlled substances offer when used appropriately. The use of clinical practice guidelines provides the opportunity to improve the quality of patient care through appropriate use of controlled substances. This is especially evident in the area of pain management, where there has been a tendency within the health care environment to allow controlled substances strict oversight and fear of abuse and diversion to hinder appropriate patient care. An example of a clinical practice guideline designed to address the appropriate management of patients with pain utilizing both controlled substances and non-controlled substances can be found at the American Geriatric Society website.[24] The state of Washington has published guidelines to assist practitioners in the safe and effective use of controlled substances for the treatment of chronic non-cancer pain.[25] Clinical practice guidelines are part of any MUE program that strives to ensure appropriate utilization of medication and can be used as a tool in a controlled substances surveillance program.

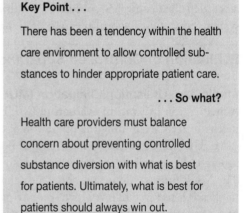

Key Point . . .

There has been a tendency within the health care environment to allow controlled substances to hinder appropriate patient care.

. . . So what?

Health care providers must balance concern about preventing controlled substance diversion with what is best for patients. Ultimately, what is best for patients should always win out.

Policies and Procedures for Controlled Substances

As with any process within the medication-use system, it is imperative that policies and procedures for controlled substances management be developed and instituted within the organization. **Policies and procedures** are a vital tool in the management of a pharmacy in any health system.[26] This is especially evident in the management of controlled substances and needs to address the entire medication management system, from selection, procurement and storage, ordering, distribution and preparation, through administration and monitoring. The following are some controlled substances subject areas that need to be addressed in policies and procedures:

■ What personnel are authorized to procure controlled substances and under what authority?

■ What are the normal and emergency procurement procedures for controlled substances?

■ What is the process for receiving controlled substances, including staff responsibilities, storage location, and procedures for handling a discrepancy?

■ How are inventory management and accountability handled in the pharmacy?

■ How are inventory management and accountability handled in patient care areas?

■ What are the procedures for distributing controlled substances within the health system from the pharmacy to patient care areas, including staff responsibilities and security of controlled substances during transfer?

■ What are the procedures for intravenous compounding of controlled substances including disposal, distribution to patient care areas, and accountability?

■ What personnel have authorized access to storage sites?

■ How are controlled substances disposed of by the pharmacy?

■ How are controlled substances returned from patient care areas handled?

■ What is the procedure for handling a patient who has a personal supply of controlled substance medications?

■ How are controlled substances managed in surgical and anesthesia services areas?

■ How are controlled substances managed in regard to automated storage and dispensing devices including staff responsibilities in stocking, quality control, discrepancies, problem solving with users, control of access codes, archiving of data, and surveillance report generation?

■ How are significant discrepancies anywhere in the health system handled? What trigger points are used to decide when to engage outside agencies (DEA, state agencies, and law enforcement)?

> ■ ■ ■
>
> **Key Point . . .**
>
> It is imperative that policies and procedures for controlled substances management be developed and instituted within the organization.
>
> **. . . So what?**
>
> The risks associated with controlled substances are too great to allow much flexibility in the process. Aside from the real risk to patients, a pharmacist's career is at risk if he or she is careless in the handling or recording of controlled substances. One of the quickest ways to be fired from a job at a pharmacy is to be lax with one's responsibility in managing controlled substances. Conscientiously following policies and procedures in this area is essential.

■ What is the process for new employee orientation and ongoing competency assessment for the staff in dealing with controlled substances?

Summary

Controlled substances medications are an integral and important component of many pharmacotherapy plans for patients. These medications have increased potential for abuse and misuse, federal and state laws require increased oversight by the health-system pharmacist. This increased oversight by pharmacy requires compliance with legal aspects of medication management. All staff must be knowledgeable, competent, and vigilant. Their vigilance in the controlled substance medication management system will enhance patient outcomes.

Controlled substances management will continue to present many challenges for the health-system pharmacist, who will continue to be counted on to provide leadership, by both health care organizations and societies in devising effective and efficient methods for the management of controlled substances.

References

1. Rich DS. New JCAHO medication management standards for 2004. *Am J Health-Syst Pharm.* 2004;61:1349-1358.

2. Fink JL, Vivuan JC, Reid KK, eds. *Pharmacy Law Digest.* 37th ed. St. Louis, MO: Facts and Comparisons; 2003: 125-167.

3. Code of federal Regulations, Title 21, Food and Drugs, Parts 1300 to 1499. Available at: http://www. accessdata. fda.gov/scripts/cdrh/cfdocs/cfcfr/CFRSearch.cfm?CFRP artFrom=1300&CFRPartTo=1499. Accessed May 17, 2009.

4. Drug Enforcement Administration's Office of Diversion Control. Pharmacy Manual, An Informational Outline of Controlled Substances Act of 1970. Available at: www.deadiversion.usdoj.gov/pubs/manu-als//index.html. Accessed May 18, 2009.

5. Drug Enforcement Administration. Drug Scheduling. Available at: http://www.usdoj.gov/dea/pubs/scheduling.html. Accessed May 17, 2009.

6. National Association of state Controlled Substance Authorities. Available at: www.nascsa.org. Accessed May 17, 2009.

7. Institute of Safe Medication Practice. ISMP's List of High-Alert Medications. Available at: http://www. ismp.org/Tools/highalertmedications.pdf. Accessed May 17, 2009.

8. Hicks RW, Cousins DD, Williams RL. Selected medication-error data from USP's MEDMARX program for 2002. *Am J Health-Syst Pharm.* 2004;61:993-1000.

9. Institute of Safe Medication Practice. ISMP Medication Safety Alert. Available at: http://www.ismp.org/Newsletter/acutecare/articles/20080828.asp. Accessed May 17, 2009.

10. Institute of Safe Medication Practice. ISMP's List of confused Drug Names. Available at: http://www. ismp.org/Tools/confuseddrugnames.pdf. Accessed May 17, 2009.

11. Institute of Safe Medication Practice. ISMP Medication Safety Alert. Available at: http://www.ismp.org/Newsletter/acutecare/articles/20040701.asp. Accessed May 17, 2009.

12. Traynor K. For opiate management, FDA pledges to balance enforcement, palliative care needs. *Am J Health-Syst Pharm.* 2009;66:968-969.

13. Cohen MR, Senders J, Davis NM. Failure mode and effects analysis: a novel approach to avoiding dangerous medication errors and accidents. *Hosp Pharm.* 1994;29:319-324, 326-328, 330.

14. Drug Enforcement Administration, Office of Diversion Control. Available at: www.deadiversion.usdoj. gov/drugreg/reg_apps.htm. Accessed May 18, 2009.

15. Title 21, Code of federal Regulations, Chapter II, Subchapter L, Part 1301-Section 1301.71. Available at: http://www.accessdata.fda.gov/scripts/cdrh/cfdocs/cfcfr/ CFRSearch.cfm. Accessed May 18, 2009.

16. Katzfey RP. JCAHO Shared visions—new pathways: the new hospital survey and accreditation process for 2004. *Am J Health-Syst Pharm.* 2004;61:1358-64.

17. ASHP guidelines on the safe use of automated medication storage and distribution devices. In: Hawkins B, ed. *Best Practices for Health-System Pharmacy. 2008–2009 Edition.* Bethesda, MD: American Society of Health-System Pharmacists; 2008.

18. Title 21, Code of federal Regulations, Chapter II, Subchapter L, Section 1306.24. Available at: http://www.accessdata.fda.gov/scripts/cdrh/cfdocs/cfcfr/ CFRSearch.cfm. Accessed May 18, 2009.

19. Cohen MR. ISMP medication error report analysis, risk of morphine-hydromorphone mix-ups. *Hosp Pharm.* 2004;39:818-820.

20. ASHP guidelines on medication-use evaluation. In: Hawkins B, ed. *Best Practices for Health-System Pharmacy. 2008–2009 Edition.* Bethesda, MD: American Society of Health-System Pharmacists; 2008.

21. Drug Enforcement Administration. Prescription opioid-related deaths increased 114 percent from 2001 to 2005, treatment admissions up 74 percent in similar period; young adults hardest hit. Available at: http://www.usdoj.gov/dea/pubs/pressrel/pr052009p.html. Accessed May 29, 2009.

22. Wellman GS, Hammond RL, Talmage R. Computerized controlled-substance surveillance: application involving automated storage and distribution cabinets. *Am J Health-Syst Pharm.* 2001;58:1830-1835.

23. O'Neal BC. Controlled substance diversion detection: go the extra mile. *Hosp Pharm.* 2004;39:868-870.

24. The American Geriatrics Society Clinical Practice Guideline Pharmacological Management of Persistent Pain in Older Persons. Available at: http://www.americangeriatrics.org/education/pharm_management.shtml. Accessed May 18, 2009.

25. Interagency Guideline on Opioid Dosing for Chronic Non-cancer Pain: an educational pilot to improve care and safety with opioid treatment. Available at: http://www.agencymeddirectors.wa.gov/Files/OpioidGdline.pdf. Accessed May 18, 2009.

26. Tomich DJ, Dydek GJ. The policy and procedure manual. In: Brown TR, ed. *Handbook of Institutional Pharmacy Practice.* 4th ed. Bethesda, MD: American Society of Health-System Pharmacists; 2006.

Chapter Review Questions

1. **The Joint Commission is the federal entity responsible with enforcing and implementing the Controlled Substance Act.**
    a. True
    b. False

    Answer: b. False. The Drug Enforcement Agency is the federal entity charged with enforcing and implementing the Controlled Substances Act.

2. **The Drug Enforcement Agency is able to carry out its mission through regulation contained in the _____.**

    Answer: Code of Federal Regulation, Title 21, starting at Part 1300.

3. **Morphine is one of the most frequent medications associated with errors that cause patient morbidity.**
    a. True
    b. False

    Answer: a. True. Morphine was second only to insulin as being associated with medication errors that cause patient morbidity.

4. **Procurement of controlled substances requires that the health-system pharmacy be registered with the Drug Enforcement Agency; this registration is required to be renewed every 2 years.**

a. True
b. False

Answer: b. False. The registration is required to be renewed every 3 years.

5. **Schedule II controlled substances are obtained through the utilization of DEA Form-106.**
   a. True
   b. False

   Answer: b. False. The official record of receipt and sale of Schedule II controlled substances is DEA Form-222. DEA Form-106 is a form used to record theft or loss of controlled substances.

6. **A biennial inventory is conducted following an initial inventory, with the same required information as in the initial inventory.**
   a. True
   b. False

   Answer: a. True. A biennial inventory is conducted following an initial inventory, with the same required information as in the initial inventory; this includes an actual count for all Schedule II controlled substances, and an estimated count for Schedule III–V controlled substances unless the container holds more then 1000 dosage units and the container has been open.

7. **Inventory of Schedule II controlled substances surrendered for disposal require the utilization of DEA Form-41.**
   a. True
   b. False

   Answer: a. True. DEA Form-41 Registrants Inventory of Drugs Surrendered "is the appropriate form to utilize when surrendering Schedule II controlled substances for disposal."

8. **Name two programs that would assist a pharmacist in proper oversight in the utilization of controlled substances.**

   Answer: A medication utilization evaluation program and a surveillance program.

9. **Name three factors that have been responsible for the increased scrutiny of controlled substances in a hospital environment.**

   Answer: federal and state laws; patient safety; complexity of pharmacotherapy.

10. **Name three key requirements for the effective management of controlled substances.**

    Answer: Appropriate inventory and record requirements; appropriate physical and storage requirements; appropriate policy and procedures in the management of controlled substances.

Chapter Discussion Questions

1. Why should pharmacists be concerned about proper management and documentation of controlled substances?
2. Discuss factors that influence the need for pharmacist involvement in controlled substances management.
3. Discuss criteria that pharmacists should consider when adding any controlled substances to the formulary.
4. Compare and contrast physical security and storage requirements for controlled substances versus non-controlled substances.
5. Compare and contrast the pharmacist involvement in the handling of controlled substances during the ordering and dispensing process in an institutional environment versus retail (outpatient) environment.

CHAPTER 9

Electronic Data Management: Electronic Health Record Systems and Computerized Provider Order Entry Systems

David A. Holdford, Stephen K. Huffines, and S. Trent Rosenbloom

Learning Objectives

After completing this chapter, readers should be able to:

1. Describe key elements of any system of electronic data, information, and knowledge management.
2. Define key terminology associated with electronic data management systems.
3. Identify major issues associated with the use of electronic data management.
4. Explain the role of pharmacists in electronic data management.

Key Terms and Definitions

- **Clinical decision support:** Clinical decision support refers to the tools providing guideline- or knowledge-based information to health care providers as they interface with the data repository. When providers enter information at the user interface, the information is checked against recommendations made by local medical libraries, national professional societies, and national governmental services. When entered information conflicts with expert guidance, an alert is sent through the interface to the provider.
- **Computer-based documentation systems:** Computer-based documentation systems prompt clinicians to provide more complete information to document their clinical decisions and patient interactions. These systems may require data fields to be filled out (e.g., allergies) before allowing clinicians to proceed with other tasks.
- **Computerized provider order entry (CPOE):** Computerized provider order entry is the process by which health care providers electronically place clinical orders (such as prescriptions, laboratory, and radiology requests) into a computerized database.
- **Data repository:** A data repository is a type of database that contains patient information, including lists of medica-

tions, allergies, laboratory and radiology testing results, clinical documents, demographic information such as age, gender, and address, and orders.

■ **Data standardization:** Data standardization defines a regular format for data entered into EHRs, the terms used to represent the data, and the data's configuration.

■ **Electronic health record (EHR) system:** An electronic health record system is an electronic version of the patient's paper-based medical record. EHRs store, manage, and display health care related records, including all clinical and administrative information entered by all practitioners involved in health care delivery.

■ **Electronic medical record (EMR):** An EMR is computerized clinical documentation of a patient's medical care over time within a single institution (e.g., hospital, physician's office).

■ **Electronic prescribing (e-prescribing):** Describes CPOE in ambulatory care settings, typically limited to electronic transmission of prescription data between prescribers, pharmacies, pharmacy benefit managers, and insurance plans.

■ **Functionality:** Functionality is defined as the sum of all things (i.e., functions) that a software program or system can do for users.

■ **Health Level 7 (HL-7):** HL-7 is one of several standards setting organizations whose mission is to provide interoperability standards for EHR systems.

■ **HIPAA:** Health Insurance Portability and Accountability Act was enacted in 1996 to improve portability and continuity of health insurance coverage in the group and individual markets, to combat waste, fraud, and abuse in health insurance and health care delivery, to promote the use of medical savings accounts, to improve access to long-term care services and coverage, to simplify the administration of health insurance, and for other purposes.

■ **Interoperability:** Interoperability is defined as the capability of information systems to exchange and use data.

■ **Personal health record (PHR):** Web-based platform accessible to and controlled by patients about their own medical care and insurance coverage. The PHR commonly contains consumer-friendly tools (e.g., weight control monitoring and guidance) to help patients manage their personal health.

■ **User interface:** The access point for information available in a patient data repository. Typically, health care providers interface with the data at a stationary computer screen or some handheld mobile device. User interfaces can permit entry of new orders or prescriptions, viewing of recent laboratory reports, scheduling clinical visits or admissions, and managing lists of diagnoses, among others.

■ ■ ■

Introduction

Electronic data management in health systems revolves around two forms of technology: electronic health records systems and computerized provider order entry systems. Both have the potential for transforming medical care in institutions and pharmacy practice by improving access to comprehensive, accurate, and timely information about patients and their care.

Electronic health record (EHR) systems are computer-based applications designed to acquire, store, manage, and display health care related records including all clinical and administrative information entered by practitioners involved in health care delivery.[1] Although the potential for EHR systems to improve health care quality and value is widely accepted, adoption remains limited.[2,3] Many reasons for limited adoption have been postulated in the scientific and lay literature. These include the high cost of developing and maintaining such systems, the unclear return on EHR investments, physician resistance, and an inadequate number of individuals trained in information technology. EHR systems can include many clinical components, including computerized provider order entry systems.

Computerized provider order entry (CPOE) is the process by which health care providers place clinical orders (such as prescriptions and laboratory testing requests) using a computerized system. At one time, the *p* in CPOE was traditionally attributed as *physician*, but *provider* is now the more accurate description since multiple health care providers serve in a prescribing role—physicians, nurse practitioners, physician assistants, and pharmacists. While only about 17% of hospitals currently use CPOE systems, the number is expected to grow due to national mandate, legislation, industry incentives, and stakeholder pressure.[3-6] Although CPOE systems support multiple order types (i.e., radiology, dietary, and laboratory), the focus of this chapter will be on the medication component.

To cover these main issues, this chapter is divided into two sections. The first section focuses on EHR systems including the evolving definition of EHR systems, the information contained in an EHR system, and the role of an EHR system in health care. The second section describes CPOE and its role in improving health care prescribing.

Electronic Health Record Systems

The history of EHR systems began in the early 1960s with early pioneers developing programs to assist in documenting patient history, physical examinations, and radiology reports.[7-9] Some of the earliest EHR systems include The Medical Record (TMR), developed in 1970 at Duke University, the Regenstrief Medical Record System (RMRS), first developed in 1972, and the HELP system in Utah.[1,9-12] Since then, many EHR systems have been developed in academic settings across the country. Examples include the COSTAR project at Massachusetts General Hospital and systems at Stanford, Johns Hopkins, Columbia, and Vanderbilt.[13] In addition, the U.S. government has developed EHR systems for the Veterans Administration, the Department of Defense, and the Indian Health Service, and many commercial vendors have been creating or licensing additional systems in the private sector.[14]

As EHR systems have evolved, the terminology associated with electronic records has too, resulting in confusion over the terms electronic health record, electronic medical record, and personal health record. An **electronic medical record** (EMR) defines the computerized clinical documentation of a patient's medical care over time within a single institution (e.g., hospital, physician's office). The EMR is essentially the electronic equivalent of a paper based medical record. In contrast, an **electronic health record** (EHR) encompasses documentation of all episodes of medical care received over time by patients within a geographic area. Information in an EHR may be compiled from data in EMRs in multiple institutions. A **personal health record** (PHR) system is typically a web-based platform accessible to and controlled by patients about their own medical care and insurance coverage. A PHR system commonly contains consumer-friendly tools (e.g., weight control monitoring and guidance) to help patients manage their personal health. To maintain consistency and avoid confusion, this chapter will only use one term, *electronic health record*, to describe the electronic medical documents in institutions whether they originate from a single institution or an integrated health system.

In general, EHR systems are designed to replicate the information found in paper-based medical records but often take on greater **functionality** (i.e., do more things for users).[15] Figure 9-1 illustrates some of the key data entered into the EHR. The value of EHR lies in how it integrates various information sources into an accessible, useful form for individuals.

EHR systems are tools that provide secure, real-time, point-of-care and patient-centered information for all health care providers.[16] This means that they make patient care information available wherever it is needed, 24 hours a day, 7 days a week. In contrast to paper medical records, EHR systems can remind and advise health care providers; provide easily retrievable information about care given days or years before, and coordinate the efforts of all parts of the health care system. Good EHR systems help clinicians manage multiple aspects of patient care (e.g., clinical documentation, medication and allergy management, laboratory results tracking) and promote better decision making by providing accurate and timely clinical information. They can enable patient care to be coordinated across different sites of health care delivery, support administrative functions related to scheduling patients' admissions or appointments, and organize information according to what is needed and when it is needed. Information extracted from EHR systems can also provide data for quality assurance monitoring and for medical research. In the United States, EHR systems must now also be designed to meet **HIPAA** patient privacy requirements.

EHR systems can include a series of linked electronic information-management sub-systems. These sub-systems consist of a range of interconnected software applications

Figure 9-1. Key data flows to electronic health record systems.

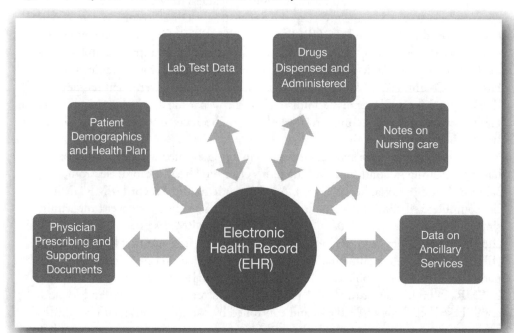

(e.g., CPOE systems, laboratory data) that provide functionality to the overall EHR system. Comprehensive EHR systems generally contain several core components: a patient data repository, user interfaces, clinical decision support tools, computer-based documentation systems, and CPOE (Figure 9-2). A **data repository** is generally a type of database that contains patient information, including lists of medications, allergies, laboratory and radiology testing results, clinical documents, demographic information such as age, gender, and address, and orders. Data can be in text, graphical, picture, or multimedia forms. The information available in a patient data repository can be displayed in or inform the functioning of other tools within an EHR system. **User interfaces** are the point of communication between clinicians and the EHR. User interfaces are stationary computer screens or mobile handheld devices that allow health care providers to interact (or interface) with the data in a patient data repository. User interfaces are essential for the basic work of medicine including the entry of new orders or prescriptions, viewing of laboratory reports, scheduling clinical visits or admissions, and managing lists of diagnoses. **Clinical decision support** tools guide and advise clinicians as they interface with the EHR. Clinical decision support tools provide feedback about the best available evidence from national professional society clinical guidelines and other expert sources. Decision support can be as simple as providing lists of the available dosage forms during order entry or as complicated as expert guidance for complex therapies such as total parenteral nutrition or chemotherapy; incorporating data on laboratory results, current diagnoses, and concurrent medications. **Computer-based documentation systems** assist health care providers in documenting their clinical decision making and patient interactions. They prompt clinicians to fill in data fields that better document their clinical decisions and patient interactions. CPOE will be discussed later in this chapter.

One of the problems often seen with EHR systems is their lack of **interoperability**: capability of information system components to exchange and use data. Interoperability is problematic because many EHR systems are made up of component tools developed in isolation from the others, and each serving one or more of the functionalities. For exam-

> ## Key Point . . .
>
> EHR systems are tools that provide secure, real-time, point-of-care, and patient-centered information for all health care providers.
>
> ### . . . So what?
>
> Paper health records are not secure—they are often left out on counters in nursing units or accompany patients to procedures (e.g., radiology). This often makes them easily accessible to unauthorized individuals. Paper health records are not available in real-time or at the point-of-care for patients because the records must be shared by everyone involved in the treatment of patients. Paper health records act more as a historical document of patient care than a real-time, point-of-care tool. In addition, the information is recorded by and designed to meet the needs of health care providers—not patients. Papers records are filled with medical jargon, scribbled notes, and technical information that can be confusing to patients.

Figure 9-2. Common components of EHR systems.

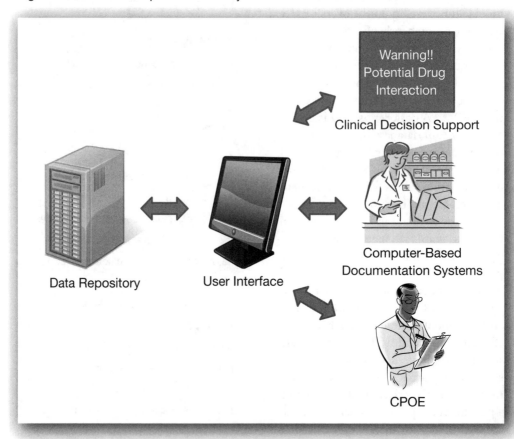

Warning!!
Potential Drug
Interaction

Clinical Decision Support

Computer-Based
Documentation Systems

Data Repository

User Interface

CPOE

ple, a system might have one software program that links the data repository to a clinical capture tool but a different system is used for clinical decision support. When different systems interact, there is greater potential for glitches to occur than when they are developed as part of an integrated system. When this occurs, additional software might be needed to integrate the EHR components and manage the data flow among them.

Benefits of EHR Systems

EHR systems provide a number of direct benefits to health care providers, including physicians, nurses, pharmacists and therapists. One key benefit results from the fact that patient information is not tied to a single location as it is with a paper chart. Access to the data is not limited either – clinicians and managers can view health record data throughout the healthcare system (e.g., ER, nursing unit, pharmacy). Another benefit is that data can be automatically captured as part of the overall workflow – information entered at keyboards or other data capture devices goes right into an EHR system. This contrasts with paper-based systems which require information to be copied and re-copied for use by individuals. Errors can be reduced with EHR systems because medical information entered into the system is immediately legible thereby reducing the potential of miscommunication between system users.

One of the major benefits of EHR systems is the wealth of automated solutions and data they can provide for quality assurance and continuous improvement efforts.[13] Clinical documentation tools, for example, can improve legibility and reduce medication and documentation errors. EHR systems can aggregate performance information by disease, by health care providers, and patient-care area. Such performance information can identify where clinical practice benchmarks are not being met. In some cases, EHR systems can be connected directly to medical devices such as infusion pumps or heart monitors and trigger alerts when patients have a significant change in status.[17] EHR systems may also help to improve compliance with regulatory society standards, such as those published by the Joint Commission by increasing the ability to manage and store data.[18]

Apart from improving medical practice and management, EHR systems can support research efforts. Patient data can be mined to answer questions such as "Which treatment works best for this patient suffering from the following medical conditions?" Without an EHR system, gathering information manually is tedious, inefficient, slow, and prone to error. With EHR systems (under ideal conditions), researchers can download information electronically from diverse locations quickly and economically. EHR systems are typically designed to improve the quality of data received by prompting clinicians to provide complete medical data (through clinical data capture tools) and that data can be made available for research shortly afterwards. Once in the EHR, systems can automatically identify patients meeting inclusion criteria for research trials, thereby improving targeted recruitment.[17]

> ■ ■ ■
>
> **Key Point . . .**
>
> EHR systems can be mined to answer questions such as "Which treatment works best for this patient suffering from the following medical conditions?"
>
> **. . . So what?**
>
> Paper medical records are static documents that have medical mysteries hidden inside. The answers must be provided by the health care professional. EHR systems can collect information from all patient records and allow professionals to combine them in useful ways. For instance, a provider might ask, "What is the probability that a specific patient's cellulitis will contain microbes susceptible to antibiotic A?" The EHR system might present laboratory susceptibility data from the institution's patients broken down by categories such as gender, age, and concurrent conditions.

Information Content and Data Issues with an EHR system

The Institute of Medicine (IOM) developed a list of potential functionalities that could be incorporated in an EHR system.[19] These functionalities can be divided into the categories of clinical documentation, test and imaging, CPOE, and decision support:[3]

- Clinical documentation
  - Medication administration records
  - Nursing assessments
  - Physician notes
  - Problem lists
- Test and imaging
  - Diagnostic-test images (e.g., electrocardiographic tracing)

- ◆ Diagnostic-test results (e.g., echocardiographic report)
- ◆ Laboratory reports
- ◆ Radiographic images and reports
- ■ CPOE
  - ◆ Laboratory tests
  - ◆ Medications
- ■ Decision support
  - ◆ Clinical guidelines (e.g., beta-blockers after myocardial infarction)
  - ◆ Clinical reminders (e.g., pneumococcal vaccine)
  - ◆ Drug-allergy alerts
  - ◆ Drug-drug interaction alerts
  - ◆ Drug-laboratory interaction alerts (e.g., digoxin and low level serum potassium)
  - ◆ Drug-dose support (e.g., renal dose guidance)

Although there is general agreement on what information/data can be contained within an EHR system under ideal circumstances, two common problems occur in real life practice settings: difficulties in data input and system information sharing limit the ability to collect and access good data.

The difficulties with data entry were articulated by McDonald in 1972 and remain to this day.[1,2,8,9,16] Most EHR systems provide a number of different ways to input patient data.[19] The earliest EHR systems permitted input using manual punch cards, which many system users believed were preferable to typed entry.[9,16] Other developers experimented with patient-entered data using simple electronic questionnaires.[20] Ultimately, the keyboard (or handheld key pad) has evolved as the primary means of data input. Other common methods of data entry include direct interfaces with other computers that generate data (e.g., digital laboratory test analyzers, some blood glucose monitors), point and click entry into a computer-form using a computer mouse or a touch-screen monitor, dictation and transcription, drawing using a specialized digital tablet, and scanning of handwritten documents.

Each method for data input has relative strengths and weaknesses. Typing, for example, may be efficient and acceptable for skilled users and relatively simple for data entry needs, but it is time consuming for others and limits the type of data that can be entered to what fits on a standard keyboard. Dictation/transcription is useful for those who cannot type efficiently, but it is expensive, error-prone, and requires a time delay before the dictated note is

Key Point . . .

The limited system interoperability of components of EHR systems has played a major role in limiting their adoption and use.

. . . So what?

The health care system is not really a system, it is a collection of independent entities that are uncoordinated, even counterproductive in their actions. One of the main reasons is the inability of systems to communicate. Imagine if your cell phone lacked interoperability with other cell phones. You might be able to use some of the applications, e.g., games, calendar, but most of its value to you would be lost. The same with EHR; lack of interoperability between systems reduces their value in coordinating and improving health care.

available in the EHR system. Point and click entry into structured forms can be very fast for simple data entry tasks, but it can become difficult and can constrain input if users have difficulty finding data fields on the form. Handwriting and scanning offer providers tremendous flexibility and ease but may lead to reduced legibility and data availability.

A more daunting problem than that of data input is that entered information cannot always be shared with other systems. This problem arises when different systems (or tools within a single system) encode the same information using different words, codes, or narrative structure. The limited system-interconnectivity (i.e., interoperability) of components of EHR systems has played a major role in limiting their adoption and use.

For example, it might be reasonable to assume that typing a patient's weight into the system might be a simple act that results in the weight being subsequently available to all connected EHR component systems. In reality, this is often not the case. One component of the system may store the data as "Weight," while another component stores it as "Wt." Still another component might store data about the patient's weight in free text, such as a physician's clinical note containing the unstructured narrative, "the patient weighs..." Sharing the patient's weight between these different systems is very difficult, if not impossible, without extensive programming this one data element into a form recognized by all system components. Indeed, the problem is multiplied for every potential piece of patient data, including medications, allergies, clinical findings, diagnoses, lab results, and orders.

The issue of non-interoperability has arisen because vendors of EHR systems have customized their products for users. This customizing has resulted in differing data categories and formats.

One solution to the problem of sharing information between systems is **data standardization**. Standardization defines a regular format for the data, the terms used to represent it, and the configuration it should take. For example, one standard would state that physical measurements, such as weight, must include the measurement name (e.g., weight), the value (e.g., 175) and the units (e.g., pounds), a corollary standard would state that weight must always be represented in EHR systems by the term "weight," and a formatting standard would state that the three must follow a certain configuration, e.g., measurement = weight, value = 175, unit = pound. A major standards organization, **Health Level 7 (HL-7)**, has been widely adopted as an industry data interchange standard. HL-7 primarily defines standards for data formatting and configuration. Data from two HL-7 compliant systems can communicate with relative ease and minimal additional programming. HL-7, however, generally stops short of defining standard terms for data exchange. The United States National Committee on Health and Vital Statistics (NCVHS) recently identified several core clinical vocabularies as terminology standards; however, these terminologies are inconsistently available or adopted by system developers.[21]

Another solution for problems with data exchange among EHR systems involves enterprise information architecture. Enterprise information architecture describes a structure for implementing information systems that takes a holistic view of system design. Rather than designing and managing information resources independently, enterprise information architecture simplifies the overall EHR system by designing interoperability into the system with compatible, logical suites of application programs. In the U.S. health care system, enterprise-information architecture is the exception rather than the rule.[4]

Promoting Expansion of EHR Systems: Issues and Solutions

At present, estimates suggest that only 5% to 39% of U.S. health care systems, office-based physician practices, hospitals, and clinics (excluding the Veterans Administration) have implemented EHR systems.[2,3] As previously discussed, there are many reasons for slow adoption, including difficulties related to data entry and interoperability. In addition, there is tremendous variability among systems in terms of functionality, ease of use, integration with other health care applications, data security, and ability to conform to clinical workflow needs. Health care providers and organizations must also expend resources to manage local knowledge-based rules and guidelines for their decision support and order entry systems. Furthermore, most EHR systems are expensive to purchase, implement, and maintain, and providers may not realize any direct benefit from their investment in such systems. To remove the negative forces created by these problems, there must be some realignment of incentives for institutions. Incentives that can help offset the EHR system purchasing costs include improved reimbursement from third-party payers and/or governmental support.

Currently, industry and the U.S. Department of Health and Human Services (HHS), Congress, Food and Drug Administration (FDA), and Centers for Medicare and Medicaid Services (CMS) have high expectations for EHR systems. The federal government plans to promote efforts to develop standards for EHR functionality, privacy, and interoperability, with the overarching goal of stimulating EHR system adoption.[22] Most health care reform proposals also aspire to make EHR systems widespread.

Computerized Provider Order Entry

Computerized provider order entry has been promoted as a major solution to the problem of medical error. In 2000, the Institute of Medicine published its first report on medical error, *To Err is Human.*[6] This report garnered a great deal of attention and galvanized many health care organizations to make patient safety the top priority. A second report, *Crossing the Quality Chasm: A New Health System for the 21st Century,* highlighted the importance of electronic health record (EHR) systems and the use of CPOE to eliminate many of the preventable adverse events in the provision of care.[25] Since medication errors are the most prevalent medical error, many CPOE systems have been designed with an emphasis on functions for reducing adverse drug events. The Leapfrog Group, a consortium of Fortune 500 companies interested in healthcare quality, made CPOE one of the three recommended goals to improve quality in hospitals.[4]

As with EHR systems, some confusion exists over the terminology associated with electronic order entry. CPOE and

> **Key Point . . .**
>
> The IOM report, *Crossing the Quality Chasm: A New Health System for the 21st Century,* highlighted the importance of EHRs and CPOE in preventing adverse events in health care.
>
> **. . . So what?**
>
> IOM reports are the basis of many of the changes in health care. Although it might be obvious to you, the fact that IOM has concluded that widespread adoption of EHRs and CPOE are needed means that government entities and professional groups are given momentum to drive that change.

e-prescribing are not synonymous terms. CPOE describes orders entered electronically into a health system's EHR anywhere within the system. **Electronic prescribing** or e-prescribing refers only to CPOE in ambulatory care settings. In addition, e-prescribing typically describes electronic transmission of prescription data between prescribers, pharmacies, pharmacy benefit managers, and insurance plans, while CPOE includes orders for laboratory, dietary, radiology, nursing, and pharmacy services.

In their earliest forms, CPOE systems date back to the mid-1970s. Early systems allowed health care providers to enter orders directly into the system but provided little decision support to alert drug-drug interactions, allergy warnings, etc. System functionality, hardware limitations, and readiness of institutions limited early adoption. Over subsequent years, technical advancement and the necessity for tools to assist professionals in delivering ever-increasing complex care to patients have led to further adoption of CPOE.

In spite of these efforts, CPOE has not yet moved far beyond the first adopters. CPOE for medications has only been fully implemented in 17% of all U.S. hospitals with 45% of hospitals having no CPOE or plans for CPOE in the near future.[3] Several reasons for not adopting CPOEs include (1) belief that physicians would not use computerized ordering, (2) products available from vendors have not been perfected, and (3) technical and process complexities of implementing CPOE translate into a significant investment with no guarantee of success.[26,27] Lack of standardization in practice across health care facilities is also cited as an additional barrier.[28]

> **Key Point . . .**
>
> In 2008, CPOE for medications had only been fully implemented in 17% of all U.S. hospitals.
>
> **. . . So what?**
>
> This fact indicates that U.S. hospitals have a long way to go to catch up with the 21st century. Lots of reasons are given: physician resistance, it costs too much, it's too hard, but these are just excuses. In truth, there is no acceptable excuse for this fact.

Implementing CPOE Systems

Advocates of CPOE systems promote their potential to reduce adverse events related to prescribing by alerting health care providers to potential errors (including drug interactions and patient allergies). Enthusiasm for CPOE has extended throughout the health care industry and into pharmacy circles in recent years. This interest comes from many different directions including health care facility leadership, standard and regulatory organizations, informatics professionals, software vendors, and within the pharmacy profession. CPOE can be expected to achieve several goals[29]:

- Improve patient safety
- Increase timeliness of care
- Facilitate use of current medical knowledge via clinical decision support
- Improve the process and coordination of care
- Limit the missed opportunities for preventive care
- Provide research capability for epidemiological studies
- Control or reduce costs

While the implementation of a CPOE system impacts every hospital department, the pharmacy often becomes disproportionately involved in the process. This is due to the complexity of the medication CPOE module, volume of transactions, and perceived value of CPOE on the medication order process.[23] CPOE implementation is generally too massive for the pharmacy to initiate; however, the pharmacy must be prepared and positioned to provide leadership in the medication component of these systems. The pharmacist is well-prepared and has historically demonstrated clinical and process skills in utilizing pharmacy computer systems.[24] These skills must be combined with innovation and a desire to provide solutions.

The process of CPOE follows the same basic steps associated with ordering any prescription (Figure 9-3). However, CPOE completes many of the routine tasks of electronically, reducing the possibility that information is overlooked or acted upon. The process starts with the prescriber signing into the computer. The sign-in verifies the identity and prescribing privileges of the prescriber thereby preventing any prescribing outside one's scope of practice. A patient is selected and the patient's medical record is reviewed for any medication therapy. Once a need is established, the process of choosing the drug occurs. After accessing the CPOE interface, the prescriber chooses a drug for the patient from a menu or by typing the drug name into a computer field. Dosage, route of administration, and other options are presented for the prescriber to select from along with any alerts or advisories relevant to the situation. When satisfied with the choice of therapy, the prescriber authorizes the order and it is sent to the pharmacy electronically or in print form.

In the pharmacy, the order is reviewed against the patient's medication profile or medical record and entered into the system. Once in the system, alerts and advisories are flagged for the pharmacist for action. After resolving any potential problems with the prescriber, the medication is dispensed with directions and sent to the nursing unit for administration to the patient.

Figure 9-3. Basic steps in prescribing and dispensing a CPOE prescription.

Assess Need for Prescription	Choose Drug	Dispense Drug
• Sign in • Select patient • Review patient data	• Access CPOE interface • Select drug • Review alerts and advisories • Authorize and sign order	• Review CPOE against medical record, alerts, and advisories • Dispense with administration directions

Clinical Decision Support

A **clinical decision support system (CDSS)** is a set of tools that facilitates the decision-making capabilities of the prescriber at the decision point of CPOE. CDS ranges from simple (reminder) to complex (algorithms) to recommend or change therapy. This is a key element of effective CPOE systems.

Pharmacies have long employed clinical decision support in pharmacy information systems. Functionality has traditionally included checking allergies, duplicate-therapies, drug-interactions, and abnormal dosage-ranges. Although an important safety tool, most pharmacists would admit that CDSS tools are not always effectively utilized in CPOE systems because many alerts are clinically insignificant while important alerts are often inadequately addressed. In addition, many systems have not allowed pharmacists access to patient demographic information, disease information, and laboratory values. This information is needed for pharmacists to effectively monitor medication therapy.

All CPOE systems provide a basic level of passive or active CDS intervention, although this functionality varies greatly with the product. Passive interventions generally present relevant patient-specific information to the prescriber without recommending a change in therapy. Examples include nonformulary alerts, drug shortages, and order sets. Active alerts utilize specific patient information combined with other content knowledge to recommend or change therapy. Examples include recommendation of dosing, allergy warnings, and safer therapy, or less expensive treatment options.

CPOE vendors provide drug-content modules (i.e., First Data Bank, Multum, Micromedex) with their products which serve as the core of medication CDS. These systems typically provide alerts for drug-drug, drug-allergy, drug-pregnancy, and other drug related problems. One critical role for pharmacists is to access these systems to ensure that the majority of alerts are clinically significant and actionable while only a minimal number are time wasters.

There are four possible outcomes for any alert (Table 9-1).[30] Ideally, alerts should only be generated for clinically significant problems. However, clinical significance is often a judgment call that is best left up to the prescribing clinician. Therefore, commercial CPOE systems often err on the conservative side by putting more alerts into a system

> **Key Point . . .**
>
> Pharmacists need to access CDS systems to ensure that the majority of alerts are clinically significant and actionable.
>
> **. . . So what?**
>
> CDS systems are rough tools for alerting providers about medical problems. By design they are conservative in their notification process, "When in doubt, notify." Pharmacists who have access to CDS systems can individualize the alerting process to the needs of their patient populations, medical staff, pharmacists, and system of medication control. For example, pharmacists at one institution might choose to only activate alerts for clinically significant, actionable drug related problems, while pharmacists at another place might decide to alert pharmacists to all potential drug related problems. Access to the CDS gives the pharmacists a choice.

than necessary, causing the problem of alert fatigue where the clinician is desensitized to warnings. Pharmacists have a particularly important role to play here in identifying nuisance alerts from relevant alerts and developing strategies for reducing them. Pharmacists also have a role of updating systems to reflect the best available evidence on therapy. Most commercial systems allow pharmacists to deactivate nuisance alerts and add new alerts deemed clinically important for an institution's patient population.

Assessing the Impact

Maintaining and improving the quality of the medication use process requires assessing the impact of CPOE. Measures of success should also be clearly defined for the CPOE system with methods to track and evaluate these measures of success. Potential areas of evaluation are the following:

- Medication safety and adverse drug events
- Response time for medication processing
- Pharmacy resource needs
- Drug cost reductions and achieving financial targets
- Downtime and availability of system
- Response time of system
- Clinical alerts and action taken by provider

Table 9-1.
Possible Outcomes for Any CDSS Alert

	Alert Generated	No Alert Generated
Correct alert	*Alert for clinically significant problem.*	*No alert generated because of no problem.*
	Example: allergy warning appears when penicillin is prescribed for a patient with a beta lactam allergy.	Example: No alert is generated when penicillin is ordered for patient with no penicillin or beta lactam allergies.
	The clinician needs to see this alert because there is risk of harm to the patient.	There is no problem so the clinician does not need to see this alert.
Incorrect alert	*Alert generated for a clinically insignificant problem.*	*No alert generated for a clinically significant problem.*
	A duplicate drug warning for a patient receiving a therapeutically appropriate two antibiotic combination.	NO allergy warning appears when a patient is prescribed penicillin but has beta lactam allergies.
	The clinician does not need to see this alert because there is no risk of harm. This is a nuisance and a time waster. It may also desensitize the clinician to clinically appropriate alerts.	The clinician needs to see this alert but does not due to a variety of causes including: the patient allergy was not recorded, the allergy warning was not in the commercial package's alert library, or the alert was blocked by the pharmacy department.

Source: Adapted from reference 30.

As with any complex system, it is imperative to monitor the performance, make needed adjustments, and provide feedback to the user. This encourages support of the system and continuous improvement of the system. A change of this magnitude will introduce new opportunities for errors. Systems must be in place to quickly identify these issues so they can be managed aggressively.

Summary

EHR and CPOE systems are likely to change institutional pharmacy practice in numerous ways.[31] Technicians are likely to oversee the process of dispensing including automated dispensing, IV pump management, and other distributive responsibilities. This will move pharmacists from distribution to clinical roles, requiring pharmacists to upgrade their clinical skills and contributions to appropriate medication use. Pharmacists who do not advance pharmaceutical care responsibilities across the continuum of care will find it increasingly difficult to justify their presence in health care institutions.

CPOE and other systems are critical tools for the effective delivery of pharmaceutical care as health care grows more complex. The pharmacy must advocate for a leadership role and provide its expertise in systems and medication therapy to ensure the success of the medication component of CPOE. It is essential that pharmacists share their experience with colleagues and advocate for standardization to enhance the successful diffusion of this powerful tool. CPOE provides new opportunities for pharmacists in the area of system integration and clinical decision support systems and demands that more formalized training for pharmacists be available. A good CPOE system properly deployed provides strategic advantages to the institution and, most importantly, improved care to patients.

Suggested Reading

Ash JS, Stavri PZ, Kuperman GJ. A consensus statement on considerations for a successful CPOE implementation. *J Am Med Inform Assoc.* 2003;10(3):229-234.

Chaffee BW, Bonasso J. Strategies for pharmacy integration and pharmacy information system interfaces, part 1: history and pharmacy integration options. *Am J Health-Syst Pharm.* 2004;61(5):502-506.

Chaffee BW, Bonasso J. Strategies for pharmacy integration and pharmacy information system interfaces, part 2: scope of work and technical aspects of interfaces. *Am J Health-Syst Pharm.* 2004;61(5):506-514.

Dumitru D. *The Pharmacy Informatics Primer.* Bethesda, MD: American Society of Health-System Pharmacists; 2009.

Gray MD, Felkey BG. Computerized prescriber order-entry systems: evaluation, selection, and implementation. *Am J Health-Syst Pharm.* 2004;61(2):190-197.

Metzger J FJ. Computerized physician order entry in community hospitals: lessons from the field. Available at: http://www.chcf.org/documents/hospitals/CPOECommHospCorrected.pdf. Accessed February 16, 2005.

Metzger J. A primer on physician order entry. Available at: http://www.chcf.org/documents/hospitals/ CPOEreport.pdf. Accessed: February 2005.

Seger AC, Hanson CM, Fanikos JR. Benefits of CPOE. *Am J Health-Syst Pharm.* 2004;61(6):626-627.

Shane R. CPOE: the science and the art. *Am J Health-Syst Pharm.* 2003;60(12):1273-1276.

References

1. McDonald CJ, Tierney WM, Overhage JM, et al. The Regenstrief medical record system: 20 years of experience in hospitals, clinics, and neighborhood health centers. *MD Comput.* 1992;9(4):206-217.

2. Ash JS, Bates DW. Factors and forces impacting EHR systems adoption: report of a 2004 ACMI discussion. *J Am Med Inform Assoc.* 2005; Jan-Feb;12(1):8-12. Epub 2004 Oct 18.

3. Jha AK, DesRoches CM, Campbell EG, et al. Use of Electronic Health Records in U.S. Hospitals. *N Engl J Med.* 2009;360(16):1628-1638.

4. The Leapfrog Group. Available at: http://www.leapfrog group.org/media/file/CPOE_FactSheet011305.pdf. Accessed February 2005.

5. Bates DW, Leape LL, Cullen DJ, et al. Effect of computerized physician order entry and a team intervention on prevention of serious medication errors. *JAMA.* 1998;280(15):1311-1316.

6. Kohn LT, Corrigan J, Donaldson MS. Institute of Medicine (U.S.). Committee on Quality of Health Care in America. *To Err is Human: Building a Safer Health System.* Washington, DC: National Academy Press; 2000.

7. Slack WV, Peckham BM, Van Cura LJ, et al. A computer- based physical examination system. *JAMA.*1967;200(3): 224-228.

8. Slack WV, Hicks GP, Reed CE, et al. A computer-based medical-history system. *N Engl J Med.* 1966;274(4): 194-198.

9. Hammond WE. How the past teaches the future: ACMI distinguished lecture. *J Am Med Inform Assoc.* 2001;8(3):222-234.

10. Stead WW, Miller RA, Musen MA, et al. Integration and beyond: linking information from disparate sources and into workflow (see comments). *J Am Med Inform Assoc.* 2000;7(2):135-145.

11. McDonald CJ. The barriers to electronic medical record systems and how to overcome them. *J Am Med Inform Assoc.* 1997;4(3):213-221.

12. Gardner RM, Pryor TA, Warner HR. The HELP hospital information system: update 1998. *Int J Med Inform.* 1999;54(3):169-182.

13. Barnett GO. COSTAR, a computer-based medical information system for ambulatory care. *Proc IEEE.* 1979;67:1226-1237.

14. Brown SH, Lincoln MJ, Groen PJ, et al. VistA—U.S. Department of Veterans Affairs national-scale HIS. *Int J Med Inf.* 2003;69(2-3):135-156.

15. Handler T, et al. *Electronic Health Record Definition Model Version 1.0. Health Information and Management Systems Society.* Chicago IL: HIMSS; 2003.

16. Collen MF. *A History of Medical Informatics in the United States, 1950 to 1990.* Indianapolis, IN: American Medical Informatics Association; 1995.

17. McDonald CJ, Tierney WM. Computer-stored medical records. Their future role in medical practice. *JAMA.* 1988;259(23):3433-3440.

18. Sado AS. Electronic medical record in the intensive care unit. *Crit Care Clin.* 1999;15(3):499-522.

19. Key capabilities of an electronic health record system. Institute of Medicine. Washington, DC. 2003. Available at: http://www.nap.edu/catalog.php?record_id=10781#toc. Accessed June 2010.

20. Stead WW, Heyman A, Thompson HK, et al. Computer-assisted interview of patients with functional headache. *Arch Intern Med.* 1972;129(6):950-955.

21. Lumpkin JR. Uniform data standards for patient medical record information. Washington, DC: National Committee on Vital and Health Statistics; 2003.

22. Brailer DJ. Decade of health information technology. Washington, DC: U.S. Department of Health and Human Services; 7/21/2004.

23. Carpenter JD, Gorman PN. What's so special about medications: a pharmacist's observations from the POE study. *Proc AMIA Symp.* 2001:95-99.

24. Gouveia WA, Shane R, Clark T. Computerized prescriber order entry: power, not panacea. *Am J Health-Syst Pharm.* 2003;60(18):1838.

25. IOM. *Crossing the Quality Chasm: A New Health System for the 21st Century.* Washington, DC: National Academy Press; 2001.

26. Poon EG, Blumenthal D, Jaggi T, et al. Overcoming barriers to adopting and implementing computerized physician order entry systems in U.S. hospitals. *Health Aff (Millwood).* 2004;23(4):184-190.

27. Doolan DF, Bates DW. Computerized physician order entry systems in hospitals: mandates and incentives. *Health Aff (Millwood).* 2002;21(4):180-188.

28. Schiff GD. Computerized prescriber order entry: models and hurdles. *Am J Health-Syst Pharm.* 2002;59(15):1456-1460.

29. Hoey P, Nichol WP, Silverman R. Computerized Provider Order Entry. In: Dumitru D, editor. *The Pharmacy Informatics Primer.* 1st ed. Bethesda, MD: American Society of Health-System Pharmacists; 2009.

30. Rose E, Jones MA. Clinical decision support. In: Dumitru D, editor. *The Pharmacy Informatics Primer.* 1st ed. Bethesda, MD: American Society of Health-System Pharmacists; 2009.

31. Sura M. A New Frontier: Impact of the Electronic Medical Record and Computerized Order Entry on Pharmacy Services. In: Dumitru D, editor. *The Pharmacy Informatics Primer.* 1st ed. Bethesda, MD: American Society of Health-System Pharmacists; 2009.

Chapter Review Questions

1. **A personal health record (PHR) is a computerized clinical documentation of a patient's medical care over time within a single institution.**
   a. True
   b. False

   Answer: b. False. A personal health record (PHR) is a web-based platform accessible to and controlled by patients about their own medical care and insurance coverage that may be available to multiple institutions.

2. **A passive CDS intervention in CPOE systems presents relevant patient-specific information to the prescriber without recommending a change in therapy.**
   a. True
   b. False

   Answer. a. True. Passive CDS interventions may include nonformulary alerts, drug shortages, and order sets. Active alerts utilize patient information and other content knowledge to recommend or change therapy (e.g., dosage recommendations, less expensive treatments).

3. **CPOE has been widely adopted and implemented in U.S. Hospitals.**
   a. True
   b. False

   Answer: b. False. CPOE for medications has only been fully implemented in 17% of all U.S. hospitals with 45% of hospitals having no CPOE or plans for CPOE in the near future.

4. **Computer-based documentation systems work by prompting clinicians to enter information in specific data fields.**
   a. True
   b. False

Answer: a. The statement is true, in many cases, but not always. There are a variety of systems available, but many computer-based documentation systems force clinicians to provide more complete information to document their clinical decisions and patient interactions by requiring certain data fields to be filled out (e.g., allergies).

5. _____ is one of several standards setting organizations whose mission is to provide interoperability standards for EHR systems.
   a. HIPPA
   b. Joint Commission
   c. Health Level 7 (HL-7)
   d. Institute of medicine

   Answer: c. HL-7 primarily defines standards for data formatting and configuration to allow HL-7 compliant systems to communicate with each other.

6. The following term describes the capability of different information systems to exchange and use data.
   a. Interoperability
   b. Data standardization
   c. Functionality
   d. None of the above.

   Answer: a. Data standardization defines the formatting, terminology, and formatting of data to be consistently entered into EHRs. Functionality refers to all of the things (i.e., functions) that a software program or system can do for users.

7. A drug interaction alert is a form of clinical decision support.
   a. True
   b. False

   Answer: a. True. Drug interaction alerts guide and advise clinicians as they interface with the EHR or CPOE system. Drug interaction notices are based upon best available evidence from national professional society clinical guidelines and other expert sources.

8. Which of the following organizations support CPOE?
   a. Centers for Medicare and Medicaid Services (CMS)
   b. U.S. Department of Health and Human Services (HHS)
   c. Leapfrog Group
   d. IOM

   Answer: a, b, c, and d. All of these governmental and private organizations support CPOE.

9. CPOE and e-prescribing are synonymous terms.
   a. True
   b. False

   Answer: b. False. CPOE describes orders entered electronically anywhere within a health system's EHR. Electronic prescribing or e-prescribing refers only to CPOE in ambulatory care settings.

10. **There are four possible outcomes for any alert associated with clinical decision support. Which of the following puts patients at greatest risk?**
    a. Alert for clinically significant problem
    b. No alert generated because of no problem
    c. Alert generated for a clinically insignificant problem
    d. No alert generated for a clinically significant problem

    Answer: d. Not being aware of clinically significant problems puts patients at greatest risk (see Table 9-1). However, an argument can be made that alerts generated for *clinically insignificant problems* can desensitize the clinician to clinically appropriate alerts and put the patient at equal risk.

Chapter Discussion Questions

1. Why is it so hard in hospitals to implement technology that is commonplace in banking, retailing, and other businesses?
2. Under what conditions should a pharmacist override clinical decision support alerts?
3. Will CPOE ever preclude a need for pharmacists? Why?
4. Is it possible to practice clinical pharmacy without access to the medical record electronically or in paper form? Why?

CHAPTER 10

Informatics

James G. Stevenson, Scott R. McCreadie, and Bruce W. Chaffee

■ ■ ■

Learning Objectives

After completing this chapter, readers should be able to:

1. Define informatics and other key terminology.
2. Contrast the terms data, information, and knowledge.
3. Describe the operational, clinical, and administrative applications of informatics.
4. Explain how pharmacists can protect the confidentiality of medical information.
5. Discuss the roles, responsibilities and necessary training of a clinical informatics pharmacist.

Key Terms and Definitions

■ **Asynchronous CDS:** Referring to clinical decision support, indicates that an alert or notification is presented at a time (or through a process) separate from the order entry process. An asynchronous alert notifies the user that potentially important information is available, but typically does not interrupt the user.

■ **Authentication:** A method of identifying a user, typically by having the user enter a valid user name and valid password before program access is granted. The process of authentication is based on each user having a unique set of criteria for gaining access.

■ **BCMA:** Bar Code Medication Administration is an information technology solution that links an electronic MAR (eMAR) with item-specific identification (bar coding) and enables the user to administer medications with general confirmation of the five rights of medication administration: right patient, right dose, right route, right time, and right medication. The system utilization at the bedside provides more precise patient and medication information resulting in improved accuracy and reduced medication errors.

■ **Biometrics:** Refers to technologies that measure and analyze human body characteristics, such as fingerprints, eye retinas and irises, voice patterns, facial patterns and hand measurements, for authentication purposes.

- **Clinical data repository:** A real-time database that consolidates data from a variety of sources to present a unified view of a single patient's clinical information.
- **Clinical decision support (CDS):** Interactive components of information systems which are designed, configured, or programmed to use diagnosis, treatment, laboratory and other information to assist prescribers and other health professionals with decision making tasks to support the clinical care of patients.
- **CDS rule:** A specific clinical decision support instruction that uses encoded health knowledge in conjunction with an event monitor to dictate that, when a certain set of circumstances is present, a specific action is initiated. For example, a CDS rule might monitor patients on gentamicin therapy and be programmed to fire an alert to a pharmacist if a patient experiences a 0.5 mg/dL increase in serum creatinine concentration.
- **CDS alert:** The specific action dictated by a CDS rule. For example, an alert may appear as a pop-up notification window within a CPOE application, a page sent to a recipient via the system application, or a flag appearing on a patient summary view.
- **Confidentiality:** Ensuring that information is accessible only to those authorized to have access.
- **Data:** Pieces of information that represent the qualitative or quantitative attributes of a variable or set of variables. Data are typically the results of measurements and are often viewed as the lowest level of abstraction from which information and knowledge are derived.
- **De-identification:** The removal of identifying information—patient name, medical record number, birth date, social security number from medical records, to protect patient privacy.

- **Encryption:** Encryption is the conversion of data into a form, called a ciphertext, that cannot be easily understood by unauthorized people. Encryption is especially important in wireless communications, but is a good idea when carrying out any kind of sensitive transaction in order to prevent unauthorized access to information.
- **Informatics:** The science of information, the practice of information processing, and the engineering of information systems.
- **Information:** Communication or reception of knowledge or intelligence.
- **Information security:** Protecting information and information systems from unauthorized access, use, disclosure, disruption, modification or destruction.
- **Interface:** A means of transmitting and translating information between entities which do not speak the same language, such as between a human and a computer (a user interface) or between two computer systems (software interface).
- **Intranet:** A private computer network that uses Internet technologies to securely share any part of an organization's information or operational systems with its employees.
- **Knowledge:** Expertise, and skills acquired by a person through experience or education; the theoretical or practical understanding of a subject.
- **Medication administration record (MAR):** Report that serves as a legal record of the drugs administered to a patient at a facility by a nurse or other healthcare professional. The nurse or healthcare professional signs off on the record at the time that the drug or device is administered. This report also documents that appropriate therapy is provided to the patient. When present electronically, this is often referred to as the eMAR.

- **Nonrepudiation:** The concept of ensuring that a party cannot repudiate, or refute the validity of a statement or information. On the Internet, a digital signature is used not only to ensure that a message or document has been electronically signed by the person that purported to sign the document, but also, since a digital signature can only be created by one person, to ensure that a person cannot later deny that they furnished the signature.
- **Pharmacy informatics:** Also referred to as pharmacoinformatics, is the application of computers to the storage, retrieval and analysis of drug and prescription information. Pharmacy informaticists work with pharmacy information management systems and automated pharmacy systems in order to help the pharmacist make excellent decisions about patient drug therapies with respect to, medical insurance records, drug interactions, as well as prescription and patient information.
- **Pharmacy information system:** Complex computer systems that have been designed to meet the needs of a pharmacy department. Through the use of such systems, pharmacists can supervise and manage how medications are used. Typically pharmacy information systems can assist in patient care by the monitoring of drug interactions, drug allergies and other possible medication-related complications, manage prescription for inpatients and/or outpatients, assist with inventory management, maintain profiles of patient medications and allergies, and communicate with other systems including automated dispensing systems.
- **Point-of-care devices:** Devices used in the delivery of health care such that they are utilized within the care process at the specific time in which the information is needed or collected.
- **Radiofrequency identification (RFID):** The use of an object (typically referred to as an RFID tag) applied to or incorporated into a product or person identifier (wrist band) for the purpose of identification and tracking using radio waves. Some tags can be read from several meters away and beyond the line of sight of the reader. There are generally two types of RFID tags: active RFID tags, which contain a battery and can transmit signals autonomously, and passive RFID tags, which have no battery and require an external source to provoke signal transmission. Today, RFID is used in supply chain management to improve the efficiency of inventory tracking and management.
- **Synchronous CDS:** Referring to clinical decision support alerts, indicates that an alert or notification is presented at the time of order entry. A synchronous alert interrupts the user's workflow and requests an action before the user can continue.
- **Verified Internet Pharmacy Practice Sites (VIPPS):** Created in 1999 by the National Association of Boards of Pharmacy (NABP), the Verified Internet Pharmacy Practice Sites (VIPPS) accreditation program provides a means for the public to distinguish between legitimate and illegitimate online drug sellers. The VIPPS program and its seal of approval assure the public that VIPPS retailers are legitimate online pharmacies appropriately licensed in each state to which they ship pharmaceuticals.
- **VeriSign™:** A provider of Internet infrastructure services that allows companies and consumers to engage in trusted communications and commerce by providing encryption and authentication services.

Introduction

Informatics is a broad term that can be defined as the application of computer and information sciences to the management and processing of data, information, and knowledge.[1] To broaden the definition, one can define **informatics** as the science concerned with the gathering, manipulation, classification, storage, and retrieval of recorded knowledge; the techniques and practices used to manage and operate information systems and technology. It covers a broad range of technologies including the ones shown in Figure 10-1.

In health care, informatics can be divided into subsets such as medical informatics, pharmacy informatics, nursing informatics, biomedical informatics, and other specialty areas.[2] Medical informatics deals with informatics supporting medical research, education, and patient care while **pharmacy informatics** is limited to those areas involving the medication management system within the health care environment.[3] The other areas focus on aspects of informatics specific to those specialties.

This chapter focuses on pharmacy informatics by exploring several topics that are pertinent to pharmacies within health care institutions. Topics include information security and confidentiality, educational applications, operations and clinical applications, systems integration, and finally opportunities and training for those interested in pharmacy informatics.

Pharmacies have been in the forefront of using technology to improve medication dispensing, ordering, record keeping, safety, and billing. Pharmacies have been using

Figure 10-1. Technologies associated with pharmacy informatics.

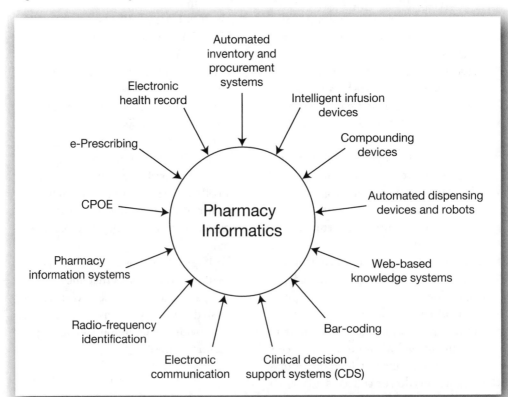

computers for profile management for many years. Computerized profiles improve the efficiency and safety of the medication-use system by reducing legibility and transcription errors. More recently, technologies have advanced to include **point-of-care devices** such as automated dispensing cabinets. Further advances in technologies have been seen in IV compounding machines and inventory management of pharmaceuticals.

Many different computing devices are used in health care environments. Behind the scenes of practice, large servers run advanced operating systems with multiple processors to power many of the software applications used in the care of patients. More visible to clinicians, a variety of devices are employed including personal desktop computers, laptops, tablet PCs, personal digital assistants (PDAs), and cell phones. In fact, most health care devices incorporate some form of informatics.

Today, information technology is increasingly integrated into the entire medication management cycle from prescribing through administration. This includes prescriber order entry, integration with pharmacy systems and dispensing devices, and electronic documentation of administration. Health systems are rapidly adopting these technologies to improve patient safety, reduce errors and improve the efficiency of the process.

With the passing of the American Recovery and Reinvestment Act of 2009, information technology has been placed center stage in the efforts to help contain health care costs. One of the primary driving incentives is financial, with providers and health care organizations ultimately receiving additional funding for demonstrating 'meaningful use' of electronic health records and having reimbursement reduced for failing to achieve these goals. While the definition of *meaningful use* is still under negotiation, private organizations such as The Certification Commission for Healthcare Information Technology (CCHIT®) will be relied on to serve as certification bodies to ensure successful adoption and interoperability of health information technologies.

Pharmacy informatics is a broad and rapidly growing field. Looking ahead, pharmacists will continue to use informatics to provide care for patients in inpatient and ambulatory environments. Electronic prescribing, currently a high priority for implementation in many health care organizations, eliminates the manual handwriting of prescriptions and significantly enhances the pharmacist's ability to partner with physicians in providing care. Pharmacists can provide more focus on the appropriateness of therapy for the patient rather than the mechanics of drug distribution.

Data, Information, and Knowledge Management

To understand informatics, one must understand the differences between data, information and knowledge.[4] **Data** are simply discrete and objective facts about a subject or an event. Good examples in health care are patient laboratory values, drug orders for a patient or the patient's weight. Data are easy to capture and store in media such as databases and files.

Information is often defined as data that has relevance and purpose. Information has meaning whereas pure data does not because information is contextualized, categorized, calculated, corrected, or condensed. In health care, an example of information is knowing that a particular laboratory result was high or low from reference values (Figure 10-2).

Knowledge is broader, deeper, and richer than data and information. Knowledge is combining information with framed experiences, norms, and contextual understanding. Information is transformed into knowledge through comparison between the current situation and another similar one, understanding the consequences of the information,

Figure 10-2. Relationship of data, information, and knowledge.

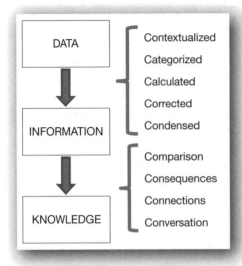

knowing how the information connects to other information, or understanding what people think about the information. Knowledge is very difficult to capture as it often resides in people's heads. In health care, having knowledge means that a clinician knows the consequences of a particular laboratory test or knows whether the drug therapy prescribed for a patient is adequate to treat the condition being treated. Knowledge is often transferred tacitly though teaching, one-on-one interactions, experience, and practice norms.

Why is this important in the field of informatics? Informatics focuses on the use of technology to improve the use of data, information, and knowledge. Tools and technologies used to improve these areas vary considerably whether the focus is on data storage, retrieval and transfer, information gathering and sharing, or knowledge sharing. Understanding the differences helps the informatics pharmacist best utilize tools and technologies to solve the business problem at hand.

Accessing Sources of Information and Knowledge Content

Historically, pharmacists have used hard-copy references to access drug information and other knowledge resources. However, today pharmacists are increasingly utilizing electronic information sources. The advantages of electronic information include availability of information from almost anywhere within the health care system and at the point of service (especially with the availability of wireless networks and mobile devices), reduced space requirements for storing information, greater ability to maintain up-to-date information, and significantly improved efficiency of information retrieval. Many pharmacy and prescriber order entry systems also embed web-based links to enable direct access of the same content from these software applications without requiring the user to open a second software program. This increased availability of information should lead to better decision making and improvements in the quality of care provided.

A wide variety of information retrieval and knowledge sources are currently available. According to an estimate in 2002, more than 100,000 websites provide health information.[8] A list of the most popular internet websites is shown in Table 10-1.[9] While it is not feasible to list all of the sources of electronic information,

Key Point . . .

To understand informatics, one must understand the differences between data, information and knowledge.

. . . So what

When dealing with informatics, it is easy to drown in the vast amounts of available data and information. Data are just meaningless facts if they are not put into some useful context. And information is useless without being transformed into knowledge than can inform and guide actions.

some of the most frequently used sites and types of sources are indicated in Table 10-2. The easy and convenient access to the literature, drug information databases, and online continuing education help enable pharmacists (even in remote areas) to maintain their professional knowledgebase and to assist them in their practice.

The next several generations of knowledge systems will likely include information availability with increased customization and decision support. That is, when a question is asked about a drug, there will be the capability of providing information within the context of the patient or clinical scenario as well. This will allow the knowledge source to return information that is specific to that particular patient or clinical situation. For example, instead of reporting the usual dosage range of a particular drug, the information provided might be a dosage recommendation specific to a patient of a given age and creatinine clearance. As these knowledge systems mature, other factors such as diagnosis, genetic profiles and a patient's history with a given medication will likely be considered.

One clear impact of the Internet is that patients will be more educated and have greater access to information than ever before. Thus, patients will be better prepared and engaged but also potentially misinformed about their conditions and medications. To help patients wade through the vast quantities of the information available on the Internet,

Table 10-1.

The Twenty Most Popular Health Websites (June 2009)

1. WebMD.com	11. everydayHealth.com
2. NIH.gov	12. RightHealth.com
3. MedicineNet.com	13. wellsphere.com
4. MayoClinic.com	14. FamilyDoctor.org
5. Drugs.com	15. QualityHealth.com
6. Yahoo!Health (health.yahoo.com)	16. HealthCentral.com
7. RxList.com	17. Prevention.com
8. RealAge.com	18. Health.com
9. MedHelp.org	19. RevolutionHealth.com
10. Healthline.com	20. eMedicine.com

Source: Reference 9.

Table 10-2.

Information Retrieval/Knowledge Sources

- Electronic databases and search engines
- Medline, International Pharmaceutical Abstracts
- Electronic journals
- Electronic drug information resources (Micromedex, Multum, ePocrates, Lexicomp, Facts and Comparisons eFacts, etc.)
- Electronic textbooks
- The Natural Medicines Comprehensive Database

some health systems are providing patients with a list of endorsed, reliable health information links.[10] Some criteria used to evaluate the quality of health-related websites are listed in Table 10-3.[8]

Practice Applications of Informatics

Operational

Informatics plays many roles in the daily operation in health care pharmacies. Computer systems manage patient drug profiles and histories allowing pharmacists to better manage care. Systems can facilitate label generation, patient billing, batch processing of workload, and other tasks that can free pharmacists to provide pharmaceutical care.

The complexity of health care systems requires that a number of interfaces be present to leverage the information stored in multiple systems. Software **interfaces** allow patient information to flow directly into the pharmacy system from a patient management system without the need for pharmacy staff to enter the data by hand. Interfaces to laboratory systems allow easy retrieval of patient laboratory results, and rules can be programmed in the systems to promote safe and effective use of drugs. In addition, interfaces to external devices such as IV compounders, automatic dispensing cabinets and robots increase the efficiency of the overall operations of the pharmacy.

Clinical

More and more, informatics plays a role in clinical pharmacy activities. A key area is in improving a pharmacist's access to information about the patient and their care. Technology helps pharmacists collect data, filter results, provide decision support and record pharmacist activities. Many applications are available for use in clinical mobility devices such as PDAs and tablet PCs.

Table 10-3.

Important Quality Criteria for Health-Related Websites

- Transparency and honesty
- Transparency of provider of site, purpose, and objective of site
- Target audience is clearly defined
- Transparency of all sources of funding
- Authority
- Clear statement of sources for all information and date of publication
- Privacy and data protection policies
- Clear and regular updating of information with date clearly displayed
- Accountability for information
- Process for user feedback and appropriate oversight responsibility
- Editorial policy has clear statement on process used for selection of content
- Guidelines on accessibility, searchability, readability

Source: Adapted from reference 8.

Another clinical area is in documentation of clinical pharmacy activities. Initial efforts to document pharmacists' interventions involved the use of paper forms and handwritten notes.[11-13] Paper documentation was cumbersome, time consuming, and the handwritten forms had the potential to be lost or unreadable and were difficult to compile.[12-13] Now technology facilitates documentation of pharmacists' interventions and patient care activities.[12,14,15] Early systems required pharmacists to record their interventions on paper and later enter them into the computer—a process that did not completely eliminate the drawbacks of manual documentation but made data interpretation more efficient.[14] Additional advantages include reduced time needed for documentation and improved ease of use, accessibility, time efficiency, and general acceptance.[15]

The better systems, however, utlize software interfaces that allow pharmacists to document their work directly into hand-held mobile devices. Popular with professionals, these mobile devices provide real-time or synchronized connections to the healthcare information systems. Mobile devices range from hand-held telephones up to wireless tablets and laptops.

Administrative

The management of pharmacy services has improved greatly through technology and informatics. Managers have information tools that allow them to better assign resources to meet workload requirements, identify opportunities for cost savings, and justify new services. Medication system automation tools have allowed managers to move pharmacists into clinical roles and increase the overall safety of the medication-use system. A number of administrative applications of informatics are in Table 10-4.

Workflow and Process Improvement

Technology improvements have had significant impacts on workflow and process improvement within pharmacies. Automation has permitted change in historically important pharmacist functions such as dispensing and has allowed these functions to be accomplished by robots, automated dispensing cabinets, and compounding devices, thus

Table 10-4.
Administrative Uses of Informatics

Item	Benefit
Drug usage reporting	▪ Compliance with policies and standard practices
Inventory management systems	▪ Control inventory costs and turns
	▪ Monitor purchasing activities
	▪ Manage recalls and drug shortages
	▪ Monitor compliance with regulatory requirements for controlled substances
Scheduling systems	▪ Manage employee schedules
	▪ Manage personnel costs
Portals	▪ Dissemination of information
	▪ Creation of knowledge sources regarding drug therapy
Workload reporting	▪ Measure efficiency and productivity of processes

allowing the pharmacist to apply their knowledge to patient-specific health issues. Pharmacists, in part due to technology improvements, are much more able to participate in patient care teams and exercise clinical skills to improve patient care.

Process improvement is also often seen through improved knowledge sharing. Technology, including email and the web, has made sharing knowledge much easier and lower in cost. Clinical guidelines, disease management approaches, formularies, and more rich content are easily accessible to the pharmacist. Perhaps the most important improvement seen with technology and automation is increased safety. Technologies such as bar coding and linking of disparate clinical systems have helped ensure that the right medication is for the right patient at the right time through **bedside bar code medication administration (BCMA)**. **Radiofrequency identification (RFID)** chips may also serve as a future technology to identify products and allow for linking of information. As technology and information systems continue to improve, health systems will continue to see improvements in safety.

Systems Integration and Interfacing

Pharmacist-Computer Interactions

There are many different types of software that are used in health care informatics, and pharmacists have varying ways in which they work with software. Software can be a simple, unchangeable system program solely designed to operate a piece of equipment or medical device, or it can be a complex application designed for data entry, storage, exchange, and retrieval. Most pharmacists generally do not get involved in software programming, especially for the complex applications required in today's health care environment. The primary interaction hospital pharmacists have with software is directing the software to perform various tasks via the user interface on the display screen of the computer or device. This interaction can consist of activities such as programming infusion rates, entering orders, entering compounding volumes, or extracting reports from various equipment, devices and systems, such as **pharmacy information systems (PIS)** or computerized prescriber order entry systems (CPOE).

> **Key Point . . .**
>
> The primary interaction hospital pharmacists have with software is directing the software to perform various tasks via the user interface on the display screen of the computer or device.
>
> **. . . So what?**
>
> To utilize computer software, pharmacists do not need to know how to program computers using complex machine language. They just need a user interface on some computer or device. The real value provided to informatics systems is the pharmacist's clinical expertise and knowledge of the medication use system.

Beyond this day-to-day interaction pharmacists have with the user interface, pharmacists and other health care professionals can get more involved in the intricacies of an information system by working with system analysts or by directly working with the system, to define the business logic required for configuring a system to meet workflow needs and/or policies using the system's software configuration options. These activities require computer skills generally acquired through specialized training and experience obtained by working with the various automation and information systems.

Access to and Use of Information

One of the most important aspects of any information system is the benefit it provides an organization in terms of accurate and efficient information storage and retrieval. Modern software applications contain three tiers: the client tier, which is where the user interacts with the system, the application tier, which is the software stored on the local machine, and a database tier, which contains the database tables where information is stored as a result of user input into the application's user interface. Depending on the complexity of the application, there may be tens of thousands of discrete data elements stored in the application's database management system including patient level data such as dispensing, billing, facility, and audit information.

While most information retrieval is conducted from within the application, some is conducted externally for functionalities other than those originally intended from the system. For example, data in a PIS contains useful historical utilization information about commonly used drugs, dose forms, doses, and frequencies of administration that can be useful for making informed decisions about drug use policies within an organization. That data may be retrieved using a vendor-supplied report writer application within the PIS database or from external report writing software that interfaces with the PIS.

A second manner in which data contained in an information system may be useful beyond its original intent is when data needs to be imported from, exported to, or exchanged with another information system. A few of the many situations where this may occur include: input of patient-specific status and location data acquired from a patient management system (e.g., patient admission, discharge, and transfer information), importation of laboratory information into the pharmacy information system for the purposes of providing pharmacists with important clinical data for use in context with medication orders, provision of pharmacy medication use information to the hospital financial system for the purposes of billing, and the clinical integration between a PIS and a CPOE system to ensure accurate and complete medication profile information.

Integrating Information Systems with Work Activities

There are several methods for integrating information systems into existing pharmacy processes. One of the most widely used is the pharmacy information system (PIS) which often serves as the backbone for pharmacy work activities. The PIS automates and organizes the daily workflow in addition to coordinating its many clinical functions. Printed cart fill lists and intravenous medication labels can be generated from the PIS database allow-

ing the pharmacy department to sort and perform work activities in batches based upon patient location, type of medication, anticipated administration time, and/or via other sorting features. Similarly, PIS-generated **medication administration records (MARs)** can help nurses organize activities related to the medication administration process. MARs provide nurses with sufficient information to safely and accurately administer medications to patients according to the time schedule desired by the prescriber. With the implementation of CPOE, electronic MARs are becoming more common compared to print MARs.

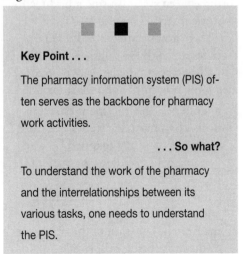

Key Point . . .

The pharmacy information system (PIS) often serves as the backbone for pharmacy work activities.

. . . So what?

To understand the work of the pharmacy and the interrelationships between its various tasks, one needs to understand the PIS.

The advantages of electronic MARs include the ability to be accessed at multiple locations, give all providers the same information in real-time, more readily audit performance in medication administration, and facilitate billing based on actual drug administration.

CPOE systems are also used to organize work activities. Most contemporary CPOE systems contain patient lists, profiles, demographic information, electronic medication administration documentation, order forms, and other features. Orders made using the system can generate electronic or printed work lists or tasks for a wide variety of departments or individual health care providers.

The pharmacy department is the recipient of a large proportion of physician orders. The format for receipt of these orders can be quite different from one hospital to another depending on a number of factors. These include work flow patterns, extent of technology deployment, physical size and layout of the hospital, type of facility, and practice-base of the physician (e.g., independent practice, group practice, hospitalist, or resident). Pharmacy orders can be: (1) handwritten or electronic; (2) individual or grouped (e.g., single sheet of paper or order set); (3) entered by physicians or a physician agent (e.g., nurse or clerk); or (4) delivered manually, via facsimile machine, via document imaging technology, or electronically from the CPOE system to the PIS. Once orders are delivered to the pharmacy, it is the pharmacist's responsibility to ensure the orders are reviewed for appropriateness of therapy and accurately placed on the patient's electronic profile in the PIS. In general, computerized prescriber-entered orders that are delivered to the pharmacy via a dedicated orders printer or an electronic interface to a PIS are more likely to be legible, complete, and delivered in a timely manner when compared to handwritten orders.

Types of Electronic Interfaces

There are several options for handling orders that are electronically delivered to the pharmacy department. The first option is for the pharmacist to take printed copies of the order and reenter the orders into the PIS. A second option is to transmit orders electronically from a CPOE system to the PIS via a one-way interface. A third option is for orders to be transmitted back and forth between systems using a bi-directional orders interface (Figure 10-3).

There are advantages and disadvantages to each of these solutions.[16] The biggest advantages to the latter two options, electronic transmittal of orders, include:

- a reduction in time spent entering orders by pharmacy staff since most orders, if correctly mapped between systems, will populate the patient profile in the PIS,
- elimination of transcription errors, entry on the wrong patient, and/or inadvertent omission of the order due to the order being misplaced

Key Point . . .

The overall strength of the integration between the CPOE system, the PIS, and the interface is only as robust as the weakest component.

. . . So what?

In informatics, everything is connected. This interconnectedness is both a strength and weakness. The weakness lies in the ability of the weakest component of the system to reduce the performance of other parts of the system. For example, an extremely fast processing system might have diminished capacity to respond to queries if it must wait for information from an outdated piece of software.

Figure 10-3. Possible computerized prescriber order entry system (CPOE) interfaces with a pharmacy information system (PIS). HL-7 indicates that the communication standards between electronic information systems are compliant with the standards set by the Health Level 7 organization, which are designed meet communication needs within a healthcare setting.

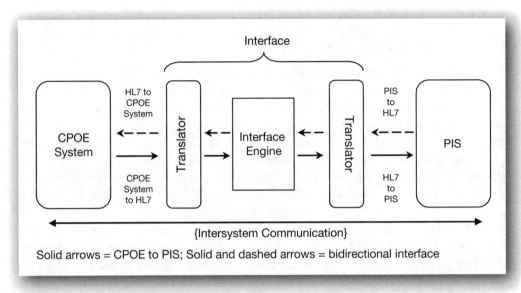

Source: Adapted from Chaffee BW, Bonasso J. Strategies for pharmacy integration and pharmacy information system interfaces, part 2: scope of work and technical aspects of interfaces. *Am J Health-Syst Pharm.* 2004;61(5):506-514.

The primary disadvantage of the electronic transmission of orders is the complexity—every component must work and work well in conjunction with each other. For example, transmission failure can result due to breakdowns in software or hardware components in the CPOE system, the PIS, and the interface itself. Indeed, the overall strength of the integration is only as robust as the weakest component.

One-way (unidirectional) order transmission interfaces have a reduced overall design complexity compared to bi-directional interfaces. Disadvantages to a unidirectional interface include the need for prescribers or the pharmacist to discontinue problem orders and then reenter the correct order in the CPOE system when order changes are required and the need for elaborate procedures in the event of CPOE system downtime.

Implementation of a bidirectional orders interface is a very complex undertaking, but it can offer some advantages over a one-way interface. For instance, any changes made in the PIS can be communicated across interfaces with other components of the system, automatically updating information stored with linked systems (e.g., the CPOE system). This eliminates the need for deletion of an incorrect order and reentry of the order in the CPOE system. Further, if either the CPOE system or the PIS system is down for significant periods of time, the interface engine can be used to queue the orders on the live system until such time as the system that is down is able to be placed back into production.

Finally, some systems can now completely integrate the PIS into the core functionality of the CPOE system. These so called "all-in-one" systems are integrated so that some of the information contained in the PIS is used by the CPOE component and vice versa resulting in the use of a single database for storing and managing information. By far, the biggest advantage is the reduction in the amount of time required to maintain the interface and test order items between systems to ensure that they match correctly. However, all-in-one systems currently contain less functionality when compared to systems built by pharmacy vendors who have several decades of experience in designing PIS to meet the complex needs of a pharmacy department.

Clinical Decision Support

The term **clinical decision support (CDS)** represents the features and functions of an information system that passively or actively convey clinical knowledge content to health care professionals so that choices can be made that are in the best interest of patient care. There are many methods for providing system users with clinical knowledge. *Passive* conveyance of clinical knowledge content occurs as a result of system design features and choices made during system configuration that may not necessarily be apparent to the user of the system.[17,18] An example of passive methods for providing basic CDS is the use of structured data elements for medication ordering in a PIS or CPOE system (Table 10-5). During system configuration, tables are built for each drug entity that define the allowable drug order choices that users of system users can select during order entry. Many systems will allow the institution to select the appearance and order of the selections and even provide default selections. By limiting the choices a prescriber can make, the institution can help prevent the errors that occur from ordering medication doses, routes of administration, or frequencies that are unsafe, subtherapeutic, excessively costly, nonstandard, or inconsistent with institutional policy. By passively directing choices in this manner, it is more likely that patients will receive safe, effective, and cost-efficient therapy.

The use of structured order entry also ensures that key clinical information contained in the PIS or CPOE system can be coded.[19] Coding of information allows the system to be used for *active* CDS. Active CDS conveys knowledge to the user of the system. Examples of active CDS include system highlighting of abnormal laboratory values and the use of pop-up alerts performed at the time of order entry, such as system-initiated clinical checking for allergy problems, drug interactions, abnormal doses, therapeutic duplication, intravenous drug admixture incompatibilities, therapeutic indication problems, and other

Table 10-5.
Examples of Basic Structured Data Elements

- Generic drug name
- Dose amount
- Unit of measure (e.g., mg, units, mg/kg, mEq/L, etc.)
- Route of administration
- Frequency or rate of administration
- Prn
- Prn reason
- Dispensing dosage form (tablet, capsule, suppository, etc.)
- Dispensing strength and amount
- Administration times

rules. For some of these basic types of decision support alerts, the clinical knowledge content is most often provided by third-party products that are designed to be easily incorporated into the CDS offerings of CPOE systems or PIS. The CPOE or PIS vendor will then imbed proprietary code or rules into their software to use this content for these basic alerts.

Clinical Data Repositories

In addition to the availability of commercial clinical knowledge content, there are other key prerequisites for expanding CDS to include rule-based alerts. The most important piece is the presence of a repository of patient-specific clinical data often referred to as a **clinical data repository (CDR)**. CDS rules often require data from other ancillary systems, such as the laboratory or dietary systems. Rather than make many system-to-system database interfaces and creating multiple, redundant repositories of these data in ancillary system databases, many institutions choose to create an organizational CDR. Data can then be imported into the CDR from ancillary systems and extracted from the CDR when necessary for use by ancillary departments. Often, organizations choose to use the CPOE system database as the organizational CDR because it already contains the largest amount of clinical data and typically contains additional storage capacity for ancillary data. Larger organizations may choose to create and maintain their own CDR using a large database management software program. In either case, having a central source of valid clinical data is key to successful implementation of rules. Data contained within the CDR is often useful beyond the CDS activities. Data within the CDR is often useful for clinical or administrative reporting purposes or for use in other applications.

A **CDS rule** is a coded program incorporated into the CPOE system, the PIS, or a standalone CDS system in order to identify specific clinical care or business-related situations for the purposes of alerting specified users of the need to address a particular situation. CDS rules can be imbedded rules created by the vendor or rules conceived by a hospital's employees. The end product of rules is most frequently seen by clinicians in the context of patient care alerts. Rules can take information from disparate systems, perform calculations, and/or incorporate logic to determine whether or not an alert should occur and then invoke that alert via a user-defined alert process.

Alerts and Knowledge Source Links

The medical literature is increasing substantially over time. It is very difficult, if not impossible, for clinicians to stay adequately informed about best practices on their own. Hospitals can utilize the collective knowledge of all of their physicians and departments to create best practice guidelines for the majority of high volume diseases. CDS alerts and links to both internal and external knowledge sources can be used to provide clinicians with warnings, supportive prompts, or access to clinical content to ensure that clinicians have the best tools at their disposal to care for their patients.

Active conveyance of clinical knowledge content is generally provided through alert and warning screens provided to the user but can also include notification of alerts via printed documents, electronic mail, and pagers. CDS alerts can be imbedded as a part of most any clinical information system, but it is most frequently seen in pharmacy information systems (PIS), inpatient or ambulatory care computerized prescriber order entry systems (CPOE), or as standalone expert systems that use data from existing clinical databases for supporting the diagnosis, surveillance, and/or treatment of disease. The proper use of CDS requires not only the wisdom and experience of health care professionals but also an understanding by these clinicians of the capabilities, limitations and deficiencies of CDS within their environment.

There are two main types of alerts that can be presented to users.[20,21] **Synchronous CDS alerts** represent pop-up warning screens that interrupt user workflow. They are generally triggered (invoked) based upon specific actions taken by a user of the system. An example of a synchronous alert might be the appearance of a drug dosing warning alert notification screen triggered when a user attempts to enter an excessive dose of a medication. The user action of submitting the order invokes a check of the dose against defined criteria within the system and interrupts the user with a request to act on the alert notification before proceeding. **Asynchronous CDS alerts** generally occur as a result of an imbedded rule and typically do not interrupt workflow unless the user chooses to do so. Asynchronous alerts can occur based on programmed logic using either data already contained within the CPOE system database resulting from user input or from data sent to the database from ancillary systems. For the former, one example might result in a notification flag being placed on a nursing patient list when the clerk documents that the patient has left the unit for a physical therapy appointment. For the latter, laboratory results introduced to the CPOE system via an interface with the laboratory information system might be examined by the CDS system to see if they are included as part of a rule. If so and if the rule criteria stipulate that an alert notification should occur, then the system will present the alert notification to a given user or category of users. An example of an asynchronous alert could be having a flag placed on a users electronic work list, patient list, or system inbox when an abnormal laboratory value is manually entered or electronically transmitted to the CPOE system for a blood chemistry test. Alternative asynchronous methods, such as e-mail notices and paging, can be used to notify staff of a needed action based upon system-defined criteria.

> **Key Point . . .**
>
> The proper use of CDS requires not only the wisdom and experience of health care professionals but also an understanding by these clinicians of the capabilities, limitations and deficiencies of CDS within their environment.
>
> **. . . So what?**
>
> CDS relies on three things—a good CDS system, clinical expertise of the professional, and an understanding of how the CDS system can be used to improve the medication use process. The CDS system can never take the place of the professional, and the professional should never rely on the CDS to make the final decision on a course of action.

Information Security/Confidentiality

Information security may be defined as reasonable protection from risk of loss, risk of inappropriate access, or doubt regarding authenticity of information. These data security concerns can be referred to as confidentiality, authentication, and nonrepudiation.[5]

Confidentiality ensures that the data is readable only by the intended recipients.

Authentication provides protection against unauthorized access or forgeries.

Nonrepudiation ensures that someone cannot deny having conducted a transaction. Vulnerabilities and threats to information security may consist of internal failures of hardware or software, human errors, deliberate attacks on information security, and natural catastrophes. Pharmacists responsible for informatics must ensure that security design in all pharmacy information systems support the prevention, detection, and correction of these vulnerabilities and threats.

Approaches to securing information and systems vary depending on the degree of sensitivity of the information. One of the first steps is to ensure that the physical location where servers are stored has been secured. Access to a network should be limited to those who need it and control must be exercised by a combination of security methods (e.g., passwords, smartcards, and/or biometric identification). These methods provide for authentication of individuals accessing information to help assure that only authorized individuals access the data. Furthermore, they provide for a history of access that can be examined if there are ever questions about who accessed certain data or was involved in specific transactions. Passwords are ubiquitous in current systems. However, a disadvantage is that they do not provide positive identification of individuals (passwords may be shared by multiple individuals). **Biometrics**, such as fingerprint recognition or retinal scanning, are becoming more prevalent due to their ability to provide a more positive authentication of an individual.

One key component of security in pharmacy systems is the ability to back up data so that it can be restored in event of internal hardware or software failures. Backing up data sets may be accomplished by replicating the data in an alternate medium and site. Media that may be used

> **Key Point . . .**
>
> Information security includes concerns about confidentiality, authentication, and nonrepudiation.
>
> **. . . So what?**
>
> Information security considers multiple issues. It must ensure that data can only be read by the intended recipients. To maintain confidentiality, individuals accessing the system need to provide some authentication that they really are allowed to access the information. After taking an action within the system, individuals have to be held accountable for their actions. These issues are the foundation of CPOE, EMRs, controlled substance medication ordering and usage, and any other critical system in an institution.

include hard drives, tapes, CDs or DVDs, or other servers, to name a few. The availability of adequate back-up systems is essential to protect against natural disasters as well as hardware or software failures. Critical applications are often created with redundancies built to protect against such failure.

Another key security issue that has arisen with the advent of electronic transmission of prescriptions between physicians and pharmacies (and, in particular, Internet pharmacies) has been the authenticity of the involved parties and the electronic signature. In response to public concern for the safety of pharmacy practices on the Internet, the National Association of Boards of Pharmacy (NABP) developed the **Verified Internet Pharmacy Practice Sites (VIPPS)** program in the spring of 1999.[6] A coalition of state and federal regulatory associations, professional associations, and consumer advocacy groups provided their expertise in developing the criteria which VIPPS-certified pharmacies follow.

Pharmacies displaying the VIPPS seal have demonstrated to NABP compliance with VIPPS criteria. To achieve accreditation, a pharmacy practice site must comply with the licensing and inspection requirements of the states in which it does business and must demonstrate to NABP compliance with VIPPS criteria including patient rights to privacy, authentication and security of prescription orders, maintenance of a quality assurance and improvement program, and provision of meaningful consultation between patients and pharmacists.

Systems such as **VeriSign™** are available to encrypt prescription or other protected health information during the electronic transmission of these data. This prevents the interception and unintended disclosure of confidential patient information during these transactions. Any pharmacy systems that involve transmission of patient data need to have a reliable and effective encryption process to assure confidentiality and authenticity.

While maintaining patient confidentiality and the security of patient information has long been a tenet of practice among pharmacists, the requirements of health care providers were increased with the passage and implementation of the Health Insurance Portability & Accountability Act (HIPAA).[7] Two goals of this legislation were to improve efficiency in health care delivery by standardizing electronic data and interchange and to protect the confidentiality and security of health data through setting and enforcing standards. The impact of HIPAA on institutions has been an increased awareness of the security and confidentiality of protected health information. Health systems must conduct detailed assessments of their computer systems to assure that appropriate privacy protections are in place and that the security of systems is adequate. In many cases this has resulted in updating information systems to safeguard protected health information (PHI) and to enable the use of standard claims and other electronic health transactions. From a security perspective, HIPAA requires institutions to ensure the confidentiality, integrity, and availability of all electronic PHI that the institution creates, receives, maintains or transmits. It requires the hospital to protect against any reasonably anticipated threats or hazards to the security or integrity of this information and to ensure that rules and safeguards are in place to prevent inappropriate disclosure of this information. Within HIPAA, disclosure of PHI is limited to the minimum needed for health care treatment, business operations, and quality improvement.

One technique that may be useful when handling protected health information is to use encryption of patient identifiers. **Encryption** involves replacing identifiers that are traceable to an individual with another set of letters or numbers which cannot be linked back to individual patients. This technique of **de-identification** is very useful when doing analyses of aggregate data sets, examining overall prescribing trends, and evaluating drug utilization when there is no need to identify patients specifically.

> **Key Point . . .**
>
> The Health Insurance Portability & Accountability Act (HIPAA) has attempted to standardize electronic data and interchange and protect the confidentiality and security of health data.
>
> **. . . So what?**
>
> HIPAA is a driving force behind many of the efforts to improve information systems within institutions. Many of informatics systems in institutions and the policies and procedures in institutions regarding informatics have been formed by HIPPA.

Clinical Informatics Pharmacist

Pharmacist positions in clinical informatics are positions that have evolved in response to contemporary pharmacy practice needs rather than ones which have a clear academic and training path. In general, pharmacists who accept these roles either have a strong interest in informatics or have developed a specific informatics aptitude on the job. The growth of the number of professionals with responsibilities related to informatics was a driving force behind the creation of a section within ASHP devoted to enhancing networking opportunities and "…improving health outcomes through the use and integration of data, information, knowledge, technology, and automation in the medication-use process" (the Section on Pharmacy Informatics and Technology). The need for pharmacists to have an understanding of pharmacy informatics has also led to the incorporation of informatics learning outcomes for both college of pharmacy and residency curriculums.

Roles and Responsibilities

Pharmacists who specialize in informatics generally are responsible for one or more of the following activities:

- Inpatient pharmacy information systems
- Outpatient pharmacy information systems
- Robotic unit-dose dispensing machines
- Automated medication dispensing machines
- Point-of-care bar code medication administration
- Automated intravenous admixture devices
- Inpatient computerized prescriber order entry systems
- Outpatient computerized prescriber order entry systems
- Clinical decision support
- Packaging machines
- Programming
- Report writing
- Inventory control systems
- Pharmacy intranets
- Customized pharmacy applications
- Desktop and application support
- Staff training and education

Education and Training

Pharmacists who wish to pursue a position in pharmacy informatics can accomplish this in several ways. One option is to take specific courses or obtain a degree in computer science, information systems, and/or business information technology. Useful coursework would include areas such as network administration, basic programming, database management, and heuristics. Another option available to pharmacists would be to complete an advanced residency in pharmacy informatics. Several sites for informatics residencies have emerged in recent years and they offer the resident a wide array of learning opportunities not generally available to most pharmacists or pharmacy practice residents. A third way is to volunteer to assume an informatics role at one's current place of employment. This can be done by indicating an interest in informatics, to volunteering to take responsibility for one or more aspects of informatics and/or obtaining as much on-the-job experience as possible, including taking coursework through local community colleges, attending certified training courses, attending vendor training courses, attending informatics-related conferences, and learning from colleagues. The field of pharmacy informatics is constantly evolving. Many pharmacists have found applying their clinical knowledge with information technology skills for the purposes of bettering patient care to be a very satisfying and rewarding career.

Summary

Pharmacy informatics is a broad and growing area. While the formal organization of pharmacy informatics is not as developed as is seen in other disciplines, pharmacists have played a leading role to date in the adoption of technologies to improve the medication-use system. Much work is yet to be done. Technology tools in the hands of properly trained pharmacists have the potential to greatly improve the safety and efficiency of the medication-use system in health care organizations.

Suggested Reading

Ammenwerth E, Schnell-Inderst P, Machan C, et. al. The effect of electronic prescribing on medication errors and adverse drug events: a systematic review. *J Am Med Inform Assoc.* 2008;15(5):585-600.

Angaran DM. Telemedicine and telepharmacy: Current status and future implications. *Am J Health-Syst Pharm* 1999;56:1405-1426.

Ash JS, Berg M, Coeira E. Some Unintended Consequences of Information Technology in Health Care: The Nature of Patient Care Information System-related Errors. *J Am Med Inform Assoc.* 2004;11:104-112.

ASHP Section of Pharmacy Informatics and Technology Executive Committee: Technology-enabled practice: a vision statement by the ASHP Section of Pharmacy Informatics and Technology. *Am J Health-Syst Pharm.* 2009;66:1573-1577.

ASHP Statement on Bar Code Enabled Medication Administration Technology. *Am J Health-Syst Pharm.* 2009; 66:588-590.

ASHP Statement on the Pharmacists Role in Informatics. *Am J Health-Syst Pharm.* 2007; 64:200-203.

Felkey BG. Health system informatics. *Am J Health-Syst Pharm.* 1997; 54:274-280.

Jha AK, DesRoches CM, Campbell EG, et. al. Use of Electronic Health Records in U.S. Hospitals. *N Engl J Med.* 2009;360:1628-1638.

Mekhjian HS, Kumar, RR, Kuehn L, et al. Immediate Benefits Realized Following Implementation of Physician Order Entry at an Academic Medical Center. *J Am Med Inform Assoc.* 2002;9:529-539.

Osheroff JA, Pifer EA, Teich TM, Sittig DF, Jenders RA. *Improving Outcomes with Clinical Decision Support: An Implementer's Guide.* Chicago: Healthcare Information and Management Systems Society; 2005.

Pedersen CA, Gumpper KF. ASHP national survey on informatics: Assessment of the adoption and use of pharmacy informatics in U.S. hospitals—2007. *Am J Health-Syst Pharm.* 2008; 65:2244-2264.

Siska MH, Meyer GE. Pharmacy informatics: Aligning for success. *Am J Health-Syst Pharm.* 2008; 65:1410-1411.

Sittig DF, Wright A, Osheroff JA, et. al. Grand Challenges in Clinical Decision Support. *J Biomed Inform.* 2008;41:387-392.

References

1. Healthnet BC Glossary. Available at: http://healthnet.hnet.bc.ca/tools/glossary/. Accessed November 12, 2004.

2. Nursing Informatics Frequently Asked Questions. Available at: http://nursing.umaryland.edu/~snewbold/sknfaqni.htm. Accessed November 12, 2004.

3. Definitions of Medical Informatics. Available at: http://www.veranda.com.ph/hermant/definitions.htm. Accessed November 12, 2004.

4. Davenport TH, Prusak L. *Working Knowledge.* Boston: Harvard Business School Press; 2000.

5. A Structure for Discussing Application Security Requirements. Available at: http://enterprise.state.wi.us/home/strategic/sec.htm. Accessed November 12, 2004.

6. Verified Internet Pharmacy Practice Sites (VIPPS) Program. Available at: http://www.nabp.net/vipps/intro.asp. Accessed November 12, 2004.

7. Tribble DA. The health insurance portability and accountability act: security and privacy requirements. *Am J Health-Syst Pharm.* 2001;58:763-770.

8. Commission of the European Communities: eEurope 2002. Quality criteria for health related websites. *J Med Internet Res.* 2002;4:e15.

9. 20 Most Popular Health Websites/June 2009. Available at: http://www.ebizmba.com/articles/health. Accessed June 29, 2009.

10. UMHS-Endorsed External Sites. Available at: http://www.med.umich.edu/pteducation/links.htm. Accessed June 29, 2009.

11. Bearce WC, Willey GA, Fox RL, et al. Documentation of clinical interactions: quality of care issues and economic considerations in critical care pharmacy. *Hosp Pharm.* 1988;23:883-890.

12. Zimmerman CR, Smolarek RT, Stevenson JG. A computerized system to improve documentation and reporting of pharmacists' clinical interventions, cost savings, and workload activities. *Pharmacotherapy.* 1995;15:220-227.

13. Haslett TM, Kay BG, Weissfellner H. Documenting concurrent clinical pharmacy interventions. *Hosp Pharm.* 1990;25:351-355,359.

14. Narducci WA, Norvell MJ. Development and use of an automated pharmacy services documentation system. *Hosp Pharm.* 1989;24:184-189,204.

15. Schumock GT, Hutchinson RA, Bilek BA. Comparison of two systems for documenting pharmacist interventions in patient care. *Am J Hosp Pharm.* 1992;49:2211-2214.

16. Chaffee BW, Bonasso J. Strategies for pharmacy integration and pharmacy information system interfaces, part 1: history and pharmacy integration options. *Am J Health-Syst Pharm.* 2004;61:502-506.

17. Teich JM, Merchia PR, Schmiz JL, et al. Effects of computerized physician order entry on prescribing practices. *Arch Intern Med.* 2000;160:2741-2747.

18. Senholzi C, Gottlieb J. Pharmacist interventions after implementation of computerized prescriber order entry. *Am J Health-Syst Pharm.* 2003;60:1880-1882.

19. Broverman C, Kapusnik-Uner J, Shalaby J, et al. A concept-based medication vocabulary: an essential requirement for pharmacy decision support. *Pharm Pract Manage Q.* 1998;18:1-20.

20. Galanter WL, Polikatis A, DiDomenico RJ. A trial of automated safety alerts for inpatient digoxin use with computerized physician order entry. *J Am Med Inform Assoc.* 2004;11:270-277.

21. Wright A, Goldberg H, Hongsermeier T, et. al. A description and functional taxonomy of rule-based decision support content at a large integrated delivery network. *J Am Med Inform Assoc.* 2007;14_489-496.

Chapter Review Questions

1. **True/False: Asynchronous CDS alerts represent warning screens that are invoked based upon specific actions taken by a user of the system and require immediate action by the prescriber.**
   a. True
   b. False

   Answer b. False. Asynchronous clinical decision support (CDS) alerts occur independently of the order entry process and do not typically interrupt the user. Synchronous CDS alerts, however, usually flag problems that must be taken care of immediately (e.g., a notice of a potentially severe drug interaction). Therefore, they usually demand immediate attention and require some action on the part of the user before further actions can occur.

2. **A clinical data repository (CDR) is used to store _____ clinical data which is often used to produce clinical or administrative reports.**
   a. Physician-specific
   b. Patient-specific
   c. Pharmacist-specific
   d. Institution-specific

   Answer b. Patient-specific. CDRs contain data on individual patients collected from interconnected databases (e.g., pharmacy and laboratory) throughout the institution. The data is consolidated in the CDR to provide decision makers with a unified view of a single patient's clinical information.

3. **Which of the following is an accreditation program that provides a means for the public to distinguish between legitimate and illegitimate online drug sellers?**
   a. CPOE
   b. RFID
   c. HIPAA
   d. VIPPS

   Answer: d. VIPPS. The Verified Internet Pharmacy Practice Sites (VIPPS) was created by the National Association of Boards of Pharmacy (NABP) to accredit pharmacy web sites to provide a seal of approval for the public to distinguish between legitimate and illegitimate online drug sellers. The VIPPS seal of approval assures that VIPPS retailers are legitimate online pharmacies appropriately licensed in each state to which they ship pharmaceuticals.

4. **Simple, discrete, and objective facts about a subject or an event is a description of:**
   a. Data
   b. Information
   c. Knowledge
   d. None of the above

   Answer a. Data. Data are pieces of information that become knowledge when they are aggregated in a meaningful way. They are often viewed as the lowest level of abstraction from which information and knowledge are derived.

5. **Which of the following are benefits of electronic information sources compared to traditional paper information sources?**
    a. Improved accessibility of information
    b. Reduced space requirements
    c. Ability to maintain up-to-date information
    d. All of the above

    Answer d. All of the above. Electronic information can be accessed by professionals anywhere inside and even outside of the health care system. The electrons used to store the information take up little space and changes can be made immediately and throughout the entire information system.

6. _____ **allow patient information to flow directly into the pharmacy system from a patient management system without the need for pharmacy staff to enter the data by hand.**
    a. Point of Care Devices
    b. Software interfaces
    c. BCMA
    d. CPOE

    Answer: b. Software interfaces. Software interfaces allow systems to talk to each other without the help of human beings. Point of care devices, BCMA, and CPOE all require human beings to allow systems to interface with each other.

7. **The intranet is often referred to as the World Wide Web.**
    a. True
    b. False

    Answer: a. False. The internet is often called the World Wide Web. An intranet is a private computer network that uses Internet technologies to securely share any part of an organization's information or operational systems with its employees.

8. **An alert that is triggered and displayed to a prescriber indicating that the dose selected is greater than normal for a patient's weight during the process of order entry is an example of:**
    a. Authentication
    b. Active clinical decision support
    c. Encryption
    d. De-identification

    Answer: b. Active clinical decision support. Clinical decision support consists of the functions of information systems that communicate useful messages to health care professionals. Active clinical decision support sends messages directly to the professional and includes pop-up alerts about clinical abnormalities or messages highlight important information in the record. Therefore, an alert about a potential dose/ patient weight problem would fall under active clinical decision support. The other options, authentication, encryption, and non-repudiation, deal with issues of data security. Authentication provides protection against unauthorized access or forgeries.

9. **Which of the following methods is best at positively authenticating individuals for purposes of enhancing information system security?**
   a. Passwords
   b. Bar code scanning
   c. Biometrics
   d. None of the above

   Answer: c. Biometrics. Authentication provides protection against unauthorized access or forgeries. It is possible for others to borrow or steal other people's passwords and bar code badges. Fingerprints and scans of the retina are harder for unauthorized individuals to acquire and use.

10. **Pharmacists who wish to pursue a position in pharmacy informatics can accomplish this by:**
   a. Obtaining a degree in computer science, information systems, and/or business information technology
   b. Completing a PGY2 residency in pharmacy informatics
   c. Assuming on-the-job responsibilities and networking with other individuals in pharmacy informatics
   d. Any of the above

   Answer: d. Any of the above. There is no single path to acquiring an informatics position. One path is to obtaining a specialized degree that offers training relevant to informatics duties. There are many different types of varying quality being offered, so it is important to choose carefully before enrolling. A less formal path is to identify a health care system offering a PGY2 residency specializing in pharmacy informatics. These are still rare but becoming increasingly common. A third option is to just do it, by volunteering to help out with informatics projects. On-the-job training and networking with experts in an institution is the way many pharmacists gained informatics expertise. When needed, they typically sign up for training offered by the health system or seek out training opportunities in the community. Ultimately, any path can be justified because the real test of an informatics pharmacist is his or her ability to manage and solve technology problems.

Chapter Discussion Questions

1. Describe the different methods by which orders can be created and transmitted to the pharmacy department.
2. Contrast the advantages and disadvantages of integration using an "all-in-one" integrated CPOE/pharmacy information system versus use of an interfaced system.
3. Explain the rationale for coding information in CPOE systems where the use of clinical decision support will be used.

CHAPTER 11

Automation in Practice

*Brad Ludwig and Jack Temple**

■ ■ ■

Learning Objectives

After completing this chapter, readers should be able to:

1. Describe how technology and automation can increase safety and efficiency within the medication use system.
2. Identify the limitations of existing automation in the medication use system and the impact of automation on the delivery of patient care.
3. Define key terms in pharmacy automation.
4. Review the role of regulations, standards and guidelines in use of technology and automation.
5. Discuss required financial, personnel, and facility resources as they relate to the safe use of technology and automation.

Key Terms and Definitions

■ **Adverse drug event (ADE):** An injury from a medication or lack of intended medication.

■ **Automation:** Any technology, machine, or device linked to or controlled by a computer and used to do work.

■ **Bar code medication administration (BCMA):** A process that encompasses the use of bar code scanning functionality into the medication administration phase of medication-use and combines a number of hardware and software components to display, receive, and chart real-time patient and medication information.

■ **Carousel dispensing technology (CDT):** A medication storage cabinet with rotating shelves used to automate medication dispensing.

■ **Computerized prescriber order entry (CPOE):** A computer application that allows physicians to type prescriptions into a computer and send them directly to the pharmacy (instead of using orders sheets or prescription pads). Also known as computerized physician order entry (CPOE) and prescriber order entry (POE).

■ **Decentralized automated dispensing devices:** Secure storage cabinets capable of handling most unit-dose and some bulk (multiple-dose) medications.

*The authors would like to acknowledge Steve Rough, M.S., Director of Pharmacy, Department of Pharmacy, University of Wisconsin Hospital and Clinics, Madison, WI, for his contributions to this chapter.

Also known as automated dispensing cabinets (ADC), automated dispensing machine (ADM), automated dispensing unit (ADU), unit based cabinets (UBC).

- **Electronic medication administration record (eMAR):** A real-time, computer displayed medication administration record.
- **Human factors engineering:** The discipline of designing workplace facilities and tasks to meet the needs and optimize the performance of human beings.
- **Interface:** A physical or electronic connection that enables otherwise incompatible computer systems to communicate and exchange data.
- **Integrate:** A process in which separate components or subsystems are combined or are designed together at the same time with a unifying architecture and problems in their interactions are addressed.
- **Medication error:** Any preventable event that may cause or lead to inappropriate medication use or patient harm while the medication is in the control of the health care professional, patient, or consumer.

- **Medication-use process:** A multi-step process consisting of five domains: (1) prescribing/medication determination; (2) medication preparation, dispensing, and counseling; (3) medication administration; (4) patient monitoring/assessment; and (5) purchasing/inventory management.
- **Radio frequency (RF) network:** Commonly used in the wireless communications industry to describe equipment using radio frequency waves to transmit sounds and data from one point to another.
- **Smart pumps:** Infusion devices with clinical decision support software and drug libraries that perform a test of reasonableness at the point of medication administration.
- **Supply chain management:** Oversight of the process of moving products, information, and money between pharmacies, wholesalers, pharmaceutical companies, and other organizations in the supply chain.
- **Technology:** Anything that is used to replace routine or repetitive tasks previously performed by people, or which extends the capability of people.

■ ■ ■

Introduction

Technological advancements are a constant in today's health care marketplace where payers and patients demand high quality, efficient, and cost-effective service. **Technology,** which is defined as anything used to replace routine or repetitive tasks previously performed by people or to extend the capability of people, is a prerequisite to the survival of the profession and the advancement of pharmacist patient care services.

Automation is a form of technology. **Automation** is defined as any machine or device linked to or controlled by a computer and used to do work. Thus, all automation is a form of technology but not all technology is automation.

This chapter provides an introduction on the use of automation in inpatient pharmacy practice. It discusses best practices for maximizing the safe and efficient use of automation and describes how automation might impact the future of pharmacy practice. This chapter is not a comprehensive review of all available automated devices and technologies, it only briefly mentions automation associated with computerized prescriber order entry (CPOE) and clinical decision support systems. Those forms of technology are discussed in more detail in Chapter 9, "Electronic Data Management," and Chapter 10, "Informatics."

History

The application of automation within the practice of pharmacy began in the early 1960s, although the pace has increased dramatically in the last 20 years. The recent demand for automation has been driven by improved technology, the need to control costs of care, and a demand for safer patient care. Automation can help pharmacy managers do more with less (i.e., provide better, faster service with fewer employees) and free pharmacists to provide patient care services to improve health outcomes.

> **Key Point . . .**
>
> All automation is a form of technology but not all technology is automation.
>
> **. . . So what?**
>
> In conversations, technology and automation are often used interchangeably but they are different. Automation is a subset of technology. It is specific only to technology controlled by computers that are used to do work.

Wholesalers have been critical to the growth of automation in many health-system pharmacies. Wholesalers are intermediary businesses that purchase pharmaceuticals from drug manufacturers for resale to pharmacies. Since the mid-1990s, major wholesalers (Amerisource Bergen, Cardinal Health, and McKesson) have expanded their technology support services for health-system pharmacies by partnering with or buying pharmacy technology and automation companies. Wholesalers now offer a range of products and support services including hand-held bar code scanners, inventory control systems, and automated dispensing devices. Pharmacies have partnered with these wholesalers because they typically do not have the expertise, personnel, or time needed to automate without assistance.

Automation and Patient Safety

Automation can help improve the safety of the medication use system. Bates et al. described four phases in the medication-use process, ordering, transcribing, dispensing, and administration, where potential and preventable adverse drug events (ADEs) could be found.[1] Bates and colleagues found that 49% of all preventable and potential ADEs occurred in the ordering phase and 26% in the administration phase. When only medication errors causing patient harm were considered (i.e., preventable ADEs), 90% of preventable ADEs occurred during the ordering and administration phases of the medication-use process.

The data suggests that technology along with automated systems aimed at improving ordering and administration in the medication-use process can have the greatest impact on patient safety in hospitals. **CPOE systems** can assist the ordering phase by guiding prescribers through the order entry process and reduce the need to transcribe orders. **Bar code medication administration (BCMA)** technology helps improve the administration phase by ensuring the five rights of medication administration: right patient, right medication, right dose, right time, and right route. Other technologies are currently in use in many health systems within various components of the medication-use process. Table 11-1 provides a list of these technologies.

Table 11-1.
Technologies and Automated Devices Applied Throughout the Medication-Use Process

Prescribing

- Clinical decision support software
- Computerized prescriber order entry

Dispensing

- Carousel technology
- Centralized robotic dispensing technology
- Centralized narcotic dispensing and inventory tracking devices
- Decentralized automated dispensing devices
- Intravenous and total parenteral nutrition compounding devices
- Pneumatic tube delivery systems
- Unit dose medication repacking systems

Administration

- Bar code medication administration technology
- Clinical decision support-based infusion pumps

Monitoring

- Electronic clinical documentation systems
- Web-based compliance and disease management tracking systems

Drug Purchasing and Supply Chain Management Systems

Drug purchasing, inventory control, and other tasks in **supply chain management** can be improved by automating the ordering process between suppliers and the pharmacy.[2,3] Automating the purchasing and inventory control systems can help simplify the medication procurement (ordering) and receiving process, reduce on-hand drug product inventory, and lower product acquisition costs. Using hand-held product reordering devices to scan bar coded product shelf labels in inventory management is an example of one technology used in supply chain management.

In order to develop an efficient supply chain management program, it is common for health-system pharmacies to partner

Key Point . . .

Automation systems aimed at improving ordering and administration in the medication-use process can have the greatest impact on patient safety in hospitals.

. . . So what?

Most preventable errors occur in ordering and administering drugs, so efforts in these areas are more likely to bear fruit. Many steps in ordering and administration can be automated, thereby providing further justification for automated systems that can improve patient safety.

with a pharmaceutical wholesaler. The largest wholesalers use state-of-the-art inventory management technology, using sophisticated computer programs to manage and track orders and deliveries, bar codes and radio frequency signals to monitor products moving through the supply chain, and robotics or other forms of technology not typically available to hospital pharmacies. Since many wholesalers also own automated dispensing technologies, they are able to **integrate** pharmacy dispensing software, prescription processing computer systems, and point-of-sale dispensing systems. Accomplishing such integration is critical in automating the procurement process. For example, if a pharmacy's computer order processing system can maintain an accurate perpetual (i.e., continually up to date) inventory of products on the shelf and account for all dispensing and crediting transactions, that system also may be able to electronically communicate real-time inventory levels to the wholesaler's order management system and automatically place an order to the wholesaler when inventory levels fall below a predetermined quantity. Such a system works best with dispensing technology that maintains a closed perpetual inventory record of drug products. When products are received in the pharmacy from the wholesaler, the same interface permits new inventory quantities received to be added to the pharmacy computer system's or automated dispensing technologies perpetual inventory.

Some wholesalers provide pharmacies with hand-held scanning devices with integrated bar code readers in order to automate the procurement process. Use of the scanners provides an automated receiving and invoice reconciliation process, thus automating the labor-intensive and error-prone product check-in process. The process begins when a pharmacy technician scans a bar code on a delivery tote from the wholesaler, which in turn generates an electronic invoice. Each product bar code is then scanned as it is removed from the tote, and the products received are electronically reconciled against the invoice. The system automatically credits product invoicing discrepancies, arranges for mis-picks (shipping errors) to be returned, and updates the pharmacy's perpetual inventory for products received. This same scanner can be used to generate new orders to be sent to the wholesaler and generate return requests to the wholesaler for damaged or unused products. After products are received, payments can be sent from accounts payable to the wholesaler via the Internet.

Health systems have been slow to implement such systems, largely due to dispensing system complexities and multiple drug inventory locations within the hospital. Some hospitals have implemented automated procurement systems for supplies of medications such as those maintained in an automated dispensing technology or in a pharmacy stockroom. Automated inventory management systems, when properly maintained, have the potential to result in dramatic one-time cost savings via reducing drug inventory on hand. It can also lead to long-term savings and efficiency by maximizing drug inventory turn rates, avoiding expired inventory and reducing labor required for the drug procurement process.

Drug Distribution and Dispensing Systems

This section briefly describes the advantages, disadvantages, and issues surrounding the use of several existing technologies, which, if appropriately deployed, may help improve the safety of the medication-use process. This section describes a sampling of technologies and is not designed to be all-inclusive. Comprehensive reviews of pharmacy automation are available elsewhere in the literature.[4-7]

Decentralized Automated Dispensing Devices

Decentralized **automated dispensing devices** are secure storage cabinets capable of handling most unit dose and some bulk (multiple-dose) medications. The devices are also referred to as automated dispensing cabinets (ADC), automated dispensing machines (ADM), automated dispensing units (ADU), and unit based cabinets (UBC). Automated dispensing devices store and electronically dispense medications in locations remote from a centralized or satellite pharmacy. They allow nurses immediate access to medications at the point of use without requiring a visit to a pharmacy. At the same time, pharmacists can control drug use by requiring nurses to access the machines by means of user identifiers and passwords. Summarized dispensing reports can also help hospitals monitor for diversion and to bill patients.

Automated dispensing devices were originally installed in hospitals in the early 1990s to provide increased control over controlled substances and floor stock medications in patient care areas. By 2008, approximately 83% of U.S. hospitals were incorporating decentralized automated dispensing devices, up from 49% only 9 years earlier.[8]

The primary focus of these automated dispensing devices is to provide prompt, real-time availability of medications for the nurse and patient. They can also help to improve controlled substance accountability, increase productivity, improve charge capture and documentation accuracy, and reduce pharmacy and nursing labor costs. Many hospitals now use these devices to store and dispense nearly all scheduled doses, thereby eliminating the manual medication cart fill and delivery process. However, the impact of these decentralized automated dispensing devices on medication errors is less clear.[9,10]

Automated dispensing devices can improve safety by incorporating bar code labeling and scanning into the replenishment process, thus improving restocking accuracy and potentially improving medication safety. Also, safety can be improved if automated dispensing devices free pharmacists to direct patient care activities including medication therapy management services.

However, automated dispensing devices can introduce medication errors if not implemented and/or managed appropriately. Some devices allow nurses to access any patient and dispense any drug they choose. This may permit the selection of inappropriate medications for administration, diversion of medications for personal use, or inadequate documentation of what drugs were administered to which patient. Problems can also occur when some nursing units have automated dispensing devices while others have manual cart fill. Mixed systems like this can cause problems as patients are moved between units and may preclude an institution's ability to maintain a well-controlled, single-dose medication dispensing system. In addition, some health systems have yet to link

Key Point . . .

Automated dispensing devices can introduce medication errors if not implemented and/or managed appropriately.

. . . So what?

Sometimes, there is a tendency to rely too much on technology. Automated dispensing devices and other technology are not perfect, nor are the individuals using them. Over-reliance on technology can lead pharmacy employees to be less vigilant to potential risks to patients. Pharmacists need to implement and manage processes that take into account the various ways that errors can arise with technology.

their pharmacy computer systems to cabinets in a way that restricts nurses from obtaining medications that are not ordered for patients. Other safety concerns include (1) retrieving of an incorrect medication because of open access to all drugs in a drawer; (2) carelessness or lack of verification of drug labels due to a belief that the system is computerized and, therefore, not as susceptible to errors (or the belief that pharmacy placed the drug there and pharmacy does not make mistakes); (3) drugs stocked in the wrong pocket either because one or more doses inadvertently fell into the wrong slot or due to a pharmacy restocking error; and (4) changing the location of the drug in the cabinet can cause errors because drugs may be selected from particular locations based upon habit rather than verifying each drug's identity.[11]

Conflicting reports exist in the literature on the impact of automated dispensing devices on medication error rates and provider efficiency.[11-14] Unfortunately, significant capital investments have been made in these systems without full understanding of their impact on operations and patient safety. Therefore, it is important for pharmacists to involve themselves in understanding the procurement, implementation, and efficient use of these systems. One way is to become familiar with the Institute for Safe Medication Practices (ISMP) interdisciplinary guidelines to help ensure the safe use of decentralized dispensing devices.[15] The guidelines were developed around twelve core processes and list approximately 100 different principles for the safe and effective use of the decentralized automated dispensing devices. Table 11-2 lists guidelines and considerations for the safe use of decentralized automated dispensing devices. Table 11-3 compares potential advantages and disadvantages of decentralized automated dispensing devices.

Automation in Centralized Dispensing

Centrally located dispensing devices help automate the entire process of medication dispensing from a pharmacy. As previously discussed in Chapter 7, "Medication Distribution Systems," the rise in the use of technology for medication dispensing can replace many of the manual tasks for medication dispensing and reduce the number of pharmacy staff needed for the process. In the past most centralized robotic systems were used to select bar coded unit dose medications for scheduled medication cart filling and such devices were interfaced with the pharmacy information system to provide access to each patient's medication profile. Today, centralized robotics are also used to automate first dose dispensing and to replenish low stock medications in decentralized automated dispensing devices. Thus, as long as the patient's medication profile in the pharmacy information system is maintained in an accurate and timely manner, the pharmacist's time spent checking medications may be reallocated to more direct patient care activities.

Perhaps one of the greatest advantages of implementing robotic technology is that all doses dispensed by the robot are bar coded, thus providing a foundation for the implementation of a bar code medication administration (BCMA) systems. Bar coding of medication doses allows dispensing accuracy to approach 100% with centralized robotics technology. However, this necessity for bar codes on all medications dispensed by the robot has the potential to introduce new error into the medication-use system. Although some manufacturers provide bar coded medications to use in centralized robotic devices, most unit dose medications must be accurately repackaged with a bar code label by the pharmacy department. A disadvantage for centralized robotic devices is the increase in labor needed to repackage medications. To offset the repackaging requirement many technology companies have developed automated packagers and even full service agreements alongside robotic devices to assist with the labor-intensive packaging requirement. Overall the use of

Table 11-2.

Guidelines for Safe Use of Decentralized Automated Dispensing Devices

■ Assign medications to devices based on the needs of the patient care unit, patient age, diagnosis, and staff expertise.

■ Create an alert system to flag high-risk medications stocked in devices (such as a maximum dose prompt).

■ Develop an ongoing competency assessment program for all personnel with access to the device; include direct observations and random restocking accuracy audits; observe dispensing accuracy as part of the assessment.

■ Develop a system to locate and remove recalled and expired medications.

■ Develop clear, multidisciplinary downtime procedures; include procedures in training and ongoing competency programs.

■ Develop systems to account for narcotic waste; routinely audit controlled substance dispense quantities against patient orders, medication administration record documentation, and waste documentation.

■ Display allergy reminders for specific drugs such as antibiotics, opiates, and NSAIDs on appropriate medication storage pockets or have them automatically appear on the dispensing screen.

■ Do not allow nurses to return medications to the original storage pockets/locations; assign a return bin to collect returned medications.

■ Establish a preventive maintenance schedule with the vendor that does not disrupt workflow.

■ Establish strict security criteria to limit unauthorized access to devices.

■ Establish stringent safety criteria for selecting medications that are (and are not) appropriate to store in devices and oversee the process for assigning new drugs to new locations in all care settings.

■ Incorporate bar code scanning for restocking and medication retrieval.

■ Limit the numbers of medications not available in profile dispense that may be overridden (dispensed without pharmacist review and verification).

■ Maximize the use of unit dose medications in ready-to-administer form, with only a few exceptions.

■ Only assign medications with minimal harm potential to open access drawers.

■ Perform routine expiration date checks, as well as concomitantly verifying inventory quantities.

■ Require all personnel to attend formal training and demonstrate competency prior to accessing the devices.

■ Require pharmacist medication order review and verification before a medication is accessed for first dose administration (profile dispensing).

■ Restrict access to provide single dose (or single drug) availability whenever possible; focus control on high-risk medications and controlled substances pocked lidded pockets).

■ Separate sound-alike and look-alike medications; do not stock these medications in the same open-access drawer.

robotics for centralized dispensing can reduce pharmacy labor costs, eliminate routine and repetitive tasks associated with dispensing, and improve medication dispensing accuracy.

Carousel dispensing technology is a dispensing device that consists of a medication storage cabinet with rotating shelves and comprehensive software that manages inven-

Table 11-3.

Potential Advantages and Disadvantages of Decentralized Automated Dispensing Devices

Advantages	Disadvantages
Ability to add extra cabinets to increase capacity	Accurate inventory quantities may be difficult with mixed distribution systems (automated and non automated)
Ability to restrict access to a single dose of a medication	Automation break downs may impact patient care
Flexible drawer configurations accommodates multiple types of dosage forms	Duplicate inventory in large numbers of dispensing cabinets may increase inventory costs and the amount of expired medications
Helps resolve discrepancies by automating controlled substance retrieval and inventory reconciliation	If devices are used to replace cart fill, several devices are needed per nursing unit
Automatically charges patients for drugs used	Inspection and removal of expired medications must be performed manually (devices do not have the software to track expiration dates)
Bar code scanning integral to system	
Reduces the time needed for patients to receive their first dose	
Improved nursing satisfaction due to fewer missing doses, fewer delays for first doses, and more nursing control over day-to-day medication distribution activities	Multiple dose access is still common in systems allowing for diversion and misuse
More pharmacy control versus traditional floor stock system	Poor integration with bedside medication storage systems
Provides detailed electronic dispensing and usage reports	Potential labor cost savings are frequently not realized
Frees pharmacists to perform patient care activities	Potential for nurses and pharmacists to take shortcuts around the system leading to errors
Saves nursing labor	Unable to accommodate all medications (limited by medication size, cabinet size, and risk level for a particular medication to be stocked in a device)
Eliminates problem of missing or misplaced narcotic drawer keys	
Eliminates narcotic counts at shift change	
Fewer narcotic discrepancies to resolve	
Less narcotic paperwork to handle	

tory and prioritizes workflow. Like other dispensing technologies, CDT utilizes bar code scanning technology to improve the efficiency and accuracy of pharmacy technicians who pick and restock medications. Likewise, the carousel must be interfaced with the pharmacy information system in order to achieve maximum benefits for safety and efficiency.[16,17] It can reduce technician travel time, bending, and reaching for medications during the filling process. Rotating shelves within the carousel place medications at easy to reach levels with a light identifying the exact location. The rotating shelves maximize rarely used vertical space to store medications. In addition, medications do not need to be stored alphabetically, so they can be arranged in any order to help increase dispensing efficiency and meet regulatory requirements for dispensing high-alert, sound-alike, and look-alike medications. Finally, CDT systems can be integrated or interfaced with decentralized unit-based dispensing cabinets to coordinate dispensing activities within the medication use system.

Narcotic Dispensing and Record Keeping Systems

As described in Chapter 8, the management of controlled substances is one of the most labor-intensive processes in health-system pharmacy. Automation helps manage the ordering, storage, dispensing, and administration of all controlled substances from the wholesaler to the nursing unit. Such systems record all doses dispensed from a central pharmacy narcotic room by scanning manufacturer's bar codes, and provides a record of the individual performing every transaction. Additionally, they can be stand-alone or interfaced with decentralized automated dispensing devices to verify that every dose dispensed from the pharmacy is stocked in the intended decentralized automated dispensing device. They generate bar-coded tracking forms for nurses to maintain accurate inventory accounting on units without automated dispensing devices and suggest reorder quantities based on past controlled substance use. Lastly, they help provide compliance and controlled substance disposal reports for the Drug Enforcement Agency. The key benefits for using automated narcotic dispensing and record keeping systems includes accurate record keeping, enhanced control of narcotics, improved regulatory compliance, and efficient ordering processes. In additional to tightening up the security of controlled substances, automated systems can help identify potential drug product diversion. Thus, it is very common to find hospitals that have moved all traditional, narcotic vault drug inventories into automated dispensing cabinets linked to narcotic inventory control software.

Medication Drug Administration Systems

Bar Code Medication Administration (BCMA) Technology

Bar code administration is a process that incorporates the use of bar code scanning functionality into the medication administration phase of medication-use. It utilizes a number of hardware and software components to display, receive, and chart real-time patient and medication information, providing caregivers (usually nurses) with the information needed to accurately administer and document medication administration. BCMA consists of a three-way check of the nurse, medication, and patient at the bedside, whereby the technology checks scanned bar codes on the nurse's identification badge, the dose of medication, and the patient's identification wristband. It also verifies the drug against the patient's **electronic medication administration record (eMAR)**, documents the time and details of administration, and can generate a charge for the drug to the billing department. If a medication is not

Key Point . . .

BCMA helps to ensure the five rights of medication administration: right patient, right medication, right dose, right time, and right route.

. . . So what?

BCMA technology can be used to verify the patient via a wrist band; the medication, dose, and route via a bar code on the package; and the time via a built-in chronometer. Things can still go wrong, but BCMA technology can significantly prevent medication errors.

given, the BCMA system requires the nurse to document the reason. BCMA helps to ensure the five rights of medication administration: right patient, right medication, right dose, right time, and right route.

BCMA can provide real-time updates to eMARs, enabling all caregivers to view updated information about the patient's current and past medication regimens and make judgments about future medication administrations. Many systems use hand-held laser bar code scanners and wireless, portable hand-held computers linked to the pharmacy information system computers via a **radio frequency network**. For all scheduled doses, the device alerts the nurse when it is time to administer the medication.

This technology offers the potential to dramatically reduce the risk of drug administration errors.[18-20] Organizations that have implemented this technology report up to 87% reductions in medication administration errors, with up to 10% of doses scanned resulting in one of the following discrepancies: wrong patient, wrong drug, wrong dose, or wrong time.[19-21]

Although improvements are being made in BCMA and other eMAR technology, effectively implementing these systems can be costly and complicated. Major limitations to implementing BCMA include (1) cost of the BCMA software; (2) cost of BCMA-related hardware such as portable scanning devices, bedside computers, centralized computer servers, bar code printing systems for patient and caregiver identification tags and bar code medication repackaging systems; (3) all medications must be bar coded in unit-of-use packaging to achieve the optimal safety benefit, usually requiring labor- intensive and potentially error-prone repackaging in the pharmacy; (4) commercially available BCMA products are still at a very early stage of development; (5) nursing workflow redesign; (6) elaborate real-time interfaces or integration between pharmacy and BCMA information systems are necessary to assure accurate patient records within the BCMA system; and (7) installation of a dedicated radio frequency network may be incompatible with certain patient monitoring devices in the hospital. These stated limitations and incompatibilities have limited the use of BCMA technology in many health care settings. Despite widespread recommendations to use BCMA technology to verify and document medication administration, it is estimated that only 24% of all pharmacies incorporate bar codes into their dispensing process and an estimated 25% of hospitals currently use BCMA technology. Although this medical error prevention technology is not yet widespread, this represents a substantial increase from the fewer than 2% of hospitals reporting the use of BCMA in 2002. (8) It is expected that implementation will increase due to efforts by the Food and Drug Administration, The Joint Commission, professional societies, and patient safety groups.

Because one of the major limitations of BCMA technology is the need to bar code all medications, a cursory understanding of the information contained in a bar code is necessary. A bar code is simply a graphic representation of data (alpha, numeric, or both) that is machine-readable. Bar codes are a way of encoding information using a combination of bars and spaces of varying widths stacked side by side. The scanner reads and interprets the rows and spaces as data. Data on medication bar codes can include information about the drug's name, dose, dosage form, route, expiration date, and lot number. Bar codes come in many varieties and symbologies (i.e., bar code languages). A scanner's ability to quickly and accurately interpret bar code data depends on the quality of the bar code print on the product, and the symbology and configuration of the bar code. Since space available on most unit-dose packages is limited, bar coding these packages is difficult although many manufacturers have been very successful in doing so.

Many pharmacies have to repackage and bar code medications because bar coded packages are not available from manufacturers. Unit dose packaging machines are available for purchase or lease that have bar coding capabilities. The cost can be substantial, but acceptable when weighed against the benefits in patient safety and added efficiency. Professional packaging systems allow pharmacies to reliably and efficiently bar code virtually all medication forms, including solids, liquid cups, vials, ampules and syringes. Much literature exists on the successful development and implementation of pharmacy-based bar code packaging operations and distribution systems.[22]

BCMA, by itself, is not an all-encompassing solution for medication safety. With any new process, there exists the potential for new sources of error including pharmacy medication repackaging errors, software interface failures, inefficient and inaccurate display of medication order information on the BCMA screen, and nursing workarounds (i.e., short cuts that subvert the safety system). In many pharmacies, individuals must be dedicated to dealing with the problems seen in BCMA technology. This additional cost is unavoidable given the potential benefits of BCMA. Table 11-4 provides a list of trade-offs associated with bar code medication administration systems.

Clinical Decision Support–Based Infusion Pumps

Errors associated with the administration of medications through intravenous infusion pumps to critically ill patients can result in adverse drug events. Variations in intravenous medication practices are also associated with increased risk of patient harm.[23] Indeed, as many as 60% of serious and life threatening errors may be associated with intravenous therapy.[24]

Intravenous (IV) infusion technology has changed tremendously over the years. **Smart pumps** (computerized infusion pumps) can now be programmed to allow infusion of several medications simultaneously and assist with complex dose calculations (i.e., loading, bolus, and maintenance doses). Devices can signal alerts when air is detected within the infusion line and be dedicated for specific needs (i.e., patient controlled analgesia, epidural pumps). Smart pumps take intravenous medication infusion safety a step further than manual pumps by performing clinical decision support at the point of care. This means a nurse can program a pump at the bedside and the pump will automatically check if the programmed doses are within acceptable ranges established by the pump's drug library. Doses outside acceptable ranges trigger an alert that must be addressed before the infusion can begin.

Smart pump software allows institutions to create individualized hospital profiles and drug libraries. Hospital profiles provide specific infusion device operating parameters, programming options, and drug libraries for specific patient populations (i.e., pediatric, pediatric intensive care, neonatal intensive care, adult critical care, or adult general care). Drug libraries are often institutional-specific medication lists that contain standard concentrations and preset dosing limits. Institutions often have the option to make dosing limits

Key Point . . .

Smart pumps take intravenous medication infusion safety a step further by performing clinical decision support at the point of care.

. . . So what?

Point of care technology allows professionals to adapt to the immediate situation at hand. Decisions can be made in response to patient needs at the bedside.

Table 11-4.

Potential Advantages and Disadvantages of BCMA Technology

Advantages	Disadvantages
■ Automated documentation	■ A number of devices are needed for busy or large nursing units, this may be cost-prohibitive for some organizations
◆ Comprehensive data and reports available "on demand"	
◆ Facilitates precise pharmacokinetic monitoring	■ All medications must be bar coded to ensure a realization of the safety benefits shown
◆ On demand view of a patient's history of administered medications	■ Lack of standard bar codes in health care
◆ Records and verifies in real time the exact time of medication administration information (eliminates missed/incomplete documentation	■ Manual printing of patient medication administration records at discharge for an organization without a fully integrated or interfaced electronic medical record
■ Improved patient safety and accuracy	■ Possible competition among nurses for access to devices (dependent on number of devices an organization can afford)
◆ Allergy checks are performed at the bedside	
◆ Bar code scanning to verify the appropriateness of a medication at the patient's bedside	■ Products are at early stages of development
	■ Radio frequency demands may be problematic for some organizations
◆ Maintains appropriate packaging and labeling of unit dose medications up to the point of administration, at the patient's bedside	■ Radio frequency devices are required for real-time updates from pharmacy computer system; may interfere with clinical patient monitoring devices
◆ Nurse is immediately alerted to discrepancies (wrong drug, dose)	
◆ Nurse is immediately alerted to missed doses	■ Short battery life requires extra batteries or frequent battery exchanges
◆ Real-time order and patient information is available to the nurse at the bedside	■ Success is dependent on nursing acceptance of the change
■ Increased charge accuracy through automation	◆ Implementation causes dramatic changes in how nurses perform their job
■ Automates tracking for controlled substances removed from decentralized dispensing devices but never scanned	
■ Marketing tool for the organization	
■ Nursing convenience	
◆ Customizable, medication administration planning reports	
◆ Easy documentation of medication administration criteria and vital signs at the bedside	
◆ Medication administration record is mobile and paperless	
◆ Small, light weight, wireless hand-held devices	

either hard limits (alerts that cannot be overridden) or soft limits (an overrideable alert with action). Once the pump is programmed, the smart pump software performs a test of reasonableness against the hospital profile and the drug library to verify the pump has been programmed correctly for the specific patient population and medication.

Smart pump software also has event recording capabilities. Data logs can track events such as the number of infusions programmed, the number of times an alert is given, the number of times an alert is overridden and detailed records for programming errors that were averted and could have caused patient harm. Depending on the vendor selected, data logs can often be accessed through direct or radio frequency downloads from each pump to a computer.

Dramatic reductions in medication infusion error rates can be seen with smart pump implementation.[25,26] However, smart pump technology is by no means foolproof, and at least one study found no measurable impact on the serious medication error rate following smart pump implementation, likely in part due to poor compliance.[27] Clinicians still have to use their own judgment. Workarounds circumventing the desired safety features of these pumps are common as the design of these pumps makes it easy for nurses to bypass the drug library which contains the drug dosing and rate limits. Alert fatigue is also a consideration if nurses are routinely prompted with alerts that are not considered clinically significant. Convincing nurses to use the safety features of this technology during time-pressed situations can be a challenge. Given that intravenous medication errors and adverse drug events are common and often very harmful, the use of this technology is likely to expand rapidly, perhaps more rapidly than BCMA and CPOE software. Although it has great promise, technological and nursing behavioral factors must be effectively addressed if smart pumps are to achieve their potential for improving medication safety.

Pharmacists must be very involved in the smart pump selection and implementation, particularly in developing the drug library and programming processes. They also need to be involved with alert analysis, quality assurance, and drug library upkeep. This technology offers a tremendous opportunity for pharmacist leadership in health systems.

Safety Issues Surrounding the Use of Automation

Ensuring System Accuracy and Reducing Errors

Although information technologies and automated dispensing systems are widely used in health systems and are integral to many regulatory and external quality reporting systems, little data exists regarding their appropriate use or impact on patient safety.[28] This is surprising given the cost and impact of technology on institutional infrastructure and practice. Nevertheless, there is consensus on the potential of technology to improve safety[1] and greater use in health systems is assured.

Automation has the potential to reduce medication errors, but technology by itself will rarely prevent medication errors. Rather, it must be effectively integrated into the existing medication-use system and appropriately managed. In fact, if implemented and used unwisely, technology can make things worse. Dedicated professionals are needed to manage and oversee implementation, training, quality assurance, and ongoing support and maintenance.

Health systems leaders can be unrealistic in what they expect from automation. Automation can instill a false sense of security and carelessness in leaders and health care professionals. For instance, it can cause professionals to neglect sound practices such as double- and triple-checking medication orders on the premise that, "The technology takes care of that." Pharmacists need to advocate for adequate processes, training of personnel, staffing, and quality control checks. The following specific features would be desirable for reducing errors:

- Bar coding of medications should be maximized throughout the medication-use process, especially the dispensing and administration phases.
- Information technologies need to be integrated to provide the necessary information about the total care of patients. For instance, CPOE systems need to be integrated or interfaced with laboratory and pharmacy systems.
- Pharmacists should have oversight of the dispensing process for automated dispensing systems.
- Pharmacists must have input into clinical decision support protocols regarding medication use.
- Automation needs to free pharmacists for clinical activities that enhance the safety of patients.
- Regardless of whether or not state regulations exist to assure safe use of technology, every health care organization needs to develop, enforce, and continuously improve multidisciplinary policies and procedures associated with patient safety.

Table 11-5 lists additional features of the use of automation in the medication-use process.

Regulatory Issues

In response to a lack of national standards and regulations for the safe use of automated dispensing systems, The National Association of Boards of Pharmacy (NABP) approved a document entitled *Model State Pharmacy Act and Model Rules* in May of 1997. The language in this act allows the definition of *dispensing* to include the use of automated technology, providing pharmacists with flexibility in the use of automation. But appropriately, it also required that such devices be used only in settings where an established program of pharmaceutical care ensures that medication orders be reviewed by a pharmacist in accordance with good pharmacy practice. The act requires policies and systems to assure safe and secure use of such devices but provides little guidance as to how. This act is intended to serve as a template for individual states to write (or rewrite) their State Pharmacy Practice Acts.

Despite the model act, some State Boards of Pharmacy erect barriers to automation. Some states require pharmacists to check every dose stocked in an automated dispensing device rather than allowing a system that incorporates technicians into the medication stocking process. Other states bog down automation initiatives with bureaucratic paperwork. Pharmacists need to play an active role in assuring that their state's Pharmacy Practice Act enables automated dispensing systems and the transfer of electronic medication (prescription) orders.

> **Key Point . . .**
>
> Automation can instill a false sense of security and carelessness in leaders and health care professionals.
>
> **. . . So what?**
>
> Technology sometimes seems almost magical. It can do so many good things that we often forget that machines are built and used by flawed human beings.

Table 11-5.
Desired Safety Features for Incorporating Automation into the Medication-Use Process

- A system must accommodate bar coded unit dose medications and utilize the bar code capability for drug restocking, retrieval, and administering medications.

- A system should force the user to specify a reason whenever medications are accessed or administered outside of the scheduled administration time or dosage range; all such events are signaled visibly or audibly to the user and are electronically documented and reported daily for follow-up.

- A unique bar code or user identification code and password are assigned to each user; audit trials of user actions must be reported in an easily viewed format and should include identification of the user, the medication, the patient for whom the drug was dispensed, and the time of the transaction.

- Bar code medication administration systems must be able to identify and document the patient, the medication, and the person administering using the scanning technology function.

- Devices are interlaced with the pharmacy computer system only allowing the nurse to view and access those medications that are ordered for a specific patient.

- Devices need electronic reminders to nurses when a medication dose is due (and by a different mechanism when it is past due).

- Hospital admit/discharge/transfer and medication order entry computer systems are interlaced with automation devices to provide caregivers with warnings about allergies, interactions, duplications, and inappropriate doses at the point of dispensing and/or administration.

- Patient specific information used in the daily care of patients must be timely, accurate, and easily accessible.

- Pertinent patient- and medication-specific information and instructions entered into pharmacy and/or hospital information systems are available electronically at the point of care (administration), and the system prompts the nurse to record pertinent information before administration may be documented.

- Real-time integration or interlaces exist for all steps in the medication-use process, starting at the point of prescribing, to order entry and dispensing, and through documentation of medication administration.

Quality Assurance

Regardless of whether or not state regulations exist to assure safe use of automated dispensing systems, it is extremely important that every organization develop, enforce, and continuously improve policies and procedures to ensure patient safety, accuracy, security and confidentiality. Specific areas that should be addressed in an organization's policies for safe use of automated dispensing systems and technology include accurate inventory and stocking controls, dispensing procedures, security and breach of security patient confidentiality reporting, documentation, training of personnel, initial and ongoing competency assessment, routine quality assurance and safety checks, scheduled (and unscheduled) hardware and software maintenance and support, and contingency plans for maintaining safe systems and service in the event of unscheduled downtime.

ASHP Positions, Statements, and Guidelines

The need for guidance in pharmacy practice has increased greatly with the changes in health care and with the influences from regulatory, accrediting, risk-management, financing, and other bodies. ASHP develops policies as positions, statements, and guidelines for pharmacy practice in integrated health systems (see www.ASHP.org/best-practices). The policies of ASHP represent a consensus of professional judgment, expert opinion, and documented evidence to provide guidance and direction to pharmacy practitioners and other audiences who affect pharmacy practice. Their content should be assessed and adapted to meet the needs of the specific organization. They are very useful in crafting departmental policies and in gaining pharmacist resources for coordination of automation projects within the organization. Policies contain varying levels of detail where positions are short pronouncements on one aspect of pharmacy practice, statements express a basic philosophy, and guidelines offer programmatic advice.

Current ASHP policy positions for automation and technology include machine-readable coding and related technology (0308), the pharmacist's role in electronic patient information and prescribing systems (0203), regulation of automated drug distribution systems (9813), automated systems (9205), and computerized prescriber order entry (0105). ASHP also provides detailed guidelines on the safe use of automated medication storage and distribution devices.

The machine-readable coding and related technology policy, for example, advocates an industry standard for the placement of bar codes and information contained in a machine-readable bar code for unit dose, unit of use, and injectable drug products. This particular policy statement was very influential in the Food and Drug Administration's final rule requiring the use of a linear bar code to encode the national data code (NDC) number on most prescription drug products by April of 2006. It is also ASHP's position that all medications be identified through machine-readable bar coding, as the use of bar code technology at the point of medication administration will help to ensure safe, accurate, and documented medication administration. ASHP also advocates pharmacist involvement when key decisions are made in the planning, selection, implementation, and maintenance of electronic patient information systems. Specific ASHP policy positions, statements, and guidelines germane to this chapter can be found at www.ASHP.org/bestpractices.

Selecting Automation Within a Health System

Historically, automation had to result in proven cost reduction, quality improvement, improved service, and/or increased efficiency in order to be funded. While expense continues to be a major barrier, various regulatory entities, external quality reporting groups, and the news media have pressured many institutions to prematurely invest heavily in new technologies based on a theoretic but unproven safety benefit.

Integrated health systems should not view automation and technology as a means to an end, but rather as a series of sophisticated tools to help them optimize the medication-use process. The value achieved by implementing new technology within organizations depends primarily upon three factors: the efficiency of the system being replaced, the level of detail applied to managing and making the most of the system following implementation, and cooperation between departments to assure success of the system. In 2008, The Joint Commission released a sentinel event alert (i.e., report of an unexpected occurrence involving death or serious injury) which provides focus to institutions on the safe implementation of health information and converging technologies. Suggested actions to help institutions prevent harm to patients include: examine workflow processes and procedures for risk and inefficiency and fixing issues prior to implementing technology; actively involve frontline clinicians, staff, and IT staff during the planning, selection, design, reassessment, and ongoing quality improvement; include a pharmacist in the planning and implementation of any technology involving medications; during implementation provide continual monitoring to identify problems and promptly address them; establish a well defined training program for all staff who will be using the technology; design a system that mitigates potentially harmful medication orders by developing standardized order sets and guidelines on paper, approve them through the pharmacy and therapeutics committee (P&T), and test them before going live; and after implementation continually reassess and enhance the safety and effectiveness of the technology.[29]

Within most hospitals, there is consensus that the inpatient medication-use process should be automated as much as possible, but there are questions and debate as to how to do so. There really is no single approach to automation and any approach can succeed or fail depending on how well it is managed.[30] Table 11-6 provides questions to consider in choosing automation vendors including considerations of desired automation system functionality, hardware and software technical requirements, installation and training support, and vendor/system reliability.

Cost Justification of Automated Systems

Historically, pharmacists could justify the costs of new automation if the technology improved the capture of medication charges or freed pharmacists to perform new billable services. This is no longer the case due to changes in hospital reimbursement from government and private payers. Now, detailed return-on-investment analyses are often needed to demonstrate that the technology makes good financial sense for the organization. The goal of a return on investment (ROI) analysis is to compare an organization's total costs before and after the implementation of automation and to demonstrate a positive ROI if a decision is made to support the automation. Chapter 13, "The Basics of Financial Management and Cost Control," provides details on what goes into conducting ROI analyses.

Automation's Impact on Pharmacy Manpower

Some pharmacists have been concerned over the years that increased use of automation coupled with expansion of the use of pharmacy technicians and prescription mail order services would reduce the demand for pharmacists. Fortunately, that has not been the case because efficiencies in automation have been offset by increased demand for pharmacy personnel due to an aging U.S. population, organizational recognition of value of clinical pharmacists, and the soaring number and complexity of medications used in hospitals. Still, the demand for dispensing pharmacists in comparison to clinical pharmacists will likely decrease as automated dispensing and patient monitoring technologies advance.

Automation will permit technicians to take over much of medication dispensing and distribution. Technicians will increasingly be expected to oversee automated dispensing systems and possibly smart IV pump and BCMA systems. This will permit pharmacists to move from distributive to clinical roles.

As technology provides pharmacists with opportunities to be more involved with direct care of patients, pharmacists will need to advocate for and promote the value of pharmacist patient care services to physicians and administrators. If not, some health-system pharmacist positions may be displaced by technology. Indeed, automation is currently forcing the issue of pharmacists' professional role in the redevelopment of health systems.

Table 11-6.
Automation Selection Criteria

- Can the vendor provide you with established policies and procedures for integrating the system into the pharmacy's daily work flow, clearly defining pharmacist and technician responsibilities, and clearly defining system downtime procedures?

- Cost-benefit analysis: Will reduced supply and labor expenses offset the cost of the automation? What is the potential increased revenue as a result of the automation?

- Does the system produce useful statistical and managerial reports, and do they provide a report writing and analysis tool?

- How does the system utilize bar code technology to improve accuracy of transactions?

- How long has the company been in business and how many units do they have in operation?

- How much space will the automation require, and is remodeling required?

- How much time is required for routine maintenance and equipment servicing? Does the company provide full service, routine and emergency software and hardware maintenance? What is the cost of this maintenance and how is it provided? Will routine maintenance disrupt workflow?

- How secure is the system?

- Is training interactive and computer-based? How will new users be trained on the system?

- Is the automation compatible with the organization's strategic goals?

- Is the company willing to guarantee a maximum percent downtime?

- Is the system compatible with existing information systems? Has the company interlaced their system with your pharmacy computer system in another organization? If not, what is the cost for building this interface? Who maintains the interface?

- What do existing customers say about the accuracy and reliability of the system, ease of use, and unscheduled downtime?

- What impact will the automation have on other departments? How are those departments involved in the selection process?

- What impact will the automation have on patient safety?

- What impact will the system have on controlled substance accountability and overall inventory control?

- What sets this company's product apart from their major competitors?

- Will the automation enable the provision of new clinical services?

- Will the vendor adapt the technology to meet your needs, goals, and objectives rather than expect your system to be redesigned to fit their product?

- Will the vendor provide you with a list of all current users?

- Will the vendor's training and implementation support meet your expectations and needs?

Given that continued automation of the dispensing process is inevitable, future work activities of pharmacists depend primarily on four things: (1) the breadth of tasks a pharmacy technician is legally allowed to perform (and/or allowed to perform by an employer); (2) the extent to which pharmacists are reimbursed for medication therapy management services; (3) the level of productivity that can be achieved through automated systems; and (4) the extent to which pharmacists are able to demonstrate improved quality and overall lower cost of patient care as a result of their role on the patient care team. Current dispensing automation clearly creates the potential for pharmacists to focus more of their time on direct patient care activities instead of product preparation.

Future Roles of Pharmacy Personnel as a Result of Automation

The transformation of the pharmacist role from distributor of drugs to cognitive provider of care has largely resulted from pharmacists' access to patient-specific information about diagnosis, laboratory results, treatment progress, and the patient's entire drug therapy regimen. Integrated delivery systems and automation will

■ ■ ■

Key Point . . .

Automation is currently forcing the issue of pharmacists' professional role in the redevelopment of health systems.

. . . So what?

Automation frees pharmacists from routine and repetitive tasks. It allows pharmacists to seek new opportunities to improve patient medication care. Indeed, if pharmacists do not identify professional roles in health systems, they risk become obsolete.

continue to provide pharmacists with opportunities to work more closely with physicians and patients to assure appropriate drug therapy decisions and outcomes. Toward this end, pharmacists must continue to assume increased accountability for understanding patient drug-related needs; identifying, solving and preventing drug-related problems; designing and initiating drug therapy plans; and continuing drug therapy plans once they are initiated. Pharmacists also have a responsibility to create systems to improve the quality and safety of drug distribution and administration. Pharmacists must possess good time management and problem solving skills and be able to focus the majority of their time on issues related to high-risk drugs and high-cost diseases, while paying particular attention to the dosing of high-cost drugs for all patients.

Pharmacists may find themselves working more in a virtual world of electronic information management where they never even touch a drug or paper prescription. Clinical pharmacists in the virtual world may have three primary responsibilities: to assess patient compliance and medication-related outcomes, drug and disease education, and intervention. The optimization of such roles in both inpatient and ambulatory environments offers opportunities to avoid displacement of pharmacists by automation.

Summary

Automation is not a panacea for the problems in pharmacy practice. There is no perfect technology, and automated systems must be well-managed to provide cost effective services and support the profession's transition to pharmacist patient care services. To be successful in the future, pharmacists must view automation-induced productivity and efficiency as desired goals, not as threats to their work. Optimized use of automation to perform distributive functions currently performed by pharmacists and technicians is essential in providing pharmacists with additional time to take care of patients. Every change must be implemented with an understanding of **human factors engineering** and safety science, as even good changes will create unexpected new hazards. In addition, policies and procedures must change as the use of technology increases to assure a safe and proper medication use infrastructure.

Pharmacy automation will continue to progress. Efficient electronic physician prescribing systems, fully automated dispensing systems, and virtual patient monitoring systems will be commonplace in the medication-use process of the future. Pharmacists have a choice to make such systems successful or to resist change. Opportunities exist for pharmacists who embrace automation, provide leadership to assure safe and efficient automation systems, and innovate through automation.

Suggested Reading

American Society of Hospital Pharmacists. ASHP statement on the pharmacist's role with respect to drug delivery systems and administration devices. *Am J Hosp Pharm.* 1993;50:1724-1725.

American Society of Health-System Pharmacists. ASHP guidelines on the safe use of automated compounding devices for the preparation of parenteral nutrition admixtures. *Am J Health-Syst Pharm.* 2000;57:1343-1348.

American Society of Health-System Pharmacists. ASHP guidelines on the safe use of automated medication storage and distribution devices. *Am J Health-Syst Pharm.* 1998;55:1403-1407.

American Society of Health-System Pharmacists. ASHP statement on the pharmacist's role in informatics. *Am J Health-Syst Pharm.* 2007;64:200-203.

American Society of Health-System Pharmacists. ASHP statement on bar code–enabled medication administration technology. *Am J Health-Syst Pharm.* 2009;66:588-590.

American Society of Health-System Pharmacists. ASHP Policy Positions: Automation and Information Technology. Available at: http://www.ashp.org/Import/PRAC-TICEANDPOLICY/PolicyPositionsGuidelinesBestPractices/BrowsebyTopic/Automation/PolicyPositions.aspx.

American Society of Health-System Pharmacists. ASHP Policy Positions: Drug Distribution and Control. Available at: http://www.ashp.org/Import/PRACTICEAN-DPOLICY/PolicyPositionsGuidelinesBestPractices/BrowsebyTopic/Distribution/PolicyPositions.aspx.

Bepko RJ, Jr., Moore JR, Coleman JR. Implementation of a pharmacy automation system (robotics) to ensure medication safety at Norwalk hospital. *Qual Manag Health Care.* 2009 April;18(2):103-114.

Dumitru D. *The Pharmacy Informatics Primer.* Bethesda, MD: American Society of Health-System Pharmacists; 2009.

Institute for Safe Medication Practices (ISMP): Guidance on the Interdisciplinary Safe Use of Automated Dispensing Cabinets. Available at: http://www.ismp.org?Tools/guidelines/ADC_Guidelines_Final.pdf.

The Joint Commission. Sentinel Event Alert: Safely Implementing Health Information and Converging Technologies. Available at: http://www.jointcommission.org/SentinelEvents/SentinelEventAlert/sea_42.htm.

Karsh, B. Beyond usability: designing effective technology implementation systems to promote patient safety. *Quality & Safety in Health Care.* 2004;13:388-394.

References

1. Bates DW, Cullen DJ, Laird N, et al. Incidence of adverse drug events and potential adverse drug events. *JAMA*. 1995;274:29-34.

2. Louie C, Brethauer B, Cong D, et al. Use of a drug wholesaler to process refills for automated medication dispensing machines. *Hosp Pharm*. 1997;32:367-375.

3. Carroll NV Changes in channels of distribution: wholesalers and pharmacies in organized health-care settings. *Hosp Phar Report*. 1997;Feb:48-57.

4. Barker KN, Felkey BG, Flynn EA, et al. White paper on automation in pharmacy. *Consultant Pharm*. 1998;13:256-293.

5. Vermeulen LC, Stiltner RS, Swearingen LL. Technology report revision: automated medication management in departments of pharmacy. Oakbrook, IL: University Hospital Consortium; 1996.

6. Thielke TS. Automation support of patient-focused care. *Top Hosp Pharm Manag*. 1994;14:54-59.

7. Perini VJ, Vermeulen LC. Comparison of automated medication-management systems. *Am J Hosp Pharm*. 1994;51:1883-1891.

8. Pedersen CA, Schneider PJ, Scheckelhoff DJ. ASHP national survey of pharmacy practice in hospital settings: dispensing and administration—2008. *Am J Health-Syst Pharm*. 2009;66:926-946.

9. Ray MD, Aldrich LT, Lew PJ. Experience with an automated point-of-use unit-dose drug distribution system. *Hosp Pharm*. 1995;30:18-30.

10. Lee LW, Wellman GS, Birdwell SW, et al. Use of an automated medication storage and distribution system. *Am J Hosp Pharm*. 1992;49:851-855.

11. Barker KN. Ensuring safety in the use of automated medication dispensing systems. *Am J Health-Syst Pharm*. 1995;52:2445-2447.

12. Sutter TL, Wellman GS, Mott DA, et al. Discrepancies with automated drug storage and distribution cabinets. *Am J Health-Syst Pharm*. 1998;55:1924-1926.

13. Borel JM, Rascati KL. Effect of an automated, nursing unit-based drug-dispensing device on medication errors. *Am J Health-Syst Pharm*. 1995;52:1875-1879.

14. Guerrero RW, Nickman NA, Jorgenson JA. Work activities before and after implementation of an automated dispensing system. *Am J Health-Syst Pharm*. 1996;53:548-554.

15. Institute for Safe Medication Practices (ISMP): Guidance on the Interdisciplinary Safe Use of Automated Dispensing Cabinets. Available at: http://www.ismp.org?Tools/guidelines/ADC_Guidelines_Final.pdf. Accessed June, 2009.

16. Oswald S, Caldwell R. Dispensing error rate after implementation of an automated pharmacy carousel system. *Am J Health-Syst Pharm*. 2007;64:1427-1431.

17. Kuiper SA, McCreadie SR, Mitchell JF et al. Medication errors in inpatient pharmacy operations and technologies for improvement. *Am J Health-Syst Pharm*. 2007;64:955-959.

18. Anderson S, Wittwer W. Using bar-code point-of-care technology for patient safety. *J Healthcare Qual*. 2004 Nov-Dec;26(6):5-l0.

19. Cummings JR *UHC Technology Report: Bar-Coded Medication Administration*. Oakbrook, IL: University Health System Consortium; 2005.

20. ASHP. Pharmacist's toolkit—implementing a bar coded medication safety program. Available at: http://www.ashpfoundation.org/MainMenuCategories/PracticeTools/BarCodeGuide.aspx. Accessed June, 2009.

21. Presentation from University of Wisconsin Hospital and Clinics. Bar coding and point of care systems: experiences at UWHC. Available at: http://www.uhc.edu/Web/COU/RX/BXDec02_mtg/AcuScan.pdf. Accessed July, 2005.

22. Ragan R, Bond J, Major K, et al. improved control of medication use with an integrated bar-code—packaging and distribution system. *Am J Health-Syst Pharm*. 2005;62:1075-1079.

23. Bates DW, Vanderveen T, Seger D, et al. Variability in intravenous medication practices: implications for medication safety. *Jt Comm J Qual Patient Saf*. 2005;31(4);203-210.

24. Eskew JA, Jacobi J, Buss WF, et al. Using innovative technologies to set new safety standards for the infusion of intravenous medications. *Hosp Pharm*. 2002;37:1179-1189.

25. Wilson K, Sullivan M. Preventing medication errors with smart infusion technology. *Am J Health-Syst Pharm.* 2004;61:177-183.

26. Williams CK, Maddox RR. Implementation of an i.v. medication safety system. *Am J Health-Syst Pharm.* 2005;62:530-536.

27. Rothschild J, Keohane CA, Cook F, et al. A controlled trial 'of smart infusion pumps to improve medication safety in critically ill patients. *Crit Care Med.* 2005;33(3):533-540.

28. Oren E, Shaffer ER, Guglielmo BJ. Impact of emerging technologies on medication errors and adverse drug events. *Am J Health-Syst Pharm.* 2003;60:1447-1458.

29. The Joint Commission. Sentinel Event Alert: Safely Implementing Health Information and Converging Technologies. Available at: http://www.jointcommission.org/SentinelEvents/SentinelEventAlert/sea_42.htm. Accessed March, 2009.

30. Darby AL. Considering a hybrid system for automated drug distribution. *Am J Health-Syst Pharm.* 1996;53:1128,1134,1137.

Chapter Review Questions

1. **Automation is one solution pharmacy departments have used to reduce the amount of pharmacist and technician labor required to perform dispensing activities.**
   a. True
   b. False

   Answer: a. True. As the profession has accepted increased responsibility for improving patient outcomes through implementation of pharmacist patient care services, automation has been relied upon to free the pharmacist from technical tasks.

2. **Medication errors resulting in adverse drug events (ADEs) only have effects on the patients that suffer from a medication error.**
   a. True
   b. False

   Answer: b. False. Medication errors resulting in ADEs (preventable ADEs) can result in significant patient harm and consumption of resources in the form of increased lengths of stay, increased cost of care, rework time, malpractice claims, and patient costs (suffering and lost productivity).

3. **Medication errors have been found to occur most often in which of the following phases of the medication-use process?**
   a. Ordering
   b. Transcribing
   c. Dispensing
   d. Administration

   Answer: a. A study by Bates et al. found that 49% of all ADEs occur in the ordering phase of the medication-use process.

4. **Inefficient processes for product procurement and inventory management can hamper a pharmacy's ability to provide direct patient care.**
   a. True
   b. False

Answer: a. True. Poor product procurement systems can result in pharmacists spending excessive time trying to locate products.

5. **Which of the following cannot be automated by centralized automated dispensing devices?**
   a. Medication storage
   b. Restocking
   c. Crediting
   d. Dispensing

   Answer: a, b, c, and d. Centrally located automated dispensing devices are designed to automate the entire process of medication dispensing including medication storage, dispensing, restocking, and crediting of unit dose medications.

6. **Carousel dispensing technology (CDT) provides the maximum efficiency and safety when dispensing medications.**
   a. True
   b. False

   Answer: b. False. Although CDT will result in improved dispensing accuracy and labor efficiency, no single technology configuration has been shown to be best.

7. **Centralized narcotic dispensing and record keeping systems provide better control, reporting, and diversion detection, than do manual record keeping systems.**
   a. True
   b. False

   Answer: a. True. It is very common to find hospitals that have moved all traditional, narcotic vault drug inventories into automated dispensing cabinets linked to narcotic inventory control software as a means to improve narcotic inventory control and dispensing accuracy within the hospital.

8. **_____ technology offers the potential to dramatically reduce the risk of medication errors during the administration phase of the medication-use process.**

   Answer: Bar code medication administration (BCMA). BCMA can reduce medication administration errors that occur as the following discrepancies: wrong patient, wrong drug, wrong dose, or wrong time. Other benefits include improved patient safety, documentation accuracy, and nurse satisfaction, as well as public and patient relations that can result from a well-designed and implemented BCMA system. These benefits dramatically outweigh BCMA implementation challenges.

9. **Once an automated system is implemented and its accuracy verified, there is no need for an institution to have double check policies and procedures in place for the automated process.**
   a. True
   b. False

   Answer: b. False. All personnel must be adequately educated so that they understand that technology cannot completely substitute for human safety checks, therefore, it absolutely critical that appropriate quality control systems exist to assure the accurate and safe use of automation. If appropriately managed and properly integrated or interfaced, all of these systems should ultimately improve patient safety and would likely be incorporated into most medication-use systems of the future.

10. **Selection of automation should include an analysis of:**
    a. Desired automation system functionality
    b. Hardware and software technical requirements
    c. Installation and training support
    d. Background checks for vendor systems
    e. All of the above

    Answer: e. All of the above. Automation selection should include a complete analysis of desired automation system functionality, hardware and software technical requirements, installation and training support, and vendor/system background reference checks.

Chapter Discussion Questions

1. Describe your ideal automation selection team in terms of the personnel needed and purpose for each member's inclusion.
2. Compare the advantages and disadvantages for the use of unit based dispensing cabinets for medication delivery.
3. Compare the advantages and disadvantages for the use of centralized dispensing automation.
4. Describe the effect automation can have on the future of health-system pharmacy practice. How will the role of the pharmacist change as a result of advances in automation?
5. Given a choice of automation products to implement, which solution would you choose to implement first and why?

CHAPTER 12

Purchasing and Inventory Control

Jerrod Milton

Learning Objectives

After completing this chapter, readers should be able to:

1. Describe the steps in purchasing medications and inventory control.
2. Define key terminology in purchasing and inventory control.
3. Discuss the processes for managing medication inventory.
4. Identify products that require special handling.

Key Terms and Definitions

- **Economic order quantity (EOQ):** A model of inventory control (also known as the Minimum Cost Quantity approach) that uses past history of inventory use, costs, and demand to develop an accounting model that predicts optimal inventory order quantities that minimizes order costs and inventory holding costs.
- **Group purchasing organizations:** Purchasing groups consisting of health systems and hospitals who join together to obtain greater collective buying power.
- **Inventory carrying costs** (or holding costs): All costs associated with inventory investment and storage. It might include interest, insurance, taxes, and storage expenses.
- **Inventory turns:** The fraction of a year that an average item remains in inventory. High inventory turnover is a sign of efficiency because inventory is constantly at work and generating revenue. Low turnover is a sign of inefficiency.
- **Just-in-time inventory management:** A philosophy of inventory management where products are ordered and delivered at just the right time—when they are needed for patient care—with a goal of minimizing wasted steps, labor, and cost. The goal is to neither over- nor under-stock products.
- **Order book:** A list of products that need to be ordered from a supplier.
- **Pareto ABC analysis:** Based on the principle that states that a relatively

small number of drugs account for a disproportionate amount drug usage in a health system. Thus, a Pareto ABC analysis groups inventory products by aggregate value and volume of use into three groupings (A, B, and C). Products in group A are the small percentage of items that make upon the greatest amount of inventory cost. Groups B and C make up decreasingly less cost.

■ **Par-level systems:** Based on the principle that individual inventory drug use falls with a predictable range or "par-level." In these systems, a range is identified and minimum and maximum order quantities are set. Inventory is ordered in a way that maintains amounts within the par-level.

■ **Perpetual inventory:** a record of inventory that is constantly updated when items are added or subtracted from inventory.

■ **Prime vendor contract:** a contract between a health-system pharmacy and a wholesaler where the pharmacy agrees to purchase most of its pharmaceuticals from a single wholesale company in return for advantageous pricing, terms of drug delivery, and support services (e.g., providing the pharmacy with electronic order entry/receiving devices and bar-coded shelf stickers).

■ **Stock rotation:** the process of placing products nearest to the time of expiration at the front of the shelf or storage unit so they will be used first.

■ ■ ■

Introduction

Purchasing and inventory control are important to all pharmacists because they are essential elements of the medication use system. They are also fundamental to patient safety because they impact the ability of the system to provide the right drug, to the right patient, in the right amount, by the right route of administration, and at the right time and frequency. Therefore, an effective purchasing and inventory control system requires the understanding and active participation of all pharmacy staff.

This chapter describes the basic principles of pharmaceutical purchasing and inventory control. It applies to all types of pharmacy settings including decentralized, centralized, home infusion, and ambulatory care pharmacy operations.

The Formulary System

The formulary is the cornerstone of the purchasing and inventory control system.[1-3] The formulary is developed and maintained by a committee of medical and allied health staff called the pharmacy and therapeutics (P&T) committee. This group generally comprises physicians, pharmacists, nurses, and administrators, although other disciplines may be present, including dieticians, medication safety officers, risk managers, and case managers. These professionals collaborate to ensure that the safest, most efficacious, and economical medications are included on the formulary.

The products on the hospital formulary dictate what the hospital pharmacy should purchase and keep in inventory. Third-party prescription drug benefit providers will also establish plan-specific formularies for their ambulatory patients. Ambulatory (retail) pharmacy staff frequently encounter insurance plan-specific drug formularies in serving their patients and adjust their inventory accordingly. Most retail pharmacies do not rigidly restrict items in their inventory, because in this setting, inventories are largely dependent on the dynamic needs of their patient population and, to some degree, their patients' respective insurance plans. Therefore, the concept of formulary management differs greatly depending on the practice setting (e.g., that of the hospital compared with that of the retail pharmacy).

The hospital formulary is generally available in print or online formats. The formulary is produced exclusively for all health practitioners involved in prescribing, dispensing, and monitoring medications, and this tool is formatted generally to inform users of product availability, the appropriate therapeutic uses, and recommended dosing of medications. Most formularies are organized alphabetically by the generic drug's name, which is typically cross-referenced with the trade name products. In most cases, the drug storage areas in the pharmacy are arranged alphabetically by either the generic or trade name of the drug. Therefore, the formulary can help the pharmacy personnel determine if a product is stocked in the pharmacy and where it would be shelved.

Drugs are added and deleted from the formulary on a regular basis with the frequency varying among organizations. Formulary publications should remain current (typically being updated every 12 to 18 months at minimum). Loose-leaf formularies and those maintained online can be updated continuously in a timelier manner, whereas bound formulary handbooks rely on supplementary updates or publication of serial editions.

Important information available in the formulary includes the dosage form, strength, and concentration; package size(s); common side effects; and administration instructions. Some institutions also indicate the actual or relative cost of a given item to guide the prescribing of the most cost effective alternatives. When selecting a drug product from inventory, the technician must consider all product characteristics, such as name, dosage form, strength, concentration, and package size. In practice settings where an electronic medical record system (**EMR**) is employed, it is possible to have real-time access to online formulary publications at the point where and when the provider places a medication order. Detailed review and consideration of each listing helps minimize errors in product selection.

Managing the Purchasing and Inventory Control System

Some pharmacies employ a few specialized individuals charged with managing the purchasing and inventory process of pharmaceuticals, while others utilize many individuals in the role.[4] Limiting the number of individuals to a specialized few permits greater expertise and efficiency, but it can also keep the remaining pharmacy staff uninformed and unengaged in purchasing and inventory control. This can be a problem if there is turnover in the specialists. It can also lead to a lack of appreciation of the importance of purchasing and inventory control by those who are uninformed and unengaged. Cross training individuals in purchasing and inventory control can help them better understand the system and make better decisions in daily practice to support patient care.

State-of-the-art practice in purchasing and inventory control uses computer and Internet technology to manage purchasing and receiving of pharmaceuticals from a drug wholesaler.[5] This technology includes using bar codes and hand-held computer devices for online procurement and purchase order generation and for electronic receiving processes. Using computer technology for these purposes has many obvious benefits, including up-to-the-minute product availability information, comprehensive reporting capabilities, accuracy, tighter inventory control and efficiency. It also helps in complying with various pharmaceutical purchasing contracts by keeping track of terms and reminding about deadlines and contract pricing deals.

Receiving and Storing Pharmaceuticals

Receiving medications from suppliers is one of the most important parts of the pharmacy operation. A poorly organized and executed receiving system can put patients at risk and elevate health care costs. For example, if the wrong concentration of a product were received by the pharmacy, it could lead to a dosing error or a delay in therapy. Misplaced products or out-of-stock products also jeopardize patient care as well as the efficiency of the department; both are undesirable and costly outcomes.

The Receiving Process

Some pharmacies follow a policy that requires the person who receives pharmaceuticals be different from the person ordering them. This process is especially important for controlled substances because it effectively establishes a check in the system to minimize potential drug-diversion opportunities.

In a reliable and efficient receiving system, the receiving personnel verify that the shipment is complete and intact (i.e., they check for missing or damaged items) before putting items into circulation or inventory.[2] The receiving process begins with the verification of the boxes containing pharmaceuticals delivered by the shipper. The person receiving the shipment first verifies that the name and address on the boxes are correct and that the number of boxes matches the shipping manifest. Many drug wholesalers use rigid plastic crates to deliver orders because they protect the contents of each shipment better than foam or cardboard boxes. These crates are also environmentally friendly because they are returned to the wholesaler for cleaning and reuse. Regardless, each box should be inspected for gross damage.

Products with a cold storage requirement (i.e., refrigeration or freezing) should be processed first. The shipper is responsible for taking measures to ensure the cold storage environment is maintained during the shipment process and will generally package these items in a shippable foam cooler that includes frozen cold packs to keep products at the correct storage temperature during shipment.

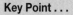

Key Point . . .

Some pharmacies require that the person who receives pharmaceuticals be different from the person ordering them.

. . . So what?

The potential to divert drugs is substantial during the process of ordering and receiving. The more steps an employee controls in the purchasing and inventory process, the more opportunities that employee has to divert products and cover up that diversion.

Receiving personnel play a critical role in protecting the pharmacy from financial responsibility for products damaged in shipment, products not ordered, and products not received. Any obvious damage or other discrepancies with the shipment, such as a breach in the cold storage environment or delivery of an incorrect product, should be noted on the shipping manifest, and, if warranted, that part of the shipment should be refused. Ideally, identifying gross shipment damage or incorrect box-counts should be performed in the presence of the delivery person and should be well-documented when signing for the order. Other problems identified after delivery personnel have left, such as mis-picks, product dating, or internally damaged goods, must be resolved according to the vendor's policies. Most vendors have specific procedures to follow in reporting and resolving these sorts of discrepancies.

The next step of the receiving process entails checking the newly delivered products against the receiving copy of the purchase order. This generally occurs after the delivery person has left. A purchase order, created when the order is placed, is a complete list of the items that were ordered. Traditionally, a purchase order will be executed in multiple copies, including an original file copy, a copy used in the receiving process, and a copy for the supplier.

The person responsible for checking products into inventory uses the receiving copy. This ensures that the products ordered have been received. The name, brand, dosage form, size of the package, concentration strength, and quantity of product must match the purchase order. Once the accuracy of the shipment is confirmed, the purchase order copy is generally signed and dated by the person receiving the shipment. At this point, the expiration date of products should be checked to ensure that they meet the department's minimum expiration date requirement. Frequently, departments will require that products received have a minimum shelf life of 6 months remaining before they expire. Otherwise, the products may expire before use and have to be destroyed or returned to the supplier. It is noteworthy to mention that on occasion, the manufacturer/wholesaler may inadvertently ship an excess quantity of an ordered product to the pharmacy. The ethical response is to notify the manufacturer or wholesaler of this situation immediately and subsequently arrange for the return of any excess quantity.

Controlled substances require additional processing on receipt.[2,6] Regulations specific to Schedule II controlled substances require Drug Enforcement Administration (DEA) Form 222 to be completed on receipt of these products and filed separately with a copy of the invoice and packing slip accompanying each shipment. If a pharmacist or pharmacy technician other than the receiving technician removes a product from a shipment before it has been properly received and cannot locate the receiving copy of the purchase order, then a written record of receipt should be created. This is done by listing the product, dosage form, concentration/strength, package size, and quantity on a blank piece of paper or the supplier's packing slip/invoice and checking off the line item received. In both cases, the name of the person receiving the product should be included, and the document should be given to the receiving technician to avoid confusion and an unnecessary call to the wholesaler or manufacturer.

The Storing Process

Once the product has been received properly, it must be stored properly.[7] Depending on the size and type of the pharmacy operation, the product may be placed in a bulk, central storage area or into the active dispensing areas of the pharmacy. In any case, the expiration date of the product should be compared with the products currently in stock. Products already in stock that have expired should be removed. Products that will expire in the near future should be highlighted and placed in the front of the shelf or bin. This is a common practice known as **stock rotation**. The newly acquired products will generally have longer shelf lives and should be placed behind packages that will expire before them. Stock rotation is an important inventory management principle that encourages the use of products before they expire and helps prevent the use of expired products and waste. It is safe to assume that the first-in, first-out (FIFO) method of inventory management is applied when it comes to pharmaceutical products.

All stock should be sorted at temperature and humidity levels recommended by manufacturers and defined by the United States Pharmacopoeia (USP). Table 12-1 identifies the optimum storage temperatures and humidity conditions. Periodic checks of refrigeration and other storage areas should be conducted to ensure they fall within recommended ranges.

Product Handling Considerations

The Role of the Pharmacy Technician

Pharmacy technicians usually spend more time handling and preparing medications than do pharmacists. This presents pharmacy technicians with the critical responsibility of assessing and evaluating each product from both a content and a labeling standpoint. It also provides the technician with an opportunity to confirm that the receiving process was performed properly.

Just as checking the product label carefully at the time a prescription or medication order is filled is important, taking the same care when receiving pharmaceuticals and accurately placing them in their storage location is essential. The pharmacy technician should read product packaging carefully, rather than rely on the general appearance of the product (e.g., packaging type, size or shape, color, logo), because a product's appearance may change frequently and may be similar to other products. Technicians play a vital role in minimizing dispensing errors that may occur because of human fallibility. They are generally the first in a series of checks involved in an accurate dispensing process.

When performing purchasing or inventory management roles, the technician must pay close attention to the product's expiration date. For liquids or injectable products, the color and clarity of the items should also be checked for consistency with the product standard. Products with visible particles, an unusual appearance, or a broken seal should be reported to the pharmacist.

Table 12-1.
Defined Storage Temperatures and Humidity[8]

Freezer	(-)25° to (-)10°C	(-)13° to 14°F
Cold (refrigerated)	2° to 8°C	36° to 46°F
Cool	8° to 15°C	46° to 59°F
Room temperature	The temperature prevailing in a working area	
Controlled room temperature	20° to 25°C	68° to 77°F
Warm	30° to 40°C	86° to 104°F
Excessive heat	Any temperature above 40°C (104°F)	
Dry place	A place that does not exceed 40% average relative humidity at controlled room temperature or the equivalent water vapor pressure at other temperatures.	
	Storage in a container validated to protect the article from moisture vapor, including storage in bulk, is considered a dry place.	

Because pharmacy technicians handle so many products each day, they are in a perfect position to identify packaging and storage issues that could lead to errors. The technician should pay close attention to these three main issues:

1. *Look-alike/sound-alike (LASA) products*—Stocking products of similar color, shape, and size could result in error if someone fails to read the label carefully. All staff members should be alerted to look-alike or sound-alike products (Figure 12-1).[9]
2. *Misleading labels*—Sometimes the company name or logo is emphasized on the label instead of the drug name, concentration, or strength (Figure 12-2).[10]
3. *Product storage*—Storing products that are similar in appearance adjacent to one another can result in error if someone fails to read the label (Figure 12-3).[11]

Alerting other staff members to products that fall into one of these categories is essential. Some pharmacies routinely discuss product-handling considerations at staff meetings or in departmental newsletters. Errors may be averted by simply relocating a LASA product or by placing warning notes (i.e., auxiliary labeling or highlights) on the shelf or directly on the product itself. Pharmacy technicians should also discuss their concerns with coworkers and advocate changes to products with poor labeling.

■ ■ ■

Key Point . . .

Pharmacy technicians have key responsibilities in assessing the labeling and ensuring the quality of each product received and placed into inventory.

. . . So what?

Some pharmacists have difficulty delegating responsibilities to pharmacy technicians. Technicians are micromanaged and discouraged from acting as independent contributors of the health care team. However, technicians are as good, or better, than pharmacists at many tasks in medication purchasing and distribution. Empowering technicians to take on tasks such as ensuring the quality of the inventory is essential for well run medication distribution.

Maintaining and Managing Inventory

An inventory management system is an organized approach designed to maintain just the right amount of pharmaceutical products in the pharmacy at all times. A key goal of inventory management is to maximize **inventory turns,** meaning simply that products should be used and not remain on the shelf. Although drugs left on the shelf could be considered assets, their useful shelf life wanes with each passing day and excessive inventory is an unproductive asset, tying up money and resources that can be used in running other elements of the pharmacy operation. Inventory turns, defined in accounting terms, are the fraction of a year that an average item remains in inventory.

A simple means of calculating inventory turns in a given period is to divide the total purchases in that period by the value of physical inventory taken at one point in time. For example, if total pharmaceutical purchases for fiscal year (FY) 2010 were $10,243,590, and the physical inventory value on 12/31/2009 was $521,550, then the calculated inventory turns for FY2010 would be 19.6 times ($10,243,590/$521,550 = 19.6). This method assumes a relatively constant volume of pharmaceutical purchases and constant residual inventory over time. If greater variability in purchasing volume exists, then the average of 2-year purchasing statistics could be used as the numerator in the formulas represented. Like any business, performing a physical inventory at approximately the same time in every fiscal period will produce more meaningful, comparable results. Seasonal variables and new drugs entering the formulary should be considered in comparative analyses.

Inventory turnover is a way of measuring the productivity of a pharmacy's inventory use and the use of invested capital. High inventory turnover is a sign of efficiency because inventory is constantly at work and generating revenue. Low inventory turnover is a sign that product (capital) is sitting unused on the shelf and is a signal of operational inefficiency.

A variety of inventory management systems are used in pharmacy practice, ranging from simple to complex. They include the order book, the minimum/ maximum (par) level, the Pareto (ABC) analysis, the economic order quantity (EOQ), and just-in-time systems.[3] Each of these systems attempt to maximize inventory turnover while at the same time minimize inventory carrying costs (or holding costs). **Carrying costs** are defined as all costs associated with inventory investment plus storage costs, which might include interest, insurance, taxes, and storage expenses, among others.

> ### Key Point . . .
> All inventory management systems attempt to simultaneously maximize inventory turnover and minimize inventory carrying costs.
>
> ### . . . So what?
> There is a fine balance going on in inventory control. Order too little, and products will not be on the shelf when needed. However, order too much, and products will set on the shelves unused. When inventory does not turn, it is like burning money. All pharmacy personnel should understand this fact.

Order Book

Many pharmacies use an order book system, also called a want list or want book. The order book is the simplest form of inventory control. When used as the sole method of inventory control, it is likely to lead to over- and under-ordering of inventory. The **order book** is a simple order list—much like a home grocery shopping list. When pharmacists or pharmacy technicians identify a product that needs to be reordered, they write the item in the order book. The listed drugs are then ordered periodically from wholesalers or other suppliers.

Although this approach is simple, it provides the least amount of organized control of inventory. One reason is that is highly dependent on the active participation of staff. Individuals must note how much drug inventory remains on the shelf, remember how much is typically used over a specified time period, forecast a need for that drug, and place a request on the order book. It is common for individuals to not notice the need for a drug or forget to note the need on the order book (causing an inventory shortage that is embarrassing and difficult to manage in the course of urgent or routine patient care). However, even the most diligent and attentive individuals can make mistakes because the order list approach relies excessively on people's memories and individual discretion. A faulty memory or poor judgment can lead to running out of drugs or ordering too much. If too much is ordered, at best, it may reduce inventory turnover, while at worst, it may remain unused on the shelf until it expires and must be returned to the supplier. Therefore, the order book system is usually not the sole method of inventory management and is often used in conjunction with one of the other systems mentioned previously.

Par-Level Systems

Par-level inventory systems are slightly more sophisticated than the order book. The par-level inventory system relies on a predetermined order quantity and an order point.

Figure 12-1. Look-alike/sound-alike products.

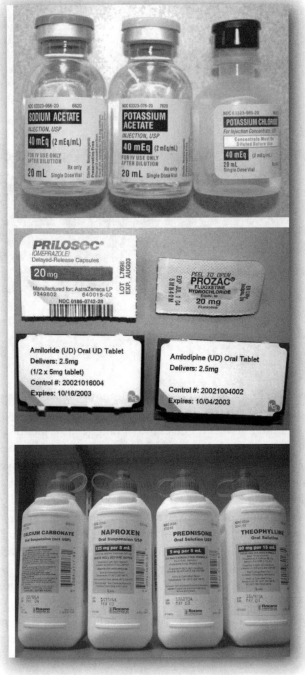

Figure 12-2. Product labeling; emphasis on manufacturer name.

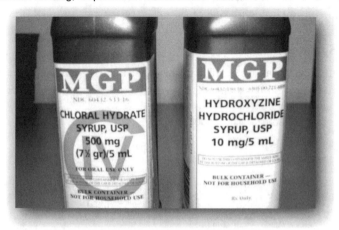

Figure 12-3. Product inventory; shelf position.

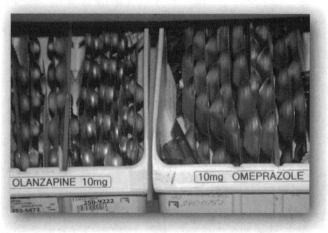

Par-level systems, also known as minimum/maximum systems, are based upon the principle that individual inventory drug use falls within a predictable range. The term "par-level" means within a standard range. If that range can be identified, then minimum and maximum order quantities can be set. Thus, a shelf-sticker is developed for each inventory product that identifies the minimum and maximum quantities of drug to be kept on hand. Shelf labels are placed on the storage bin or shelf to alert all staff to the minimum stock quantity (Figure 12-4). These shelf stickers act as a general guide for staff to avoid running short on a product or overstocking. In more sophisticated models where real-time inventory quantity is maintained, a computerized database may be employed to manage a par-level system as opposed to shelf stickers and manual accounting. When the inventory is reduced to, or below, the order point, designated pharmacy personnel initiate a purchase order, or electronically transmit a purchase order, to a drug wholesaler. The amount of drug ordered should be of a sufficient quantity to bring the amount to a level within the min-max range, but should generally not exceed the maximum level established. This system requires pharmacy staff to routinely scan inventory levels, often using a hand-held bar-code scanning device, and place orders accordingly.

Figure 12-4. Shelf labels.

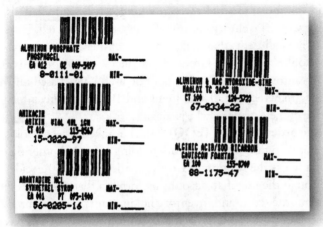

The par-level system can be either managed manually or electronically. Frequent reassessments of the par levels must be conducted to respond to the diversity of patient needs. In the fully computerized inventory system, each dispensing transaction is subtracted from the **perpetual inventory** log that is maintained electronically; conversely, all products received are added to the inventory log. When the quantity of a pharmaceutical product in stock reaches a predetermined par-level point, a purchase order is automatically generated to order more of the product. The system does not depend on any one employee to monitor the inventory or to reorder pharmaceuticals. The technology is available to have a computerized inventory in most pharmacies, but interfacing a computerized inventory system with existing pharmacy computer systems designed for dispensing and patient management is often difficult. In addition, other variables, such as product availability, contract changes, and changing use patterns (either up or down), make relying on the fully computerized model challenging. Consequently, even the most sophisticated electronic or automated systems require careful human oversight.

Economic Models

Economic models of inventory control attempt to use economic and statistical methods to predict the need for drugs over time. One time-tested model is the Pareto ABC analysis. The **Pareto ABC analysis** is based on the 80/20 principle that states that approximately 80% of most problems can be attributed to roughly 20% of their potential causes. Applied to inventory control, the Pareto principle highlights the fact that a relatively small number of drugs account for a disproportionate amount of drug usage (and often times cost) in a

> **Key Point . . .**
>
> The Pareto ABC method of inventory control is based on the 80/20 principle which highlights the fact that a relatively small number of drugs account for a disproportionate amount drug usage and expense.
>
> **. . . So what?**
>
> The 80/20 principle is useful in prioritizing almost any action in medicine, business, or other aspect of life. Knowing that focusing on the 20% of the things causing 80% of the variability associated with a problem can save time and improve performance.

health system. Thus, a Pareto ABC analysis essentially groups inventory products by aggregate value and volume of use into three groupings (A, B, and C). This analysis is useful in determining where inventory control efforts are best directed. For example, group A may include 10% of all items that make up 70% of the inventory cost. Tight control over these items would be sensible. Group B may include 20% of items and 15% of the inventory cost. An automatic order cycle might be useful here based on well-established par levels. Group C may include 70% of items and 10% of the inventory cost. Less aggressive monitoring of these items may be justifiable.

The **economic order quantity (EOQ)** model of inventory control is another method that attempts to minimize inventory holding costs and ordering costs. The EOQ approach (also known as the Minimum Cost Quantity approach) decides inventory order quantities through the use of an accounting formula that calculates the point where the combination of order costs and inventory holding costs are minimized.

The exact details of the EOQ approach is beyond the scope of this chapter but some details are relevant. EOQ relies heavily on the accuracy of various data inputs, such as annual product usage, fixed costs associated with each order (including processing the purchase order, receiving, inspection, processing the invoice, vendor payment, and inbound freight costs), and the annual cost per average on-hand inventory unit. If calculated accurately, it results in the most cost-efficient order quantity. It can be argued that anytime one has repetitive purchasing tasks, EOQ should be considered. However, applying EOQ universally is relatively difficult in pharmacy practice because of the wide variability of the individual patient's pharmaceutical needs. Therefore, some pharmacies may find it useful to use EOQ with a combination of the other systems mentioned here.

A sophisticated system for inventory management is an automated or computerized system that supports a just-in-time product inventory.[12] **Just-in-time inventory management** is a philosophy that simply means products are ordered and delivered at just the right time—when they are needed for patient care—with a goal of minimizing wasted steps, labor, and cost. Pharmaceuticals are neither overstocked nor under-stocked. The pharmacy's productivity "pulls" the inventory required into the system at just the right time. In pharmacy, this business philosophy couples responsible financial management of pharmaceutical purchasing with the clinical aspects of patient care.

The use of automated dispensing devices in inpatient hospital nursing units, clinics, operating rooms, and emergency rooms has facilitated the use of computers for inventory management. These devices are essentially repositories, or pharmaceutical vending machines, for medications that will be dispensed directly from a patient care area. A variety of manufacturers of automated dispensing devices are in the market today. The Pyxis Medstation and Omnicell suppliers are examples of products available to institutions today. These machines generally are networked via a dedicated computer file server within the facility, and they allow both unit-dose and bulk pharmaceuticals to be stocked securely on a given patient care unit location. The machines are capable of tracking perpetual inventory at the product level. They also limit access to only authorized personnel, record the identities of those who access inventory, and record how much of a specific drug was removed for a given patient. A useful feature in many of these systems allows pharmacy personnel to automatically generate a fill-list of what needs to be replenished on the basis of a par-level system. In essence, the nursing and medical personnel who use these automated dispensing devices have a computerized inventory and billing system that the pharmacy staff manages. Medications used to restock these devices may be taken from the pharmacy's main inventory, or a separate purchase order may be executed for each device on a periodic basis.

Drug Recalls

A manufacturer, on its own or at the direction of the Food and Drug Administration (FDA), will occasionally recall pharmaceuticals for such reasons as mislabeling, contamination, lack of potency, lack of adherence to the acceptable Good Manufacturing Practices, or other situations that may present a significant risk to public health. A pharmacy must have a system for rapid removal of any recalled products.[2]

Role of the Food and Drug Administration in Recalls

The FDA plays an active role in initiating the drug-recall process. It coordinates drug recall information, helps manufacturers and distributors develop specific recall plans, and performs health hazard evaluations to assess the risk facing the public by products being recalled. It also classifies recall actions in accordance with the level of risk and formulates recall strategies on the basis of the health hazard presented by the product in addition to other factors, including the extent of distribution of the product to be recalled. It decides on the need for public warnings and assists the recalling agency with public notification about the recall as needed. The following are top reasons for drug recalls[13]:

1. Deviations in good manufacturing processes at the manufacturer
2. Subpotency
3. Stability data does not support expiration date
4. Generic drug or new drug application discrepancies
5. Dissolution failure
6. Label mix-ups
7. Content uniformity failure
8. Presence of foreign substance
9. pH failures
10. Microbial contamination of nonsterile products

Key Point . . .

Pharmacies must have systems in place to rapidly remove any recalled products.

. . . So what?

A proactive system of removing recalled products protects patients and saves time for pharmacy employees. Without a system to easily identify drugs for removal, employees have to comb through the inventory every time a recall occurs.

Role of Manufacturer/Distributor in Recalls

Because of their responsibility to protect the public consumer, manufacturers or distributors typically implement voluntary recalls when a marketed drug product needs to be removed from the market. This method of recall is more efficient and effective in ensuring timely consumer protection than an FDA-initiated court action or seizure of the product. Recall notices are sent in writing to pharmacies by the manufacturer of the product or by drug wholesalers. These notices indicate the reason for the recall, the name of the recalled product, the manufacturer, all affected lot numbers of the product, and instructions on how to return the product to the manufacturer. On receipt of the recall notice, a pharmacy staff member, usually a pharmacy technician, will check all pharmaceutical inventory stores to determine if any recalled products are in stock. If none of the recalled products are in stock, a note indicating "none in stock" is written on the recall notice and filed in a recall log to document that the recall was properly addressed. If a recalled product is in stock, all products should be gathered, packaged, and returned to the manufacturer according to the instructions on the recall notice. The package should be reviewed by the pharmacist in charge before returning it to the manufacturer. If patients have received a recalled product, the pharmacist in charge must take actions recommended by the institution's policies and procedures. On completion of all activity regarding the product recall, a summary of actions taken should be documented on the recall letter and filed for later access. The FDA has been known to request documentation of all recall activities to ensure compliance and, ultimately, patient safety. Pharmacy personnel should keep in mind that it may be necessary to order replacement stock to compensate for recalled items that were removed from stock. In some instances, the recall may encompass all products, and it will be impossible to order replacement stock.

The pharmacist in charge should be notified in this case because he or she will need to decide which, if any, alternative products may need to be placed into inventory as therapeutic alternatives to the out-of-stock items.

Drug Shortages

Occasionally, manufacturers will be unable to supply a pharmaceutical because of various supply and demand situations. This may involve the inability of the manufacturer to obtain raw materials, manufacturing difficulties related to equipment failure, or simply the inability to produce sufficient quantities to stay ahead of the market demand for the pharmaceutical. Although unfortunate, drug shortages are a reality that must be dealt with to avoid compromising patient care. As with drug recalls, the pharmacist in charge should be notified so he or she can communicate drug shortages and recommend alternative therapies effectively to prescribers.

Ordering and Borrowing Pharmaceuticals

Pharmaceutical Purchasing Groups

Most health-system pharmacies are members of a **group purchasing organization** (GPO).[4,14] Health systems, hospitals, and ambulatory practices can join together in a purchasing group to leverage collective buying power and take advantage of any lower prices manufacturers offer to large groups that can guarantee a significant volume of orders over long periods of time (typically 1 to 2 years). Contracts may involve sole-source or multisource products. Sole-source products (typically brand-name drugs) are available from only one manufacturer, whereas multisource products (often generics or substitute products) are available from numerous manufacturers.

GPOs negotiate purchasing contracts that are mutually favorable to members of the group and to manufacturers. Members benefit from lower drug prices and reduced need for staff to spend time establishing and managing purchasing contracts with product vendors. Manufacturers benefit from a steady demand for products from the purchasing organization.

A typical contract works as follows. A GPO guarantees the price for pharmaceuticals over the established contract period, which may be 1 year or more. With the purchase price predetermined, the pharmacy can order the product directly from the manufacturer or from a wholesale supplier. Occasionally, manufacturers are unable to supply a given product that the pharmacy is buying on contract, which may require the pharmacy to buy or substitute a competing product not on contract at a higher cost. Most purchasing contracts will include language to protect the pharmacy from incurring additional expenses in the event this occurs. Generally, the manufacturer will be liable to rebate the difference in cost back to the pharmacy when this occurs. Therefore, it is important that the pharmacy technician documents any resulting off-contract purchases and shares these with the pharmacist in charge for reconciliation with the contracted product vendor.

Direct Purchasing

Direct purchasing from a manufacturer involves the execution of a purchase order from the pharmacy to the manufacturer of the drug instead of indirectly through a wholesaler. The advantages of purchasing direct rather than from a middleman include not having to pay handling fees to a third-party wholesaler, the ability to order on an infrequent basis (e.g., once a month), and a less demanding system for monitoring inventory. Disadvantages include the need to order larger quantities to take advantage of manufacturer discounts, the need for more capacity to store the additional inventory, more cash tied up in inventory, more complicated drug return and crediting, and the need to spend more time to prepare, process, and pay purchase orders to many different companies. Other disadvantages have to do with the likelihood that the manufacturer may be distant to the pharmacy creating problems with long lead times and product delivery.

For most pharmacies, the disadvantages of direct ordering outweigh the advantages. As a result, most pharmacies primarily purchase through a drug wholesaler. Some drugs, however, can be purchased only directly from the manufacturers. These products generally require unique control or storage conditions. Consequently, most pharmacies will have a combination of direct purchases from manufacturers and drug wholesalers.

> **Key Point . . .**
>
> For most pharmacies, the advantages of purchasing from wholesalers outweigh the advantages of ordering direct from manufacturers.
>
> **. . . So what?**
>
> There is a misconception, often promoted by advertisers, that "buying direct" or "cutting out the wholesaler" saves money. However, when one considers the purchasing costs, carrying costs, and other costs associated with ordering direct from a large number of suppliers, purchasing from wholesalers often provides better value.

Drug Wholesaler Purchasing/Prime Vendor Purchasing

Purchasing from a drug wholesaler permits the acquisition of drug products from different manufacturers through a single vendor. When a health-system pharmacy agrees to purchase most (90% to 95%) of its pharmaceuticals from a single wholesale company, a **prime vendor contract** arrangement is established, and, customarily, a contract between the pharmacy and the drug wholesaler is developed. Usually, wholesalers agree to deliver 95% to 98% of the items on an acceptable schedule and offer a 24-hour/7-day-per week emergency service. They also provide the pharmacy with electronic order entry/receiving devices, a computer system for ordering, bar-coded shelf stickers, and a printer for order confirmation printouts. They may also offer highly competitive discounts including those for prepayment. These wholesaler services make the prime vendor contracts appealing and result in more timely ordering and delivery, less time spent creating purchase orders, fewer inventory carrying costs, less documentation, computer-generated lists of pharmaceuticals purchased, and overall simplification of the credit and return process.

Purchasing through a prime vendor customarily allows for drugs to be received shortly before use, supporting the just-in-time ordering philosophy mentioned earlier in this chapter. Purchasing from a wholesaler is a highly efficient and cost-effective approach toward pharmaceutical purchasing and inventory management.

Borrowing Pharmaceuticals

No matter how effective a purchasing system is, there will be times when the pharmacy must borrow drugs from other pharmacies. Most institutional pharmacies have policies and procedures addressing this situation. Borrowing or loaning drugs between pharmacies is usually restricted to emergency situations and limited to authorized staff.

Borrowing is also limited to commercially available products, thus barring any borrowing of compounded products or investigational medications. Most pharmacies have developed forms to document and track borrowed or loaned merchandise (Figure 12-5). These forms also help staff document the details imperative to error-free transactions.

The pharmacy department's borrowing and loan policies and procedures should provide detailed directions on the process, which products may be borrowed or loaned, sources for the products, and reconciliation of borrow-loan transactions (the pay-back process). Securing the borrowed item may require the use of a transport or courier service or may include the use of security staff or other designated personnel. This information is vital for pharmacy personnel to understand and fulfill their responsibility when borrowing and loaning products.

Products Requiring Special Handling

Most pharmaceuticals will be handled and processed in the inventorying and purchasing systems described above, with the exception of controlled substances, investigational drugs, compounded products, repackaged drugs, and drug samples.

Figure 12-5. Borrow/loan form.

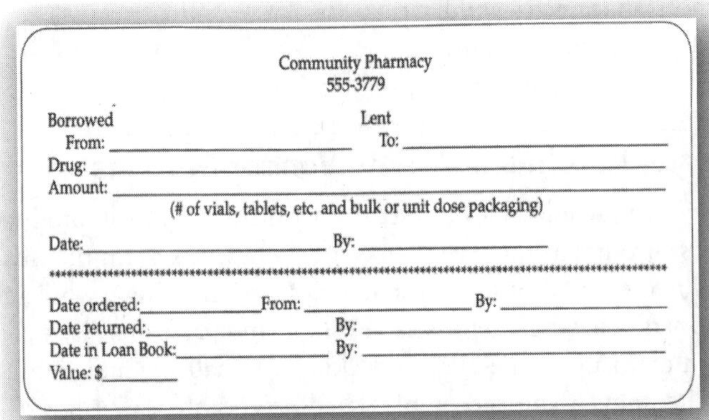

Community Pharmacy
555-3779

Borrowed From: ______ Lent To: ______
Drug: ______
Amount: ______
(# of vials, tablets, etc. and bulk or unit dose packaging)

Date: ______ By: ______

Date ordered: ______ From: ______ By: ______
Date returned: ______ By: ______
Date in Loan Book: ______ By: ______
Value: $______

Controlled Substances

Controlled substances have specific ordering, receiving, storage, dispensing, inventory, record-keeping, return, waste, and disposal requirements established under the law (see Chapter 8: Controlled Substances Management). The Pharmacist's Manual: An Informational Outline of the Controlled Substances Act of 1970 and the ASHP Technical Assistance Bulletin on Institutional Use of Controlled Substances also provide detailed information on the specific handling requirements for controlled substances.[6]

In some pharmacies, pharmacy technicians work with pharmacists to manage inventory and order, dispense, store, and control narcotics and other controlled substances. The pharmacy technician should know two principles regarding controlled substances: (1) Ordering and receiving Schedule II controlled substances requires special order forms and additional time (1 to 3 days), and (2) these substances are inventoried and tracked continuously via a perpetual inventory process, whereby each dose or packaged unit is accounted for at all times.

Investigational Drugs

Investigational drugs also require special ordering, inventorying, and handling procedures. Generally, the use of investigational drugs is categorized into two distinct areas: (1) in a formal protocol approved by the institution, and (2) for a single patient on a one-time basis that has been authorized by the manufacturer and the FDA. In both cases, the physician may be responsible for the ordering, and the pharmacy staff handles the inventory management of the investigational drug.

Some pharmacies associated with academic affiliations or institutions conducting clinical research may have formally organized investigational drug services managed by a pharmacist principally dedicated to pharmaceutical research activities. In these cases, the investigational drug service pharmacist may be responsible for the ordering, dispensing, and inventory management of investigational drugs according to the research protocol.

Compounded Products

Compounded pharmaceuticals are another type of product handled by pharmacy personnel, and unlike drugs ordered from an outside source, compounded products are extemporaneously prepared in the pharmacy as indicated by scientific compounding formulas and processes. These products may include oral liquids, topical preparations, solid dosage forms, or sterile products.

The use of these products requires that prescribing patterns and expiration dates be monitored closely because many compounded products have short shelf lives. Pharmacy technicians will likely be the ones charged with monitoring patient use of compounded drugs, product expiration dates, and identifying additional stock needs. Specific pharmacy technicians may initiate compounding activities, but this may vary according to departmental procedures.

Repackaged Pharmaceuticals

Although manufacturers supply many drugs in a prepackaged unit dose form, the pharmacy staff is responsible for packaging some products. These items are generally unit-dose tablets and capsules, unit-dose oral liquids, and some bulk packages of oral solids and liquids. Each pharmacy establishes stocking mechanisms for these products and relies on pharmacy technicians to identify and respond to production and stock needs. Generally, designated technicians coordinate repackaging activities, but some pharmacies may integrate repackaging with other pharmacy technician responsibilities. Knowledge of the department's procedures for repackaging is required to prevent disruptions in dispensing activities.

Nonformulary Items

Nonformulary items also require special handling. No matter how much planning is devoted to formulary management, some patients will legitimately need medications not routinely stocked in the pharmacy. The pharmacist usually determines when a nonformulary medication should be ordered into stock. However, the pharmacy technician is often in the best position to monitor the supply and determine when and if additional quantities should be ordered. Nonformulary medications generally are stored separately from formulary products and have separate inventory mechanisms. Manual tracking mechanisms and computer system queries of active nonformulary orders are the two most common techniques used to monitor and order these products.

Medication Samples

Storage and use of medication samples in institutions is controversial and requires special handling procedures. Traditional inventory management and handling practices do not work well with medication samples for two reasons. First, medication samples are not ordered by the pharmacy; they are usually provided to physicians on request by the drug manufacturer free of charge. This often occurs without the pharmacy's knowledge. Second, samples are not usually dispensed by the pharmacy. These factors make it difficult to know whom to contact if a medication sample is recalled and to ensure that medication samples are not sold. Because of difficulties in controlling samples, organizations may allow samples to be stored and dispensed in ambulatory clinics only after being registered with the pharmacy for tracking purposes. These difficult logistical and control factors have led many organizations to adopt policies that simply disallow medication samples altogether.

If an organization allows samples, they will probably be stored outside the pharmacy, and pharmacy personnel will be required to register and inspect the stock of medication samples. Pharmacy technicians are sometimes involved in inspecting medication sample storage units. These technicians are often responsible for determining if a sample is registered with the pharmacy, stored in acceptable quantities, labeled with an expiration date that has not been exceeded, and, generally, stored under acceptable conditions.

Proper Disposal and Return of Pharmaceuticals

Expired Pharmaceuticals

The most common reason drugs are returned to the manufacturer is because

Key Point . . .

The logistical and control problems associated with medication samples has caused many pharmacies to prohibit their use in institutions.

. . . So what?

Samples are not "free." They encourage use of new, more expensive drugs for patients—often in opposition to pharmacy efforts to provide the most cost effective medications to patients. Samples also require a separate inventory control and distribution system that adds to pharmacy personnel and overhead costs.

they are expired. Each year, approximately 2% of all drugs shipped to pharmacies are returned to the manufacturer.[15] The process for returning drugs in the original manufacturer packaging is relatively simple and not particularly time-consuming when done routinely. Returning expired products to the manufacturer or wholesaler prevents the inadvertent use of these products while enabling the department to receive either full or partial credit for them. Some wholesalers limit credit given on returns of short-dated products. Generally, wholesalers will not give full credit on returns of products that will expire within 6 months. To return products, pharmacy personnel must complete the documentation required by the product's manufacturer or wholesaler and package the product so it can be shipped. Many wholesalers have implemented electronic documentation systems to further simplify the return process.

Technicians often perform these duties under the supervision of a pharmacist. Some pharmacies contract with an outside vendor who completes the documentation and coordinates the return of these products for a fee. In that case, the pharmacy technician need only assist the returned goods vendor with the location and packaging of expired pharmaceuticals.

Pharmaceuticals compounded or repackaged by the pharmacy department cannot be returned and must be disposed of after they have expired. Proper disposal prevents the use of sub-potent products or products without guaranteed sterility. The precise procedure for disposal depends on the type and content of the product. Some products, such as expired repackaged solids, can be disposed of using the general trash removal system, whereas others, such as expired compounded cytotoxic products, must be disposed of according to hazardous waste removal procedures. Each pharmacy has detailed procedures for hazardous waste removal, and pharmacy personnel should be familiar with these procedures. Disposal of expired compounded or repackaged pharmaceuticals by the pharmacy technician should be completed under the supervision of the pharmacist.

Other products requiring disposal rather than return are chemicals used in the pharmacy laboratory. Most pharmacies will stock a supply of chemical-grade products used in extemporaneous pharmaceutical compounding. Examples of chemical products include sodium benzoate or sodium citrate (preservatives), lactose or talc (excipients), buffers, and active ingredients, such as hydrocortisone, triamcinolone, neomycin, or lidocaine powders. When such products expire, they should be disposed of in accordance with the pharmacy's hazardous waste procedures.

Expired controlled substances are disposed of uniquely. These products may not be returned to the manufacturer or wholesaler for credit. They must be destroyed, and the destruction must be documented to the satisfaction of the DEA.[6] The DEA provides a specific form, titled "Registrant's Inventory of Drugs Surrendered" (Form 41), for recording the disposal of expired controlled substances (available at ww.FDA.gov). Ideally, the actual disposal of expired controlled substances should be completed by a company sanctioned by the DEA or by a representative of the state board of pharmacy. In other cases, the DEA may allow the destruction of controlled substances by a pharmacy provided the appropriate witness process is followed and documented. The DEA disposal of controlled substances form should be completed properly and submitted to the DEA immediately after the disposal. A copy of the record of disposal form will be signed by a DEA representative and returned to the pharmacy, where it is kept on file. Previously, the DEA allowed for shipment of expired controlled substances and the completed disposal form to the regional DEA office, but this practice is no longer permitted.

The disposition of expired investigational drugs must also be documented carefully. Expired investigational drugs should be returned to the manufacturer or sponsor of an investigational drug study according to the instructions they provide. Investigational drug products that expire because of product instability or sterility issues should never be discarded. These doses should be retained with the investigational drug stock and be clearly marked as expired drug products because the investigational study sponsor will need to review and account for all expired investigational drug products.

Pharmaceuticals that need to be returned because of an ordering error require authorization from the original supplier and the appropriate forms. The Prescription Drug Marketing Act mandates that pharmacies authorize and retain records of returned pharmaceuticals to prevent potential diversion of pharmaceuticals. The pharmacy personnel must be familiar with pharmacy department procedures for returning medications to a supplier. Typically, a pharmacy will have a process for returning mis-ordered medications to the prime drug wholesaler on a routine basis, which prevents the need for storage in the pharmacy of overstocked or mis-ordered products. The pharmacy technician may be responsible for relevant documentation, filing paperwork, and packaging returned products under the supervision of the pharmacist.

Summary

Figure 12-6 summarizes the main issues covered in this chapter. A wide variety of drugs requiring unique handling procedures are purchased and stored in institutional pharmacy inventories. These include controlled substances, investigational drugs, and norm-formulary medications. Inventory of these drugs is managed with one or more forms of inventory control, from the simple (order book) to the complex (EOQ). Drugs are purchased

Figure 12-6. The medication purchasing and inventory system.

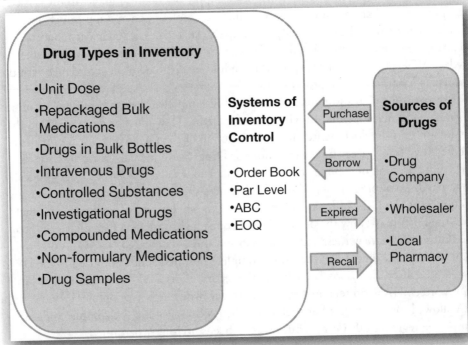

directly from companies or indirectly through wholesalers in most cases, although they are sometimes borrowed from other pharmacies in emergency situations. The movement of pharmaceuticals into and out of the pharmacy through purchase, borrowing, recall, or expiration requires an organized, systematic, and cooperative approach. Each pharmacy staff member plays a role in the management of his or her pharmacy's system.

Suggested Reading

Carroll N. "Accounting for inventory and cost of goods sold." In: *Financial Management for Pharmacists: A Decision-Making Approach.* Philadelphia: Lea & Febiger; 1991.

West DS. "Purchasing and inventory management." In: Desselle SP, Zgarrick DP, eds. *Pharmacy Management.* New York: McGraw-Hill/Appleton & Lange; 2004:373-388.

References

1. American Society of Hospital Pharmacists (ASHP). ASHP statement on the formulary system. *Am J Hosp Pharm.* 1983;40:1384-5.

2. Soares DP. Quality assurance standards for purchasing and inventory control. *Am J Hosp Pharm.* 1985;42:610-620.

3. Bicket WJ, Gagnon JP. Purchasing and inventory control for hospital pharmacies. *Top Hosp Pharm Manage.* 1987;7(2):59-74.

4. Yost DR, Flowers DM. New roles for wholesalers in hospital drug distribution. *Top Hosp Pharm Manage.* 1987;7(2):84-90.

5. Roffe BD, Powell MF. Quality assurance aspects of purchasing and inventory control. *Top Hosp Pharm Manage.* 1983;3(3):62-74.

6. U.S. Department of Justice Drug Enforcement Administration. Pharmacist's manual: an informational outline of the Controlled Substances Act of 1970. Washington, DC: DEA; April 2004. Available at: http://www.deadiversion.usdoj.gov/pubs/manuals/pharm2/pharm_manual.htm. Accessed May, 2005.

7. Joint Commission on Accreditation of Healthcare Organizations (JCAHO). *Hospital Accreditation Standards 2005.* Oakbrook Terrace, IL: JCAHO; 2005: MM11-13.

8. United States Pharmacopeia (USP). *USP 28/The National Formulary 23.* Rockville, MD: USP; 2004:10.

9. Joint Commission on Accreditation of Healthcare Organizations (JCAHO). *Hospital Accreditation Standards 2005.* Oakbrook Terrace, IL: JCAHO; 2005.

10. Cohen MR. *Medication Errors.* Washington, DC: American Pharmaceutical Association; 1999:13.1-13.22.

11. Cohen MR. *Medication Errors.* Washington, DC: American Pharmaceutical Association; 1999:9.1-9.9.

12. Hughes TW. Automating the purchasing and inventory control functions. *Am J Hosp Pharm.* 1985;42:1101-1107.

13. U.S. Food and Drug Administration/Center for Drug Evaluation and Research. Report to the nation—improving public health through human drugs. Washington, DC: FDA; 2003. Available at: http://www.fda.gov/cder/reports/rtn/2003/Rtn2003.pdf. Accessed May, 2005.

14. Wetrich JG. Group purchasing: an overview. *Am J Hosp Pharm.* 1987;44:1581-1592.

15. Orey M. Cottage industry finds niche in expired drugs. *WSJ (Eastern Ed).* New York: Aug 29, 2001:B.1.

Chapter Review Questions

1. **The _____ is developed and maintained by the P&T committee and the cornerstone of the purchasing and inventory control system.**

   Answer: formulary. The formulary determines what is purchased and stored in pharmacies. An overly lenient formulary leads to a large number of products to be purchased and inventoried. This leads to greater inventory carrying costs and less efficient use of inventory.

2. **Pharmacies frequently require that medications received from suppliers have a minimum shelf life of _____ remaining before the medications expire.**
   a. 2 years
   b. 1 year
   c. Six months
   d. 1 month

   Answer: c. Actually, the answer to this question is dependent on the policies of each individual pharmacy. Six months is a good answer because it allows enough time for pharmacies to use the drug, but still allows suppliers to use up their supply of medications with longer expiration dates.

3. **The process of placing newly acquired products behind currently stocked medications of the shelf is called _____.**

   Answer: stock rotation. Stock rotation tries to ensure that drugs with the shortest shelf expiration date will be used first. This assumes that the drugs currently on the shelf have shorter expiration dates than those being received from the supplier.

4. **If total pharmaceutical purchases for fiscal year (FY) 2010 are 10 million dollars and the physical inventory value on 12/31/2009 was 1 million dollars, the calculated inventory turns for FY2010 would be _____.**
   a. 5
   b. 10
   c. 15
   d. 20

   Answer: b. ($10 million/$1 million = 10).

5. **Which of the following inventory control systems is the least sophisticated and most prone to poor inventory control?**
   a. Order book
   b. Par-level
   c. Pareto ABC analysis
   d. EOQ approach

   Answer: a. The order book is similar to a home shopping list and relies on the memories, attentiveness, and conscientiousness of busy pharmacy staff members. This is a recipe for poor inventory management.

6. **Which of the following systems of inventory control system is also known as the maximum/minimum method of inventory control.**
   a. Order book
   b. Par-level
   c. Pareto ABC analysis
   d. EOQ approach

Answer: b. The par-level inventory system sets minimum and maximum order quantities based upon the principle that individual inventory drug use falls with a predictable range.

7. **Voluntary recalls of products initiated by the FDA are more efficient and effective in ensuring timely consumer protection than FDA recalls or seizures initiated through court action.**
   a. True
   b. False
   c. Answer: a. True. Recalls initiated by the courts are slow and costly. That is why active participation by pharmacists in voluntary recalls is essential for ensuring the safety of patients and the drug distribution system.

8. **Purchasing drugs direct from the manufacturer saves pharmacies money in comparison to ordering from wholesalers.**
   a. True
   b. False

   Answer: b. False. In most cases, the potential lower prices seen in ordering directly from manufacturers is more than offset by the increased administrative and carrying costs.

9. **_____ contracts are agreements between a health-system pharmacy and a wholesaler where the pharmacy agrees to purchase most of its pharmaceuticals from a single wholesale company.**

   Answer: Prime vendor. Prime vendor contracts give the pharmacy better drug prices, terms of drug delivery, and support services in return for using a single wholesaler for most purchases.

10. **Which of the following drug classes can be returned to suppliers after expiration?**
    a. Prepackaged drugs
    b. Chemical-grade products used in extemporaneous compounding
    c. Investigational drugs
    d. Controlled substances

    Answer: c. Investigational drugs are typically returned to the manufacturer or sponsor of the research although investigational protocols may indicate otherwise. Drugs from the other drug categories must be disposed of using various procedures described in the chapter.

Chapter Discussion Questions

1. How do hospital formularies influence the process of inventory control?
2. How does a hospital formulary differ from a formulary seen in community pharmacy settings?
3. Should inventory control be delegated completely to specific individuals or should all employees be involved in the process?

4. What are the positive and negative consequences of outsourcing inventory control to local wholesalers?
5. Compare the advantages and disadvantages of order book, economic model, and just-in-time inventory management systems.

CHAPTER 13

The Basics of Financial Management and Cost Control

Andrew L. Wilson

■ ■ ■
Learning Objectives

After completing this chapter, readers should be able to:

1. Identify the role of pharmacists in financial management of institutional resources.
2. Define key financial terms.
3. Describe the pharmacy and hospital budget process and the different budget components that comprise a pharmacy budget.
4. Discuss the purpose of productivity measurement and benchmarking in controlling operating costs.

Key Terms and Definitions

■ **Accounting:** A standard method for reporting the expenses, revenues, and accumulation of assets, and other financial results.

■ **Acuity:** Variations in the healthcare needs of a patient based on their severity of illness.

■ **Assets:** The real, intangible, and financial items that are owned by the health system.

■ **Balance sheet:** A financial statement which lists the wealth of the institution at a specific point of time.

■ **Budget:** A plan for future expenses and revenue, typically over a 12-month period.

■ **Capital budget:** The part of the budget typically comprised of items that cost more than a fixed threshold (e.g., an expense >$5,000) and have a useful life greater than 5 years.

■ **Capital expense:** Costs of a physical improvement or a piece of equipment that will provide benefit over a number of years. Capital expenses are typically significant in size and scope.

■ **Case mix index (CMI):** An indicator of the average diagnosis related group (DRG) weight for all patients at an institution.

■ **Case rate:** A negotiated payment that is based on a diagnosis-related group, a per diem (daily) amount, or other benchmark method to determine the hospital's payment. The hospital receives the case rate payment for the complete patient care episode, irrespective of the individual charges posted to the patient's account.

■ **Chief executive officer (CEO):** The highest ranking executive in a health system, in charge of the total management and making the major corporate decisions.

■ **Chief financial officer (CFO):** A corporate officer primarily responsible for managing the financial risks of a corporation.

■ **Diagnosis related group (DRG):** A system to classify hospital cases into one of approximately 500 groups, also referred to as DRGs, expected to have similar hospital resource use. The patient's primary diagnosis is typically the basis for payment.

■ **Direct expense:** Expenses that are incurred by the pharmacy to deliver services and products.

■ **Double entry bookkeeping:** A bookkeeping technique of entering a transaction on both sides of the balance sheet (as a debit on one side and a credit on the other) to keep income and expenses balanced.

■ **Equity (also called net worth):** The net of assets and liabilities.

■ **Expense:** A payment made by the health system to others for value received.

■ **External benchmarking:** A process of measuring costs, services, and practices and comparing them to the organization's peers or to industry leaders.

■ **Fixed expense:** A category of direct expense that does not vary significantly in the short-term with the volume of activity.

■ **General ledger:** A detailed record of each financial transaction of the hospital.

■ **Income statement:** A statement that lists the Revenue, Expense, and Profit (or loss) of the institution over a period of time.

■ **Indirect expense:** (also called overhead): Payments for services that support the pharmacy but are not directly paid by the pharmacy.

■ **Internal benchmarking:** The process of measuring costs, services, and practices against the organization's prior performance.

■ **Liabilities:** The debts, i.e., unpaid bills the hospital owes to creditors, loans, and bonds issued.

■ **Operating budget:** The part of the budget that represents a forecast of the daily expenses required to operate the pharmacy.

■ **Return on investment (ROI) or return on equity (ROE):** A mathematical model that measures how effectively funds invested in the firm by its owners or stockholders have been used.

■ **Revenue:** Money received for products or services provided to customers.

■ **Time and motion study:** A review of the activities and resources required to produce a good or service. A time and motion study is used to determine the resources necessary to complete a task or set of tasks and can be the basis to set goals for improvement or change.

■ **Variable expense:** A category of direct expense that varies in the short-term with the level of activity.

■ **Variance:** The difference between the budgeted amount and the actual amount spent for a period, typically a month or for the fiscal year to date.

■ **Volume budget:** The number of admissions, patient days, CMI, outpatient visits, emergency department visits, and other activities. The volume budget is prepared by the CFO and is the basis for budget calculations.

■ **Work volumes:** Work units and paid hours are generally used to describe pharmacy work volume. Health-system pharmacy workload volume may include prescriptions filled, orders processed, or doses dispensed and combinations of these components.

Introduction

Financial management and cost control are key activities for pharmacists in leadership roles in institutional practice. The high cost of pharmaceuticals, high pharmacist salaries, combined with the compelling need for pharmacy services and medication therapy in hospital care require thoughtful, cost-conscious management to ensure success. The growth of support systems and technology to manage medication use process safety and effectiveness, including automation and information systems add to the scope of financial management and cost control responsibilities of pharmacists. Pharmacy directors and managers encounter tension between their patient care leadership and their management roles as they work to balance costs, benefits and patient care outcomes in delivering pharmaceutical care. A working knowledge of financial management is essential to ensure that high quality pharmacy services are effectively delivered, and that the patient care mission of the pharmacy and the hospital are carried out optimally.

Pharmacists in hospitals are charged with developing and maintaining a medication use system that provides the highest quality of care and one that serves the medical and pharmaceutical needs of the patient to their fullest. However, in a health care delivery system where resources are finite, the pharmacy leadership role requires monitoring, prioritizing, and actively managing pharmaceutical and professional resources to use them to their greatest advantage. Building working relationships with administration, physicians, nurses and others is based on an understanding of key relationships in cost management and finance. Figure 13-1 is a schematic representation of the financial relationships and key terms which underlie the discussion later in the chapter. In some instances, resource limitations and the balance between cost and benefit for pharmacy services and medication therapy may not be well-defined by senior hospital management or medical staff leadership, adding the burden and the opportunity to develop a broader, financially responsible plan for the hospital or health system to the pharmacy director.

An active, engaged pharmacy director is well-versed in clinical and professional disciplines surrounding medication use and pharmaceutical care. The director also possesses a keen understanding of the financial and productivity performance for his or her areas of responsibility and works to understand the role of the pharmacy service in the context of the institution. A knowledgeable pharmacy manager works to communicate the impact of pharmacy services and medication therapy, and secure the necessary resources to accomplish these goals. Audiences and forums for these discussions include the medical staff, in pharmacy and therapeutics committee meetings, and other discussions and senior hospital leadership in budget review and other administrative meetings. Because of the scope, magnitude, costs and outcomes associated with medication therapy, health-system boards of trustees and corporate leaders rely on pharmacists to contribute to understanding the impact of medication costs. Increasingly, a key role of pharmacy leadership is to articulate a coherent plan for clinical pharmacists and other pharmacy staff to understand the balance of cost, benefit, and outcome in their daily professional decision-making.

Thoughtful financial management and cost control strategies allow institutional pharmacy directors to ensure that their department receives appropriate resources to meet patient care needs and the organizational mission. The controls and reporting mechanisms that the institutional and pharmacy leadership put in place and maintain, ensure that these goals are met and that patient care quality and outcomes are optimized.

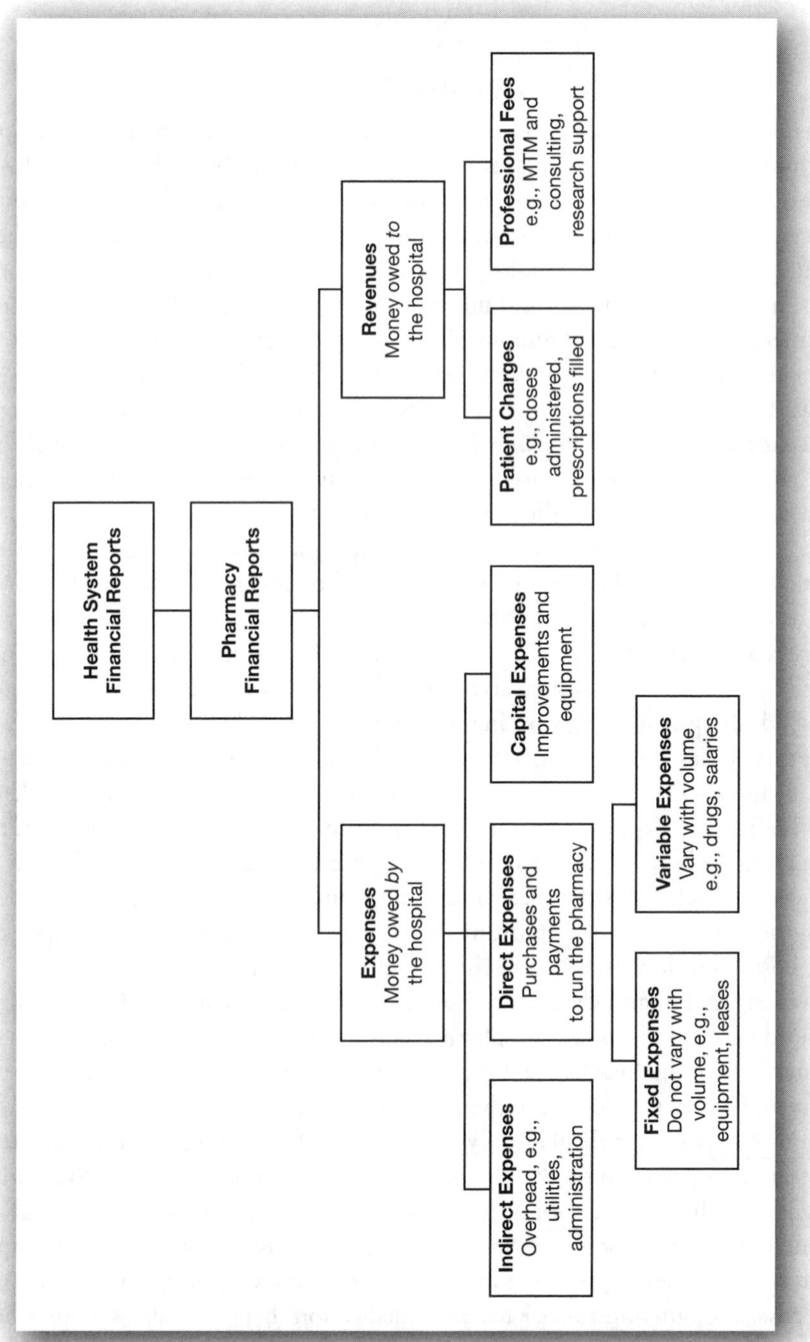

Figure 13-1. The financial structure of a health system pharmacy.

This chapter presents the basics of financial management in institutions for pharmacy students and newly practicing pharmacists. The purpose is to provide them with sufficient working understanding of financial principles to let them participate in management and leadership decisions that impact the success of the pharmacy practice. This chapter is presented in the belief that pharmacists and other pharmacy employees should see themselves as professional leaders and partners with hospital administration, rather than hired employees. If pharmacists understand financial concepts such as revenue, profit, and expense and incorporate them into their decision-making and professional work, they will make better decisions that have a positive impact on the long term viability of the pharmacy and the institution. Pharmacists that participate as partners are encouraged to be more engaged in managing the pharmacy and more accountable for providing efficient distribution and clinical services.

Practice Standards

ASHP Practice standards and guidelines refer to the leadership responsibilities of pharmacists and identify key roles and responsibilities related to financial management of a pharmacy service[1,2]:

- *Budget Management*—The pharmacy budget should be sufficient to meet the hospital's scope of pharmacy services and patient care needs.
- *Workload and Productivity Management*—Workload and financial performance should be managed effectively as a part of the hospital's overall financial management requirements.
- *Analysis and Control Methods*—Hospital and pharmacy management should have resources to (1) assess pharmacy service costs, (2) analyze variance from the planned pharmacy budget, (3) provide for purchasing pharmacy equipment and facilities, (4) project pharmacy revenue, and (5) assess pharmacy personnel requirements to meet workload and productivity targets.

- *Financial Decisions*—Management should be able to analyze financial ratios (e.g., cost per patient day, cost per prescription filled, patients counseled, drug cost by therapeutic class, pharmacy service cost by clinical service) to assess the efficiency of resource use.
- *Drug Expenditures*—Pharmacy policies and procedures for managing drug expenditures should address such methods as competitive bidding, group purchasing, medication utilization review programs, inventory management, and cost-effective patient services.
- *Revenue, Reimbursement, and Compensation*—The pharmacy director should be knowledgeable about revenues for pharmaceutical services including reimbursement for the provision of drug products and related supplies and compensation for pharmacists' cognitive services.

Key Point . . .

Pharmacists and other pharmacy employees should see themselves as partners with management, rather than hired employees. Understanding the financial management objectives of the institution provides them with skills to participate as partners.

. . . So what?

Many pharmacists have little interest in the management of pharmacy finances or people. Indeed, some even take an adversarial stance toward management, "They are just paper pushers and bean counters! They have no idea what it is like to be on the front line!" However, all pharmacy employees have some responsibility in managing people or products written into their job descriptions and expectations of performance. Understanding financial management objectives and terminology helps employees meet their responsibilities.

■ Processes should exist for routine verification of patient healthcare insurance benefits and for counseling patients about their anticipated financial responsibility for planned medication therapies. A process should also exist for providing pharmacy support to uninsured, underinsured, and medically indigent patients.

Financial Terms

Medical terminology is precise, and so is financial terminology. Pharmacists are trained to value thoughtful, direct, and evidence-based evaluations of medications, procedures, policies and programs. They work to communicate professional assessments and directions in a precise manner to ensure that appropriate actions are undertaken. Leadership colleagues of pharmacists including the institution's **chief executive officer (CEO)** and **chief financial officer (CFO)** use similar precision in descriptions of the financial and operational performance of the hospital. Pharmacists need to embrace these financial terms, concepts and metrics when describing the financial performance of the pharmacy service.

Financial terms and performance expectations must be understood within the context and goals of each institution. For-profit hospitals; not-for-profit hospitals; HMOs; integrated health systems; state, federal and other types of institutions each have different financial goals, reporting needs and management structures. A pharmacist must learn the full meaning and implications of each of these terms in the context of their organization. The use and importance of each term will vary with the goals of the institution and with the financial status of the organization. Key terms to understand in all types of organizations include the following:

Expense

An **expense** is a payment made by the health system to others for value received. Pharmacy expenses fall into several categories. **Direct expenses** are those expenses that are incurred by the pharmacy to deliver services and products. Supplies are the largest category of direct expense; predominately pharmaceuticals. Other categories of supplies managed by pharmacy include blood products, intravenous fluids, syringes and needles, administration sets, and *nonpatient care* supplies such as packaging materials, paper, labels, and other office supplies. Human resources are generally the second largest category of direct expense. Human resource expenses consist of the salary and benefit costs for pharmacists, pharmacy technicians, pharmacy managers, and others.

Other direct expenses incurred by the pharmacy include the following:

■ Leases for hardware and software to manage medication delivery, including automated medication cabinets, dispensing robots, pharmacy computer systems, and intravenous pumps.
■ Services including hood certification, service agreements for technology and equipment, and maintenance and repairs for pharmacy facilities.
■ Professional education and development expenses including meetings, travel, and competency programs.
■ Licenses, taxes, and other fees associated with accreditation, including pharmacy residency program accreditation.

Direct expenses can be further classified as fixed or variable. **Fixed expenses** are defined as costs that do not vary significantly in the short-term with the volume of work. Property and equipment are examples; their cost does not change as the number of prescriptions filled rises and falls. **Variable expenses** are costs that vary in the short-term with the level of activity. Purchase costs for pharmaceuticals are an example; costs rise and fall as the number of patients served and the number of prescriptions filled change. Pharmacy work volume may be counted based on the number of patient days, prescriptions or orders processed, or as the number of doses dispensed. Most health-system budgets base variable expense budgets for pharmacy supply and manpower on a combination of inpatient days, emergency department visits, and clinic visits or other ambulatory volumes.

Indirect expenses are payments for services that support the pharmacy but are not directly paid by the pharmacy. These include housekeeping, heat and air-conditioning, electricity, hospital administration salaries, hospital purchasing services, information systems support, the human resources department, the hospital finance department, and others. The cost of these indirect services is also referred to as overhead. In the modern health system the magnitude of these costs is substantial.

■ ■ ■

Key Point . . .

The magnitude of indirect expenses is substantial in institutions but generally beyond the control of the pharmacy manager.

. . . So what?

Pharmacy departments share the expenses of many facilities and supportive services with other departments in institutions although pharmacists have little influence on these expenses. These indirect expenses are a cost of doing the business of pharmacy and should be considered when conducting cost-benefit analyses and return-on-investment calculations for new pharmacy programs or other major spending.

Because indirect expenses are beyond the control of the pharmacy manager, they are not generally a part of regular financial reports. However, indirect costs are considered when business plans and profitability of a service or program are reviewed, including pharmacy services.

An additional expense category in which a pharmacy service is increasingly involved is capital expenses. **Capital expenses** are defined as the cost of a building improvement or a piece of equipment that will provide benefit over a number of years. Health systems budget and manage capital expense separately from regular operating expenses. Accounting methods allow capital expenses to be spread across several years. Capital expenditures are typically significant in size and scope. Pharmacy examples of capital expenses might include new IV admixture hoods, remodeling of a pharmacy, or building a new pharmacy satellite. Health systems typically specify a financial test (e.g., an expense >$5,000) and a duration of useful life of the purchase (e.g., >5 years) to identify an item or project as a capital expense.

Revenue

Revenue is defined as money received for products or services provided to customers. Pharmacy revenues consist primarily of patient charges. Patient charges may result from doses administered in an inpatient setting or from prescriptions dispensed in an outpatient pharmacy. Pharmacies may also generate revenue by providing professional services, including consultation, management of research studies, providing education and other support services, and for medication therapy management (MTM).

Inpatient pharmacy revenues appear on patients' hospital bills as charges. A total of all charges posted by the pharmacy to all bills for an accounting period (e.g., a month), are reported as the pharmacy's gross revenue.

Although charges for medications and for pharmacy services are a focus for pharmacy managers, they are typically not the payments received by the hospital. Most inpatient care is paid at a case rate. A **case rate** is a payment that is negotiated based on a diagnosis-related group (DRG), a per diem (daily) amount, or other benchmark method to determine the hospital's payment. The hospital receives the case rate payment for the patient's care, irrespective of the individual charges posted to the patient's account. Some hospital contracts pay a discounted percentage of billed charges, and most payers provide supplemental payments for patients whose care substantially exceeds the negotiated amount. However, almost no payer, including the federal government pays full charge. Patients without insurance often are unable to pay their hospital bill, requiring the hospital to "write off" all or part of their bill, considering the cost of care as a charitable loss.

The case rate payment method is designed to encourage hospitals to provide care economically. It also allows the hospital to be the beneficiary of savings and efficiencies that it develops or to incur the cost of inefficient care delivery. Although this approach works well in theory, it creates challenges for pharmacy managers in understanding the impact of therapy selection and the management of the medication use process. Because case rates are diagnosis-specific, diagnoses where medications are a significant expense are of the greatest financial and cost control interest to pharmacists. Formulary decisions, practice guideline development, and therapeutic decisions at the bedside may have a significant impact on the health system's ability to meet financial objectives treating these patients. This is discussed later in this chapter.

When the hospital receives payment for services, the case-rate based payment is matched to the charge-based patient bill, and the "discount" is calculated and subtracted; the resulting payment is the net revenue. The net revenue consists of the gross revenue minus the discounts resulting from case rate-based payment. The hospital's accounting system allows the deductions from the gross revenue to be applied to the charges posted by the pharmacy and other departments. The resulting adjustment determines the net revenue to each department. The pharmacy's overall net revenue is calculated by subtracting the pharmacy's share of discounts, contractual allowances, and nonpayment for all patient bills to the hospital from the pharmacy gross revenue.

Outpatient prescriptions are typically charged in the same fashion. The pharmacy contracts with a third party (insurance provider, state Medicaid program, or pharmacy benefits manager [PBM]) to fill prescriptions at a fixed rate based on medication costs and service fees. Rate structures are typically based on a percentage of average wholesale prices for the medication plus a filling fee. Outpatient prescription payment methods are typically handled electronically at the time of dispensing; generally referred to as adjudication at the point of service. Each prescription claim is electronically verified and payment posted through access to a centralized information system. These systems provide record-keeping and revenue tracking systems for outpatient pharmacy in real time.

Assets

Assets are the real, intangible and financial items that are owned by the health system. These include land, buildings, equipment, and the value of inventory. Assets also include cash, accounts receivable (unpaid bills owed by patients, insurance companies and others) for services delivered but not yet paid. In the case of pharmacy, the majority of assets of interest are equipment and the inventory of drugs and supplies. Assets are offset by **liabilities**, the debts (unpaid bills the hospital owes to creditors, loans, bonds issued) owed against them. The net of assets and liabilities is equal to the **equity** held by the institution. In a for-profit organization, equity is a form of liability representing what the corporation owes to the stockholders.

Work Volumes

The amount of work done by pharmacies is represented by **work volumes**. Work volumes consist of a sum of the work units accomplished by the pharmacy, such as the number of orders processed, number of doses dispensed, the number of consults completed, or the number of patient counseling sessions completed. The total hours paid for pharmacy employees is also a volume measure. Work volume for a hospital is generally reported as adjusted discharges or patient days. Health-system pharmacy workload calculations may use a denominator of patient counts such as inpatient admissions or discharges and a numerator of prescriptions filled, orders processed, or doses dispensed and combinations of these components to describe pharmacy workload. Typical indicators for pharmacy workload are adjusted using **case-mix-index (CMI)** or another indicator of patient acuity to recognize the additional cost and resources required to care for sicker patients. Outpatient pharmacy workload is generally reported as prescriptions filled and may include patient counseling, MTM and other direct patient care activities. Institutional pharmacy workload should also be adjusted to reflect the significant amount of effort and cost required to support outpatient surgery, emergency department activity, outpatient infusion services, and other areas that are not reflected in patient day or inpatient discharge count.

As pharmacy has evolved from a primary focus on medication dispensing to include more substantial clinical and cognitive services, workload models based on doses charged, or doses dispensed have fallen out of favor. Workload models based solely on medication doses handled do not reflect the full range of pharmacy service activities, and their use is discouraged.

Health Care Institution Accounting Methods

Accounting is a standard method for reporting the expenses, revenues, and accumulation of assets, and other financial results. An institution maintains a balance sheet that lists its assets, liabilities, and equity. The **balance sheet** is a financial statement which lists the wealth of the institution at a specific point of time. Traditionally, assets appear on the left side and liabilities on the right and the two must be in balance. The balance sheet is described by the equation:

$$\text{Assets} = \text{Liabilities} + \text{Equity}$$

Double entry bookkeeping ensures that both sides of the equation remain balanced at all times. **Double entry bookkeeping** enters any transaction on both sides of the balance sheet (as a debit on one side and a credit on the other) to keep the equation balanced. As an example, a purchase of an IV hood creates a liability but creates and asset of equal value. Table 13-1 is a simplified example of a balance sheet for a health system.

The second part of an organization's periodic financial review is the income statement. The **income statement** lists the revenue, expense, and profit (or loss) of the institution over a period of time. Traditionally, revenue appears on the right and expenses on the left. The income statement and balance sheet together comprise the financial

Table 13-1.

Hospital Balance Sheet

Balance Sheet Community Hospital June 30, 2010

Assets		Liabilities and Equity	
Cash	$1,000,000	Accounts payable	$250,000
Accounts receivable	$3,000,000	Long-term debt	$12,000,000
Inventory	$200,000	Equity	$5,950,000
Land	$1,000,000		
Buildings	$10,000,000	Total	$18,200,000
Equipment	$3,000,000		
Total	$18,200,000		

statement. Hospitals prepare financial statements monthly and generally report results to a board or other oversight body on a monthly, quarterly, and annual basis.

The balance sheet and income statement are fed by data maintained in the hospital's general ledger. The **general ledger** is a record of each transaction of the hospital. Balances on the general ledger are referred to as trial or unaudited balances, as corrections and changes may be made through an audit process. Reports generated from the general ledger provide significant detail about the institution's activities and finances. A monthly report comparing the actual expenses and activities to the budget for the same period provides pharmacy managers and administrators with information to understand the financial status of the department. These monthly activity reports or responsibility summaries are a key to understanding the financial performance of the pharmacy. Table 13-2 is an example of a monthly operations report.

Financial Planning

The annual budget is an important part of the pharmacy manager's financial responsibility. A **budget** is a plan for future expenses and revenue, typically over a 12-month period. A budget does not represent the actual amount of money available to be spent. The pharmacy budget is a thoughtful forecast of future expenses and revenue and a benchmark for measuring financial performance.

The Budget Process

Each year the institution develops an annual plan. The institutions CEO, CFO, and Board of trustees develop goals for services, activity levels, expenditures, and revenues. This is typically done 6–9 months before the fiscal year begins. Forecasts are developed for admissions, service activity, growth, expansion, and other program changes. The director of pharmacy receives these forecasts and begins the process of developing the pharmacy budget. Each institution's budget process varies slightly. However, the CFO provides a budget manual or other instructions, including a calendar for budgeting and an outline of the required approvals and reviews. Instructions may also specify the projections for forecasting inflation and other price increases to be used in budget development. As discussed earlier in the chapter, parts of the budget represent fixed costs that will not vary with activity while others are variable costs, requiring the manager to carefully review forecasts for admissions, patient days and other volume indicators.

Table 13-2.

Example Monthly Operating Statement—Inpatient Pharmacy

Community Hospital Pharmacy

Current Month Actual	Current Month Budget	Difference	Revenue
$8,485,475	$8,315,766	$169,710	Inpatient pharmacy services
$1,385,651	$1,357,938	$27,713	Outpatient pharmacy services
$9,871,126	$9,673,703	$197,423	Total patient services revenue
$(5,653,838)	$(5,540,761)	$(113,077)	Contractual adjustments
$4,217,288	$4,132,942	$84,346	Net patient revenue
			Personnel Expenses
$32,485	$31,835	$650	Salary: management and supervision
$386,939	$379,200	$7,739	Salary: pharmacist and technician
$16,764	$16,429	$335	Salary: support staff
$10,360	$10,153	$207	Overtime
$9,146	$8,963	$183	Shift differential
$262	$257	$5	On call
$114,935	$112,636	$2,299	Employee benefits
$570,891	$559,473	$11,418	Total personnel expense
			Non-personnel Expenses
$2,042,204	$2,001,360	$40,844	Drugs
$32,401	$31,753	$648	Intravenous supplies
$13,512	$13,242	$270	General medical/surgical supply
$792	$776	$16	Office and general supplies
$46,910	$45,972	$938	Purchased services
$2,136,346	$2,093,619	$42,727	Total non-personnel services
$2,707,237	$2,653,092	$54,145	Total operating expenses
$1,526,967	$1,496,428	$30,539	Net excess

Capital Budget

The budget cycle typically begins with the development of a capital budget. The **capital budget** is usually comprised of items that cost more than a fixed threshold (e.g., an expense >$5,000) and a useful life greater than 5 years. These thresholds are set by the institution's Board. Capital expense budgets are generally set several years in advance because many capital expenses can be forecast. The need to replace equipment, renovate or build facilities or to incur expenses for a new program lends themselves to forward planning.

Capital budget needs are typically larger than the institution can afford, so some prioritization of need may be undertaken, normally a focused review of the expense (Is it required by a new regulation or standard? Is the current equipment broken or nonfunctioning? Is the equipment necessary to support a new patient care program?). A review of the **return on investment (ROI)** is also generally used to prioritize or determine the wisdom of making capital purchases. ROI is a structured calculation of the operating cost and revenue changes that the institution with incur with the new capital expense (Will fewer employees be needed due to increased productivity? Will additional patient volume be available due to increased capacity? Will more revenue be collected?). ROI answers the question, "How quickly will it take to earn back the investment made on a capital purchase?" ROI calculations are generally stated in terms of the number of months or years that a capital purchase takes to pay back its purchase cost. Shorter payback periods are generally more favorable, and capital expenses that do not result in payback of their costs may not be easily approved and budgeted, unless they are required to meet a legal or accreditation standard.

■ ■ ■

Key Point . . .

ROI calculations answer the question, "How quickly will it take to earn back the investment made on a capital purchase?"

. . . So what?

ROI calculations are not just used for capital purchases: they can demonstrate the return on new pharmacist services and clinical programs. Pharmacists are often told that they need to demonstrate their value to administrators, payers, and other professionals, and ROI calculations are a way of doing so. In an ROI calculation, the costs of pharmacy investments must be balanced against the benefits accrued from those investments. Pharmacists need to think about ROIs when proposing any major spending in institutions because it is certain that administrators and other key decision makers will be doing so.

Operating Budget

The **operating budget** represents a forecast of the daily expenses required to operate the pharmacy. Development of the health-system budget generally takes advantage of the fact that most expenses are similar in size and scope to prior years. In many organizations, the pharmacy director is presented with a preliminary budget based on the activity for the prior fiscal year. Even when this is not done, the pharmacy director should perform a detailed review of the proposed expenses and revenues by comparing them to the pharmacy's experience over the past 1–2 fiscal years. Further he should test the proposed changes based on institutional and industry trends, news, and other information. The budget review and approval process generally uses this method to ensure continuity and prevent errors.

Volume Budget

The **volume budget** is prepared by the CFO and supplies the number of admissions, patient days, CMI, outpatient visits, emergency department visits, and other activities. The Pharmacy director should examine historical relationships between these volume statistics and pharmacy activity to develop a pharmacy volume budget. Table 13-3 is an abbreviated example of a pharmacy volume budget developed based on the CFO's base statistics.

Table 13-3.
Pharmacy Volume Budget

LOCATION	JUL	AUG	SEP	Monthly Average
Inpatient Pharmacy	369,392	369,392	357,476	365,420
Inpatient Pharmacy Total	**369,392**	**369,392**	**357,476**	**365,420**
Orders/Day	*11,915.87*	*11,915.87*	*11,915.87*	*11,915.87*
Outpatient Pharmacy #1	16,557	15,869	16,180	16,202
Outpatient Pharmacy #2	9,617	9,885	9,916	9,806
Outpatient Pharmacies Total	**26,174**	**25,755**	**26,097**	**26,008**
Rx/Day	*1,106*	*1,088*	*1,140*	*1,111.32*
Home Infusion Pharmacy	11,935	11,935	11,550	11,807
Rx/Day	*385.00*	*385.00*	*385.00*	*385.00*
GRAND TOTAL:	**407,501**	**407,082**	**395,123**	**403,235**

Expense Budget

Pharmacy expenses can be divided into three categories: human resources, supplies, and other expenses.

Human Resource Expense

Human resource expense includes the salaries for all professional, technical, and support staff, and their benefits including insurance, workers compensation, disability, etc. The benefit cost is typically stated as a percentage of the annual salary. Benefits cost can run as high as 25% to 30% in some markets. The benefit percentage for a pharmacy budget calculation is typically provided by the CFO in the annual budget instructions. The pharmacy manager takes the number of approved positions in each job category (pharmacist, pharmacy technician, secretary, etc.) and multiplies them by the number of paid hours for the fiscal year and the hourly rate for the year to arrive at the salary cost. Benefits are added as a percent of the final salary figure. A spreadsheet detailing the calculation for each incumbent employee and with vacant positions listed ensures a correct calculation. Projected raises and salary increases for the coming budget year should be included

Key Point . . .

Cost of employee benefits can run as high as 25% to 30% of an employee's salary.

. . . So what?

Costs of employee benefits are often overlooked by pharmacists when thinking about personnel costs. When pharmacists negotiate employment contracts with their employers, they need to realize that benefits are a major part of the job offer. When they calculate ROI for new programs, benefits should be added to any salary totals.

in this calculation. New positions added to the pharmacy service are typically added to this calculation during the budget review and approval process as they are approved.

Supply Expense

The vast majority of pharmacy supply expense is for drugs, and the size and scope of drug expense have substantial impact on the hospital's overall budget. A thoughtful, well-supported supply budget for drugs is crucial for the pharmacy department's success. Forecasting drug and other supply expense requires knowledge of four factors: (1) level of price inflation, (2) amount of drug utilization, (3) drug mix (i.e., what drugs are used), and (4) a blend of utilization and mix representing expensive, innovative medications. The authors of a continuing series of articles examining trends in hospital drug cost recommend that the pharmacy director and his management team follow a nine-step process to ensure success in forecasting drug expense[3]:

- *Step 1*—Collect data. Historical purchase data can be gathered from wholesaler data systems and utilization data can be pulled from hospital and pharmacy information systems. Group purchasing organizations (GPO) provide reports on anticipated contract price changes and an annual forecast that serves as a resource for predictions of new drug approvals, adoption of recently approved drugs, generic drug introductions, and overall trends.
- *Step 2*—Review financial history. Evaluate the pharmacy's performance against budget for the most recent full fiscal year and for the current fiscal year (annualizing current fiscal year-to-date data). Compare actual fiscal year data to identify inflationary trends by drug and, when possible, by disease, diagnosis, or clinical service. Identify areas of exceptional variance for more detailed assessment. Review the performance of current pharmacy cost containment efforts.
- *Step 3*—Build a high-priority drug budget. A relatively small number of drugs (<100 products out of the 3,500+ purchased by a typical hospital pharmacy) represent 80 to 90% of total purchases and utilization in most hospitals. Create a drug product-specific budget for these drugs based on historical utilization, and project changes in volume of use.
- *Step 4*—Build a new-product budget. Consider new drugs expected to be approved during the period covered by the budget. Work with prescribers and the P&T Committee to identify which new drugs will be added to the formulary, how they will be used, and how often.
- *Step 5*—Build a non-formulary drug budget. Budget commonly used non-formulary products separately for financial monitoring purposes.
- *Step 6*—Build a low-priority drug budget. The low-priority drug budget represents a small portion of the total drug budget and can be safely budgeted as a lump sum. This component of the budget should be predicted as a variable cost based on the consideration of any anticipated change in overall patient volume. Other medical supplies and general supplies can also be forecast using this method.
- *Step 7*—Establish a drug cost containment plan. Include consideration of drug-use-evaluation results indicating inappropriate prescribing, drug classes with multiple competing products, and reports of successful cost-containment efforts published by other institutions. For each cost-containment target identified, produce a targeted forecast that includes the scope of the plan, what the intervention will entail (e.g., guideline implementation, formulary change), the timing of intervention implementation, and an estimate of the costs for a fully successful plan.

- *Step 8*—Finalize and present the total drug budget. The total drug budget is the sum of expected expenditures on the high priority list, new products, non-formulary agents, and low-priority products minus the total cost impact expected from the cost-containment plan. In many cases, the initial estimate of expenditures may be higher than hospital leadership is able to support. Using this budgeting model, requests for cuts can be met in a variety of ways.
- *Step 9*—Vigilance. Budgets established using the eight steps above provide a level of detail and a robust basis for comparison with actual performance and variance reporting.

Other Fixed Expense

Other non-supply expense is generally fixed, and varies only in response to inflation and price changes. Non-supply expense consists of a full range of expenditures including salaries, benefits, and overhead.

Revenue Budget

The development of a revenue budget remains an important component of the pharmacy budget, even though few payers actually pay full charge for pharmacy items and services, Pharmacy charges offer an opportunity to track the operations of the pharmacy and serve as a proxy for net revenue after discounts and allowances.

Pharmacy revenue can be predicted from workload volume and from supply expense. Because a detailed volume budget has been developed, the charges associated with this work volume can be forecast. However, since most pharmacy charges are derived from the cost of service, including drug cost, it is important to account for the influence of changes in the mix of drugs used and the influence if increased drug supply cost. Further, revenue targets set by the CFO may be set as an overall pharmacy department gross revenue figure. The pharmacy manager must develop a detailed plan that meets the CFOs target using the expense budget.

Budgeting for a New Program

New pharmacy programs that add operating expense should be considered carefully. New drug and supply expense, additional personnel, new equipment, software and other expenses merit careful consideration. The budget for a new pharmacy program is a smaller version of the budget process described above. Rather than including these new expenses "buried" in the entire budget, a spreadsheet identifying the costs by budget category should be prepared. A narrative supporting the new program including objectives, program description, advantages, resources required, and a bottom line should be developed. Many organizations also consider indirect costs for new programs, although they are generally not a significant part of the annual budget process for the pharmacy.

Budget Negotiation, Review, and Approval

After all departments develop their budgets, they are returned to the CFO or budget office for a "roll-up" where the individual department budgets are aggregated and a first version of a working budget for the health-system is created. Because the budget development process takes place at the department level, the resulting budget draft generally needs substantial work. The CFO and Finance team work to balance the budget, to identify errors and problematic assumptions, and to develop a workable budget plan.

The institution's administration, led by the CEO and CFO set priorities for funding and ask departments to change, cut, reduce, or otherwise modify their initial budget proposals. Some requests for change or new programs may be deferred to future years or denied outright. Budget development is both a rational and a political process; negations revolve around the organization's highest priorities and the quality of preparation and presentation made by the respective department leaders.

Pharmacy budgets developed as described above are evaluated against prior fiscal year experience to ensure that they are realistic and reasonable. The integrity of the development process and the level of support for key assumptions such as pharmacy volumes, drug price increases, and new drug adoption are also a factor in considering how the pharmacy budget is considered and accepted. The track record of the pharmacy and the pharmacy director in meeting prior budgets often has significant influence on the outcome of the current budget review. A thoughtful, well-developed budget supported by data has the greatest chance of success and provides the health system with the best forecast of the future.

Monitoring the Budget

During the fiscal year, the hospital finance team collects information and manages the hospital's expenses and revenues to meet the objectives set in the budget process. Volume, expense, and revenue data are collected in real time by the institution's financial management data systems. Monthly activity reports are provided to pharmacy managers. These reports provide a summary of expenses in each of the areas where the pharmacy spends and receives money, and compare it to the target set for the month and for the fiscal year to date. The pharmacy director should review the reports and take action to address financial issues in the pharmacy to ensure that the pharmacy department meets targets set during the budget process. Alternatively, if the report shows changes that were not anticipated in the budget process (e.g., a new high cost drug is introduced earlier than anticipated), and the pharmacy will not meet the budget target, regular review will ensure that action is taken to resolve the problem, or appropriate action is taken to alter the budget to reflect the new reality.

Variance Analysis

Variance analysis can be illustrated using the pharmacy department monthly operating statement shown in Table 13-2, A **variance** is a difference between the budgeted amount and the actual amount spent for a budget period, typically a month. Variances are generally evaluated monthly: examining monthly changes and variance from the start of the fiscal year to date. Variances can be described as positive (expenses lower than forecast; revenues higher than forecast) or negative (expenses higher than forecast; revenue lower than forecast). A positive variance is one that allows the hospital to retain more cash, while a negative variance causes the hospital to have less cash than the budget forecast. Variances can be absolute—the total actual spent amount is higher irrespec-

Key Point . . .

Some variation in expense and revenue is expected. It is the unexpected that should catch the pharmacy manager's attention.

. . . So what?

Basic knowledge of computer spreadsheets and their graphing capabilities are an essential skill for pharmacists. These programs allow data to be manipulated in ways that allow pharmacists to pick up data patterns that are otherwise not visible. They help differentiate the unexpected from the expected.

tive of volume—or adjusted by volume; the variance in cost cannot be explained solely by changes in activity volume.

Some variation in expense and revenue is expected—human resource cost should hover within 2% of that forecast while drug expenses might have a 5% to 10% acceptable variance. It is the unexpected that should catch the pharmacy manager's attention, considering both the magnitude of variance and the ability to influence it. The absolute variation in expense may also be considered cause for review. Each hospital sets the acceptable limits for budget variance; typically a threshold is set by the CEO or CFO.

Determining the Cause of Variance

Operating statements like that in Table 13-2 are designed to identify the nature of expense variance. To determine the sources of variance, the pharmacy manager must look at each category of expense that meets the threshold for investigation. A human resource expense might have a positive variance if a job opening exists for a position resulting in salary savings. A negative variance in human resource expense might result from additional overtime expenses required to meet a specific patient care need. Supply expense variance might be positive if a high-cost drug was released onto the market later than expected. On the other hand, supply expense might show a negative variance if an outbreak of an infectious disease caused a higher than anticipated use of a costly antibiotic, if a shortage of medication caused the pharmacy to switch to a more costly drug, or if drug prices rose faster than forecast. Both human resource and supply cost might be higher than anticipated if the hospital census was higher than budgeted resulting in negative variances for both categories.

Pharmacy leaders are expected to have a continuing, current understanding of the nature and source of expense variance. Their understanding should include both the business and clinical therapeutics understanding for which they are trained. The regular discipline of monthly analysis provides an opportunity to understand and to take action to ensure that the hospital's funds are expended wisely.

Integrating Cost and Revenue Analysis

As reimbursement for health care services has become more competitive, pharmacy managers have had to make hard choices based upon profitability of services. Cost alone is insufficient for deciding the most appropriate course of action in managing drug use and pharmacy costs. The payment system for patient care services and DRGs often creates the need to ask a more fundamental question: does the hospital make or lose money on treating this type of case?

Most case rates are determined based on the current standard practice or on some other current norm. However, introduction of a costly new drug or treatment onto the market or when treatment protocols or standards change, the cost of medications may exceed the amount paid and the profitability of the case can change. Therefore, decisions about whether to add drugs to the Formulary, new practice guidelines, and other choices made by P&T committees and pharmacists should consider not only the cost and cost-benefit relationships associated with a particular drug therapy, but also the reimbursement received by the hospital. Revenues and costs are time-consuming to track in a health system. However, a thoughtful pharmacy leader must consider the implications of revenue and margin in choosing a course of action. This is a critical skill, particularly when high cost and high impact drugs are considered for use in a hospital.

Productivity Measurement and Benchmarking

The budgeting process helps hospitals measure productivity. Productivity is defined using the following equation:

$$\text{Productivity} = \text{Output}/\text{Input}$$

Because the budget develops indicators of input (supply costs, hours worked, salary costs) and outputs (doses dispensed, patients treated, patients discharged) a baseline for calculating productivity is created. Although productivity measured in this way is a key management indicator, movement to an assessment of the impact of pharmacy services based on patient outcomes has added an additional dimension to the role of workload and productivity measures.

Productivity measures can also be designed using detailed time and motion studies or through the use of benchmarking. **Time and motion studies** consist of a detailed analysis of the time it takes to complete various tasks. These studies determine the resources necessary to complete tasks and the results are used to set goals for improvement or change. Benchmarking uses data collected from some comparator (e.g., peer institutions, past performance) to set standards for productivity.

External benchmarking is a process of measuring costs, services, and practices against the organization's peers or against industry leaders. The goal of external benchmarking is to find and implement the best practices of peer organizations. External benchmarking presents a significant challenge. The idea behind external benchmarking is attractive, but because there is limited information about peer institutions, incorrect or inappropriate comparisons may be made. The real cause of differences indicated by key external benchmarking indicators may result from factors outside the scope of the data being collected and compared. As examples, differences in hospital information systems, the size, layout and logistics support in the hospital facility, or even the allocation of medication delivery tasks between pharmacy and nursing may have substantial impact on the reported productivity indicators across two hospitals. External benchmarking does offer an opportunity to identify variation in performance across a group of industry peers and to target opportunities for investigation. But excessively rigid or overly casual use of external cost and labor benchmarks can create significant problems by identifying false improvement opportunities or setting performance goals that are unreachable or are inappropriately low.

> **Key Point . . .**
>
> The payment system for patient care services and DRGs requires pharmacists to ask a fundamental question: does the hospital make or lose money on treating this type of patient case?
>
> **. . . So what?**
>
> The answer to this question can influence strategies for serving patients within institutions. Health systems might target patients with conditions associated with profitable DRGs, seeking to attract these patients with innovative services or other offerings. Alternatively, interventions could be developed to reduce the costs of treating patients associated with unprofitable DRGs. For instance, patients could be tracked as they move throughout the health care system, identifying inefficiencies and unnecessary costs.

In contrast, **internal benchmarking** is the process of measuring costs, services, and work volumes and activities against the organization's prior performance. The goal of internal benchmarking is to refine and improve the organization's performance incrementally over time. Internal benchmarking does not assist in identifying best practices. It assesses the impact of changes in systems, practices and procedures in a standard set of measures. Internal benchmarking against prior department and health-system performance offers a different analysis of improvement opportunities and assesses them in a more data-rich fashion. A full understanding of quality and safety issues, combined with a broad assessment of changes in case mix, programs, and other variables make internal benchmarking a more robust methodology. Because productivity and operational benchmarking lack a quality of care and outcome dimension, they are being displaced by *dashboard* and *scorecard* methodologies that incorporate indicators of quality and outcome into efficiency and effectiveness review. Because internal benchmarking data is a high level assessment, typically department-wide, it may not be sensitive enough to detect small but important internal improvements in pharmacy processes. Further, cross-functional and interdepartmental productivity improvements (e.g., implementation of computerized physician order entry [CPOE]) require collaboration and separate analysis.

Budgeting, time and motion, and benchmarking all seek to develop a ratio of input to output expressed as monetary cost/unit of output or hours worked/unit of output. Table 13-4 lists examples of productivity measures that are in use in evaluating pharmacy services and medication therapy. Some productivity measures do not measure the full range of pharmacy service activities. For instance, productivity measures based on the number of doses charged or dispensed by a pharmacy ignore the application of pharmacist's knowledge and skills complexity of complexity of resolving clinical care issues.

Summary

Thoughtful financial management by pharmacists and pharmacy leaders is critical to the success of the organization's pharmaceutical care plan. A working knowledge of financial management supports the effective delivery of high quality pharmacy services, and supports optimal achievement of the patient care mission of the pharmacy and the hospital. Pharmacy leaders can balance costs, benefits and patient care outcomes in

Table 13-4.

Example Pharmacy Productivity Ratios

Labor Productivity Ratios

- Hours worked per adjusted patient day
- Hours worked per adjusted discharge
- Hours worked per 100 orders processed
- Hours paid per adjusted patient day
- Hours paid per adjusted discharge
- Hours paid per 100 orders processed

Cost-Base Productivity Ratios

- Drug cost per 100 orders processed
- Supply cost per 100 orders processed
- Labor cost per 100 orders processed
- Total cost per 100 orders processed
- Drug cost per adjusted patient day
- Supply cost per adjusted patient day
- Labor cost per adjusted patient day
- Total cost per adjusted patient day
- Drug cost per adjusted discharge
- Supply cost per adjusted discharge
- Labor cost per adjusted discharge
- Total cost per adjusted discharge

delivering pharmaceutical care using an organized data-based budget, monitoring variance, assessing and managing costs and revenues.

Suggested Reading

Cleverly WO, Cameron AE. *Essentials of Healthcare Finance.* Sudbury, MA: Jones & Bartlett; 2007.

Finkler SA. *Finance & Accounting for Nonfinancial Managers.* New York: Aspen; 2003.

Schumock GL, ed. *How to Develop a Business Plan for Clinical Pharmacy Services: A Guide for Managers and Clinicians.* Kansas City, KS: American College of Clinical Pharmacy; 2007.

Wilson AL, ed. *Financial Management Basics for Health-System Pharmacists.* Bethesda, MD: American Society of Health-System Pharmacists; 2007.

Zelman WM, ed. *Financial Management of Health Care Organizations: An Introduction to Fundamental Tools, Concepts and Applications.* Malden, MA: Blackwell; 2003.

References

1. American Society of Health-System Pharmacists. ASHP guidelines: minimum standard for pharmaceutical services in ambulatory care. *Am J Health-Syst Pharm.* 1999;56:1744-1753.

2. American Society of Health-System Pharmacists. ASHP guidelines: minimum standard for pharmacies in hospitals. *Am J Health-Syst Pharm.* 1995;52:2711-2717.

3. Hoffman JM, Shah ND, Vermeulen LC, et al. Projecting future drug expenditures—2005. *Am J Health-Syst Pharm.* 2005;62:149-167.

4. Murphy JE. Using benchmarking data to evaluate and support pharmacy programs in health systems. *Am J Health-Syst Pharm.* 2000;57(suppl 2):S28-31.

5. Knoer SJ, Could RJ, Folker T. Evaluating a benchmarking database and identifying cost reduction opportunities by diagnosis-related group. *Am J Health-Syst Pharm.* 1999;56(11):1102-1107.

Chapter Review Questions

1. **What is a direct expense?**
   a. Monies received by the hospital based on pharmacy services
   b. Expenses incurred by the pharmacy to deliver services and products
   c. Expenses covered by 3rd party plan payments such as a PBM
   d. Expenses paid by the hospital to support the pharmacy such as hospital administration salaries

   Answer: b. Direct expenses result directly from the delivery care to patients. Answer a describes a source of revenue. For answer c, direct expenses can be part of expenses covered by 3rd party plans, but not all. Answer d is a type of indirect (or overhead) expense.

2. **Flaws of external benchmarking include:**
   a. The real cause of differences may result from factors outside the scope of the data collected and compared
   b. Because there is limited information about peer institutions, incorrect or inappropriate comparisons may be made
   c. External benchmarks can identify false improvement opportunities or set inappropriate performance goals

d. a and c

e. All of the above

Answer: e. All of the above. External benchmarking consists of comparing one's organization with an outside organization. Answers a, b, & c are all flaws of external benchmarking because comparing oneself with others is problematic if the wrong data is collected, the collected data is not accurate, and attempts to mimic others may not be the right strategy for your institution.

3. **Which of the following statements is NOT true of a hospital pharmacy variable direct expenses in hospital pharmacies?**
   a. They are costs that rise and fall in the short term with the level of activity.
   b. Purchase costs for drugs is an example of a variable direct expense.
   c. The number of orders processed and prescriptions dispensed affect work volume and may drive variable expenses.
   d. Most hospitals do not consider pharmacy supply cost to be variable based on volume.
   e. Pharmacy manpower is generally budgeted as a variable expense.

Answer: d. Pharmacy supplies, including drugs, vary based upon the number of patients in the hospital because they are directly associated with the treatments of these patients. Answers a, b, c, and e all describe variable direct expenses of a hospital pharmacy.

4. **A case rate is a negotiated payment that is based on a diagnosis-related group (DRG), a per diem (daily) amount, or other to determine the hospital's payment. Which of the following is a correct statement about case rate reimbursement?**
   a. Most case rates are determined based on standard practices or current practice norms
   b. When a costly new drug treatment is introduced, the costs of pharmacy services and the profitability of the case can change
   c. P&T committees should consider reimbursement when considering adding new drugs to a formulary
   d. All of the above
   e. a and c only

Answer: d. All of the above. Answer a is correct because case rates are determined by current standards of practice. Answer b is correct because new expensive treatments and drugs can cause treatment costs to exceed revenue and affect the profitability of treatment. Answer c is correct because P&T need to consider profitability along with other concerns when making formulary decisions.

5. **The case rate payment method is designed to do which of the following?**
   a. Encourage hospitals to provide care economically
   b. Limit cost overruns in pharmacy spending
   c. Allow the hospital to be the beneficiary of improved savings and efficiencies
   d. Encourage the use of costly medications when they limit the length of a hospital stay
   e. a and c
   f. b and d

Answer: e. Answer a is correct because a case rate payments cap the amount of money received for treating patients and c is correct because case rate payments also allow hospitals to keep any money left over. Answer b is incorrect because higher pharmacy spending may result in lower treatment costs because of the relative cost effectiveness of drugs compared to other treatment alternatives. Answer d is incorrect because use of costly medications is unprofitable if lower cost alternatives are available.

6. **A variance is a difference between the budgeted amount and the actual amount spent for a budget period. Which of the following descriptions of a variance is NOT true?**
   a. Positive variance: expenses lower than forecast
   b. Positive variance: expenses higher than normal
   c. Negative variance: revenue lower than forecast
   d. Negative variance: revenue lower than normal
   e. a and c
   f. b and d

Answer: f. Answer b and d are not true because variance is the difference between the budgeted and actual amounts, not "normal" amounts. What is "normal" and what is "budgeted" may be different. Answers a and c are true because the budget is a form of forecast and a positive variance is one that causes the hospital to retain more money.

7. **Forecasting drug expense is a combination of four factors. Which of the following correctly identifies these factors?**
   a. Formulary status, medication error review, new drug factors and generic substitution
   b. Price inflation, drug utilization, drug mix and a blend of utilization and mix of high-cost medications
   c. High-hazard medications, MTM requirements, clinic and hospital visit volume, and a mix of high-cost medications
   d. Clinical service factor, medication utilization review , price inflation and drug utilization

Answer: b. Price inflation, drug utilization, drug mix, and a blend of utilization and mix of high-cost medications are all functions of overall drug expenses. Drug expenses are determined by price multiplied by the amount used. Price inflation refers to price increases while drug utilization, drug mix, and the blend of utilization and drug mix refer to the amount used.

8. **The operating budget is a forecast of the daily expenses required to operate the pharmacy. Which of the following is a correct statement regarding the operating budget?**
   a. The operating budget is only a suggestion, it can be treated casually when considering the pharmacy operation.
   b. The pharmacy operating budget may include high-cost equipment items that have an extended useful life, typically beyond 5 years.

c. The pharmacy director is typically presented with a preliminary budget based on the prior year's operating expense.

d. The pharmacy operating budget does not include drugs. They are included in a special supply budget.

Answer: c. The operating budget starts with what was used last year. Then adjustments are made by determining how the current year differs from last year. Considerations about the rate of drug price inflation, increases in pharmacist salary, new programs started, impact of cost savings initiatives, and so on will determine the new budget.

9. **What is an asset?**
   a. Anything of positive value about the operations of the health system, including reputation, employee staff, and key programs such as oncology or transplant.
   b. A statement of an amount of money owed to the health system by a payer or patient.
   c. Real, intangible, and financial items owned by the health system, including buildings, equipment and inventory, cash and accounts receivable.
   d. Unpaid bills the hospital owes to suppliers, loans and bonds issued.

Answer: c. Assets can be either things that can be touched (buildings, inventory) or not (promises to pay, electronic totals of money in the bank).

10. **The balance sheet is a financial statement that lists the wealth of the institution at a specific time. Which equation describes the financial statement correctly?**
    a. Assets = Liabilities + Equity
    b. Wealth = Assets – Equity
    c. Wealth = Assets + Liabilities
    d. Wealth + Equity = Assets + Liabilities

Answer: a. The sum of liabilities (what is owed) and equity (what is owned) equals total assets or wealth. The balance sheet is an accounting of the relative balance of liabilities and equities.

Chapter Discussion Questions

1. What advantage would a clinical pharmacist gain by understanding general accounting principles?
2. What advantage would a pharmacist with operations and distribution responsibilities gain by understanding general accounting principles?
3. What types of impact does the use of case rates in reimbursing hospitals have on the way hospital pharmacy is practiced?
4. Which is better: external benchmarking of the efficiency of a pharmacy or internal benchmarking? What are the advantages of the method that you selected?
5. How might pharmacists contribute to the budgeting process?

CHAPTER 14

Sterile Preparations and Admixture Programs

Philip J. Schneider and E. Clyde Buchanan

■ ■ ■

Learning Objectives

After completing this chapter, readers should be able to:

1. List national standards that apply to compounding sterile preparations.
2. Differentiate among uses of laminar airflow workbenches, biological safety cabinets and compounding isolators.
3. Discuss the importance of a buffer room to compounding sterile preparations.
4. Describe how a person should cleanse and garb before compounding sterile preparations.
5. List the information that must appear on a label for a compounded sterile preparation.

Key Terms and Definitions

■ **Ante area (or anteroom):** An ISO Class 8 or better air quality area where personnel perform hand hygiene, and garbing procedures, staging of components, order entry, compounded sterile preparation (CSP) labeling and other high particulate-generating activities.

■ **Aseptic technique:** The methods used to manipulate manufacturer-supplied sterile products so that they remain sterile as compounded sterile preparations.

■ **Biological safety cabinet (BSC):** A primary engineering control device that is a ventilated cabinet for CSPs, personnel, product, and environmental protection having an open front with inward airflow for personnel protection, downward high-efficiency particulate air (HEPA)-filtered laminar airflow for product protection, and HEPA-filtered exhausted air for environmental protection.

■ **Buffer area (or room):** The area where the primary engineering control (PEC) is physically located. Activities that occur in this area include the preparation and staging of components and supplies used when compounding CSPs.

■ **Clean room (or buffer room):** A room in which the concentration of airborne particles is controlled to meet a specified airborne particulate cleanliness class. Microorganisms in the environment are monitored so that a microbial level for air, surface, and personnel gear are not exceeded for a specified cleanliness class.

- **Cold storage conditions (refrigerator):** 2–8°C (36–46°F).
- **Components:** The individual ingredients, containers and closures that are used to compound sterile preparations.
- **Compounded sterile preparation (CSP):** A dose or doses of medication that are prescribed for a patient(s) that must be prepared for administration and is sterile.
- **Compounding aseptic containment isolator (CACI):** A primary engineering control that is designed to provide worker protection from exposure to undesirable levels of airborne drug throughout the compounding and material transfer processes and to provide an aseptic environment for compounding sterile preparations. Air exchange with the surrounding environment should not occur unless the air is first passed through a microbial retentive filter (HEPA minimum) system capable of containing airborne concentrations of the physical size and state of the drug being compounded. Where volatile hazardous drugs are prepared, the exhaust air from the isolator should be appropriately removed 100% by properly designed building ventilation.
- **Compounding aseptic isolator (CAI):** A primary engineering control that is a form of isolator specifically designed for compounding pharmaceutical ingredients or preparations. It is designed to maintain an aseptic compounding environment within the isolator throughout the compounding and material transfer processes. Air exchange into the isolator from the surrounding environment should not occur unless the air has first passed through a microbially retentive filter (HEPA minimum).
- **Critical site:** A location that includes any component or fluid pathway surfaces (e.g., vial septa, injection ports, beakers) or openings (e.g., opened ampuls, needle hubs) exposed and at risk of direct contact with air (e.g., ambient room or HEPA filtered), moisture (e.g., oral and mucosal secretions), or touch contamination. Risk of microbial particulate contamination of the critical site increases with the size of the openings and exposure time.
- **Direct compounding area (DCA):** A critical area within the ISO Class 5 primary engineering control (PEC) where critical sites are exposed to unidirectional HEPA-filtered air, also known as first air.
- **First air:** The air exiting the HEPA filter in a unidirectional air stream that is essentially particle free.
- **Garb:** Clothing worn by personnel during the compounding of sterile preparations to minimize particulates being shed from body and clothing into the buffer room and primary engineering control.
- **Hazardous drugs:** Drugs are classified as hazardous if studies in animals or humans indicate that exposure to them has potential for causing cancer, developmental or reproductive toxicity, or harm to organs.
- **Laminar air flow workbench (LAFW):** A primary engineering control that is a controlled environment created by a high-efficiency particulate air (HEPA) filter to retain airborne particles and microorganisms. Its use decreases the chance of microbial contamination during the compounding of sterile preparations.
- **Media-fill test:** A test used to qualify aseptic technique of compounding personnel or processes and to ensure that the processes used are able to produce sterile product without microbial contamination. During this test, a microbiological growth medium such as Soybean–Casein Digest Medium is

substituted for the actual drug product to simulate admixture compounding.

- **Primary engineering control (PEC):** A device or room that provides an ISO Class 5 environment for the exposure of critical sites when compounding CSPs. Such devices include, but are not limited to, laminar airflow workbenches (LAFWs), biological safety cabinets (BSCs), compounding aseptic isolators (CAIs) and compounding aseptic containment isolators (CACIs).
- **Pyrogens (bacterial endotoxins):** Metabolic products of living microorganisms, or the dead microorganisms themselves, that cause a pyretic (rise in body temperature) response upon injection.
- **Risk levels**
  - **Low risk:** Involves only transfer, measuring, and mixing manipulations using not more than three commercially manufactured packages of sterile products and not more than two entries into any one sterile container or package (e.g., bag, vial) of sterile product or administration container/device to prepare the CSP.
  - **Medium risk:** Multiple individual or small doses of sterile products are combined or pooled to prepare a CSP that will be administered either to multiple patients or to one patient on multiple occasions. Or the compounding process includes complex aseptic manipulations other than the single-volume transfer. Or the compounding process requires an unusually long duration.
  - **High risk:** Contains nonsterile ingredients, including manufactured products not intended for sterile routes of administration (e.g., oral). Or a nonsterile device is employed

before terminal sterilization. Or any of the following are exposed to air quality worse than **ISO Class 5** for more than 1 hour: a) sterile contents of commercially manufactured products, b) CSPs that lack effective antimicrobial preservatives, and c) sterile surfaces of devices and containers for the preparation, transfer, sterilization, and packaging of CSPs. Or compounding personnel are improperly garbed and gloved. Or nonsterile water-containing preparations are stored for more than 6 hours before being sterilized. Or it is assumed, and not verified by examination of labeling and documentation from suppliers or by direct determination, that the chemical purity and content strength of ingredients meet their original or compendia specifications in unopened or in opened packages of bulk ingredients.

- **Secondary engineering controls:** The ante area and buffer area (see definitions above).
- **Standard operating procedures (SOPs):** A set of instructions or steps someone follows to complete a job safely, with no adverse impact on the environment (and which meets compliance standards), and in a way that optimizes operational and production requirements.
- **USP Chapter <797>: Pharmaceutical Compounding—Sterile Preparations:** A pharmacy-related general chapter in the *United States Pharmacopeia-National Formulary* that is among those chapters numbered below 1000 so as to be enforceable by the Food and Drug Administration, The Joint Commission, and some State Boards of Pharmacy.

Introduction

Patient safety is a crucial component to patients receiving the most benefit from their medications. Pharmacists have historically played a critical role in protecting patients from harm that may result from drug therapy. Increased attention has been devoted to the use of high-risk medications—those that have the greatest potential to cause adverse drug events when used. High-risk medications are most commonly defined according to drug toxicity but may also be defined by the route by which they are administered. Focusing on both high-risk medications and high-risk methods of administering these medications can narrow the scope of work. There is an excellent chapter titled "High- Alert Medications: Safeguarding against Errors" in the text *Medication Errors*.[1] Sixteen medications or drug categories are listed, 14 of which can or are administered by the intravenous route. Kaushaul et al. found that the intravenous route of administration was the most common in medication errors detected in pediatric inpatients.[2] In one of their annual reports, the United States Pharmacopeia (USP) reported that "the intravenous route of administration often results in the most serious medication error outcomes" based on the reports submitted to MEDMARX[SM].[3] We do not need a formal failure mode analysis to know that intravenous drug administration is a high-risk area of medication use, and needs the full attention of pharmacists and other health care providers.

The intravenous route of administration bypasses three physiologic safeguards—the gut, liver, and skin. The gut may break down medications before they are ever absorbed, or the drug may not even be absorbed through the gastrointestinal tract. The liver protects patients from many toxic doses of medications and can safeguard patients through the first pass effect when medications are administered orally. The skin protects patients from infections that might be caused by pathogenic microorganisms that are in the environment, especially the hospital. Thus, preventable adverse medical events resulting from medications administered by the intravenous route may result from either infections from contamination, toxicity from the medicine, or both.

Reports about problems with the safety of intravenous drug therapy were reported in the late 1960s. Patterson et al. expressed concerns about drug incompatibilities and the length of time between preparation and administration of medications prepared at the bedside after finding that 60% of intravenous fluids used at their hospital contained more than one drug, and many were administered more than an hour after preparation.[4] These authors recommended that pharmacy assume responsibility for compounding intravenous admixture doses to resolve these problems. Flack et al. reported being asked for "technical help from the pharmacy service" by the surgeons investigating the effectiveness and safety of parenteral nutrition to resolve problems of contamination and incompatibilities with the formulas that were being "hand mixed in open laboratory surroundings."[5] Thur et al. observed nurses preparing parenteral admixtures in patient care areas and reported an error rate of 21%. The rate of wrong doses prepared was 9%, incompatible drugs mixed was 6%, wrong drug or solution used was 3%, and preparation of drugs not ordered was 3%. Deviations from accepted sterile technique were observed, with counters not being cleaned (99%), hands not washed (97%), touching sterile areas of the IV container (47%), and vial or bottle tops not being cleaned (31 %).[6] O'Hare et al. used a disguised observer method to evaluate error in preparation and administration of intravenous medications by physicians and nurses. They found that physicians made at least one error in 98% of the doses prepared and 83% of these doses were administered by nurses.[7] Taxis and Barber also observed nurses who prepared and administered intravenous drugs on 10 wards in a hospital in the United Kingdom. Of 249 errors identified, at least 1 error occurred in 212 of the 430 doses observed. Most errors occurred when bolus doses were prepared and administered or for doses requiring multiple steps to prepare. One strategy recommended to decrease errors was to reduce the amount of preparation on the ward.[8]

Even if properly ordered, errors can occur in preparation that can cause harm to patients. Thompson et al. evaluated the concentrations of admixed medications delivered to patients and found evidence of incomplete mixing of medications in IV solutions prepared at the bedside. They also found that there was more uniformity of concentrations of potassium chloride when these doses were prepared in the pharmacy.[9] Calculation errors are also a root cause of error in preparing medications. Perlstein et al. found that one of 12 doses calculated by nurses had an error that resulted in a tenfold dose compared to that ordered. Pediatricians made errors in one of 26 computations. Pharmacists made fewer errors than nurses and physicians.[10]

As a result of these reports, pharmacy-based centralized intravenous admixture programs have emerged as a fundamentally safer medication-use system. According to ASHP National Surveys of Pharmacy Practice in hospital settings, this system has been shown to be present in the vast majority of U.S. hospitals. In 2008, only 10 % of U.S. hospitals relied on nurses to prepare intravenous medications as the primary method. Most hospitals used the **minibag system** (i.e., small volume parenterals; see Chapter 15) to administer medications by the intravenous route and doses are prepared in the pharmacy.[11]

In spite of this, there is some evidence that complacency can arise in pharmacies undermining the potential benefits of a pharmacy-based intravenous admixture program. Sanders et al. reported that pharmacists had an error rate of 7.24% and a contamination rate of 7%.[12] These errors and contamination rates were higher than that observed for pharmacy technicians. Pharmacists made fewer errors and contaminated fewer IV preparations when they knew they were being observed, suggesting the emergence of compla-

cency and the need for continuing vigilance. High error rates in pharmacy-based intravenous admixture programs were also reported by Flynn et al. They found an error rate of 9% in five hospital pharmacies studied using an observation-based method.[13] Trissel et al. evaluated the aseptic technique of pharmacists and technicians when compounding complex USP medium-risk sterile preparations using media fill tests. Pharmacist compounding resulted in a contamination rate of 4.4% compared to a rate of 6.2% for technicians. The overall contamination rate was 5.2%.[14]

Recent reports of patients being harmed by pharmacy-compounded sterile medications, including intravenous admixtures have resulted in public concern

> **Key Point . . .**
>
> USP Chapter <797> Pharmaceutical Compounding—Sterile Preparations establishes a national enforceable standard for compounding both non-hazardous and hazardous sterile preparations.
>
> **. . . So what?**
>
> This document guides much of the activities for handling sterile preparations. Failure to follow the recommendations could lead to problems with accreditation and licensing.

about patient safety. The publication of an enforceable standard, **USP Chapter <797>**[15] and attention to this by The Joint Commission (TJC) and State Boards of Pharmacy mandates pharmacists taking responsibility for competently compounding sterile preparations. The intent of this chapter is to summarize the requirement for doing this.

Quality Assurance in Compounding Sterile Preparations

Preparations to be used for parenteral, ophthalmic, and irrigation purposes must be free from chemical and physical contaminants, accurately and correctly compounded, sterile and free of **pyrogens**, stable until their beyond use date, and properly packaged and labeled for use.

Components

The majority of **compounded sterile preparations (CSPs)** are comprised of **components** that are clean, sterile, and pyrogen-free as purchased from pharmaceutical manufacturers. High-risk compounding involves the use of components that are not sterile and may not be pyrogen-free. The extemporaneous compounding of concentrated morphine sulfate injection from the powder is an example. In high-risk compounding, it is essential to use a USP grade chemical or to obtain a certificate of quality analysis from the supplier of the chemical, since the pharmacy is usually not equipped or qualified to perform chemical analyses. Assuming that the certificate is judged to be reliable and the substance meets acceptable standards, like those of the USP, the pharmacist can take the responsibility for compounding with the chemical. Compounding policies and procedures (i.e., **standard operating procedures**) must be developed so that the final preparation meets the standards required for a sterile preparation, including sterility, freedom from pyrogens, and an acceptable particulate level. For high-risk preparations, the pharmaceutical characteristics must be produced as a consequence of the compounding and processing steps. Sterility must be achieved, usually by appropriate filtration, through sterile, disposable, nonreactive, 0.2-micron porosity membrane filter devices. During filtration, particulate matter is removed to very low levels, below visible sizes, rendering the solution clear. Removing pyrogens is more difficult; the best approach is to obtain raw materials that are free from pyrogens as supplied.

For low- and medium-risk preparations, assuring that the preparation has the required characteristics is primarily a matter of maintaining the quality level built into the product by the commercial manufacturer.

Compatibility and Stability

Responsibility for the compatibility and stability of formulated preparations rests with the pharmacist. Detailed compatibility and stability information may not be readily available for high-risk compounding. Lacking the facilities to perform research and testing, pharmacists are challenged to draw upon their basic chemical and physical knowledge, experience in compounding, and awareness of available literature resources. Probably the most widely used reference is Trissel's *Handbook of Injectable Drugs.*[17] Other information may be available from the commercial supplier of a component and from other literature resources.

Unexpected compatibility problems may be visible immediately or within a few hours after compounding, but not all incompatibilities are visible. All incompatibilities affect the stability of a preparation. However, stability considerations are broader and include overall assurance that the activity and chemical/physical integrity of the formulation is maintained until the preparation is administered to a patient.

Batch Formulas and Records

Batch compounding of CSPs requires strict adherence to standard operating procedures. Any failure in the process of compounding can lead to waste and/or pose a threat to patient safety. Master formula sheets and batch control records establish a uniform approach to the compounding process. The master formula sheet provides exact directions on the standard compounding of the batch preparation. See Figure 14-1. The batch control record then documents the completion of these tasks and identifies that each step has been followed for each individual batch of CSPs.

■ ■ ■

Key Point . . .

A pharmacist is responsible for the stability and compatibility of compounded sterile preparations and should be consulted when a CSP is made outside the pharmacy.

. . . So what?

Just because a CSP might be compounded outside of the pharmacy does not mean that the pharmacist is no longer responsible for its impact on patient outcomes. Pharmacists need to ensure that processes are established and supported for ensuring stability and compatibility of compounded products.

Environmental Controls

The facilities and equipment in which the compounding of sterile preparations is performed must be designed and operated in a manner conducive to achieving/maintaining intended quality characteristics of the finished preparations.

Primary Engineering Controls

USP Chapter <797> requires that all sterile compounding, regardless of risk level, be done in an ISO Class 5 environment (i.e., fewer than 100 airborne particles larger than 0.5 microns per cubic foot) that is maintained in a horizontal **laminar airflow workbench (LAFW)**, a suitable **biological safety cabinet (BSC)** or a suitable **compounding aseptic isolator**.[15] These are key engineering control devices designed to continuously sweep the **direct compounding area** with High Efficiency Particulate Air (HEPA)-filtered air, i.e., **first air**. The 99.97% efficiency of a HEPA filter should render the air stream clean and approaching sterility. Still, this relatively slow air flow can easily be overcome with adverse air currents, even by the expelled breath from compounding personnel talking; thus, the direct compounding area must be protected from inappropriate activities of personnel (to be discussed

■ ■ ■

Key Point . . .

Primary engineering control devices provide the HEPA-filtered first air that bathes critical sites of syringes, needles, vial tops, and ampul openings to prevent microorganisms from entering the final compounded sterile preparation.

. . . So what?

Any barriers to the laminar flow of HEPA-filtered air can introduce the potential for contamination.

Figure 14-1. Example of a master formula sheet. *Source:* McCluskey SV. Sterilization of glycerin. *Am J Health-Syst Pharm.* 2008;65:1173–1176.

Sterile Glycerin for Injection 100% 3 mL KEEP REFRIGERATED Lot No.: 08122007-01 Prepared by: VB/RDP Beyond-use Date: February 12, 2008 **XYZ Pharmacy Department**	**Pharmacy Department** **Master Formula Sheet**	Attach Batch Label Here

Sample Label (above)

Preparation: Sterile Glycerin for Injection 100% **Control No:** 09182008-01 **BUD:** 3/18/2009

Equipment:

Peristaltic Pump—Baxa Repeater Pump
Clean depyrogenated glass beaker, 500 mL
Sterile tubing set—Baxa fluid transfer tube set no. 11
Sterile extension set—Baxa extension set no. 87

Hydrophilic filter—Baxa Supor capsule 0.2 micron filter
 (H938 24102 3)
Sterile fluid dispensing connector—B. Braun No. 415080
Sterile disposable syringes, 6 mL and 60 mL
Sterile latex-free Luer tip caps—Becton Dickinson

Ingredient	NDC, Lot No. & Expiration	Ingredients	Amount	Measured by & date	Checked by & date
1		Synthetic Glycerin, USP	400 mL		
2					
3					

Procedure: (Caution: This is a high-risk sterilization procedure.)

1. Pour 400 mL of glycerin into a 500-mL clean depyrogenated glass beaker.
2. Working in appropriately cleaned compounding aseptic isolator, attach fluid transfer tube set to inlet end of filter. Attach extension set to outlet end of filter. Attach fluid dispensing connector to free end of extension set.
3. Place the free end of the fluid transfer tube into the beaker containing the nonsterile glycerin.
4. Place fluid transfer set tubing into the peristaltic pump.
5. Prime tubing by setting pump at lowest possible setting (low, 1). When glycerin reaches the filter, allow 100 mL to pass by the pump. Turn the pump off and allow the filter to become wet (about five minutes).
6. Continue to pump glycerin at lowest setting; a faster pumping rate will cause failure of tubing inside pump head.
7. After air is out of the tubing sets and filter, aseptically attach a 60-mL sterile syringe to the fluid dispensing connector.
8. Set pump for 500 mL. Remove and inspect the extension tubing around the pump head every 500 mL to make sure it is not stretched, as this will lead to tubing failure.
9. When approximately 50 mL of glycerin has filled the 60-mL syringe, remove syringe and fluid dispensing connector. Attach another clean sterile fluid dispensing connector to the extension set. Attach a clean, sterile 60-mL syringe to the fluid dispensing connector. Repeat procedure until all glycerin is filtered.
10. After glycerin is filtered, perform the filter integrity test on the used filter.
11. After the filter passes the integrity test, attach a 6-mL sterile syringe to the 60-mL syringe containing the filtered glycerin using the fluid dispensing connector. Fill syringe with 3 mL of sterile glycerin.
12. Aseptically place a Luer tip cap on all syringes.
13. Repeat filling process until all glycerin is packaged. Theoretical yield = 166 syringes; Actual yield = _____
14. Test sterility by USP Chapter <71> and visually test for color, clarity, particulate matter, and syringe integrity.
15. Perform bacterial endotoxin test according to USP Chapter <85>.
16. Label filled syringes. Quarantine filled syringes for 14 days under refrigeration.

Approved by: _____ **Date:** _____ **Time:** _____

later). The HEPA filter should be protected from damage during use and its efficiency certified at least every 6 months. BSCs and **Compounding Aseptic Containment Isolator (CACIs)** must be used to maintain sterility of the preparation and to protect compounding personnel when **hazardous drugs** are being compounded.

Secondary Engineering Controls

Because primary engineering controls draw air from the surrounding room, USP Chapter <797> requires a **buffer area** around these devices that meets ISO Class 7 (i.e., fewer than 10,000 airborne particles larger than 0.5 microns per cubic foot). Low- and medium-risk preparations may be compounded in facilities where there is no physical separation between the **ante area** and the buffer area. High-risk preparations require an anteroom separate from the buffer room. See schematics in Figures 14-2 and 14-3.

The surfaces of all ante and buffer area ceilings, walls, floors, shelving, cabinets, and work surfaces should be smooth, impervious, free from cracks and crevices, and nonshedding, making them easy to clean and disinfect. Junctures of ceilings to walls, walls to walls, and floors to walls should be coved (i.e., angled to prevent a crevice) or caulked to make them easier to clean. There should be no dust-collecting ledges, pipes, or similar surfaces. Work surfaces should be constructed of durable, smooth, and impervious materials, such as stainless steel or molded plastic. Carts should be of stainless steel wire or sheet construction with good quality, cleanable casters.

Clean air flow should be outward from the direct compounding area through the buffer area, then through the ante area by means of cascading differential air pressures.

Figure 14-2. Schematic example of clean room floor plan suitable for low- and medium-risk level compounded sterile preparations. *Source:* Reference 15. Used with permission from <797> *Pharmaceutical Compounding - Sterile Preparations*, United States Pharmacopeial, 2008.

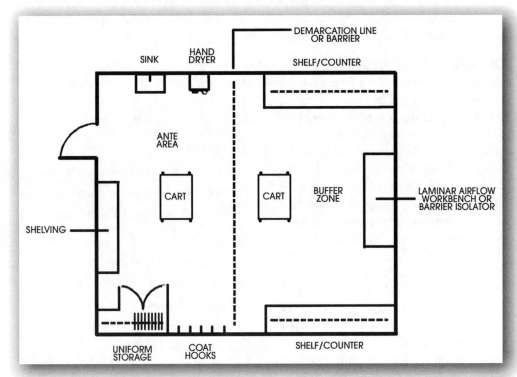

Figure 14-3. Schematic example of a clean room floor plan suitable for high risk level compounded sterile preparations. *Source:* Reference 15. Used with permission from *<797> Pharmaceutical Compounding - Sterile Preparations*, United States Pharmacopeial, 2008.

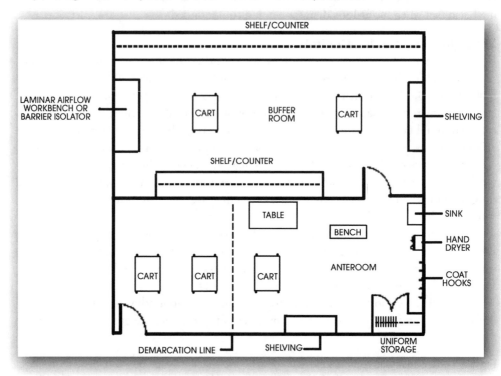

These or similar structural design considerations, along with planned cleaning programs, disinfecting of all surfaces, and traffic control of personnel and supplies, make it possible to protect the direct compounding area.

Cleaning and Disinfecting

Surface contamination can be expected, even within the LAFW, BSC, or compounding aseptic isolator. Therefore, written standard operating procedures should be followed for cleaning and disinfecting all surfaces within the ante and buffer areas. Cleaning of floors, walls and ceilings should be performed with a mild detergent solution (i.e., "hospital disinfectant") using a nonshedding, absorbent mop, wipe or sponge. This should be followed by wiping work surfaces with an effective disinfectant like sterile 70% isopropyl alcohol (IPA). All shelving, supply carts, and countertops in the remainder of the ante and buffer areas should be cleared of supplies, cleaned and disinfected in a similar manner at least monthly. Floors in

Key Point . . .

Secondary engineering controls provide a very clean environment within which the primary engineering controls work best.

. . . So what?

The best aseptic conditions consist of layers of engineering controls. If an aseptic environment exists within a very clean environment, chances of contamination are lessened.

these areas should be cleaned and disinfected daily, working from the cleanest area outward. All reusable cleaning tools should be restricted to use in the ante and buffer areas and thoroughly cleaned and sanitized after each use. Cleaning in the LAFW, BSC or compounding aseptic isolator should be done with a sterile, nonshedding wipe dampened with sterile 70% IPA.

Traffic Control

The flow of supplies and personnel through the ante and buffer areas must be rigidly controlled to prevent carrying contamination inward. No personnel should be allowed to approach the primary engineering control device unless properly **garbed** and adequately trained. This includes housekeeping personnel. All supplies should be externally cleaned and disinfected during transition through the ante area to the buffer area.

An arrangement in which supplies are brought into the ante area external to the demarcation line is preferred (see Figures 14-1 and 14-2). At this point, they are unboxed, cleaned, disinfected and transferred to a clean cart restricted to the buffer room. This step serves as a barrier to many of the natural contaminants on the outside of large volume parenteral (LVP) bags, vials, syringe pouches, transfer set packages and other required supplies.

A further transfer barrier step should occur as supply items are introduced into the LAFW, BSC or compounding aseptic isolator. Whenever possible, an external wrap would be removed (such as peeling back syringe pouches) at the edge of the LAFW or BSC. Vials and other items not packaged in an outer wrap should be carefully disinfected by wiping with a wipe dampened with sterile 70% IPA. The supply items introduced into the primary engineering control device should be limited to those required for the planned procedure and should be arranged so as not to obstruct the HEPA airflow pattern and to provide for efficient processing—that is, to the right and left of the work site in a horizontal LAFW and around the perimeter in a BSC or compounding isolator.

These barrier steps during the introduction of supplies should be recognized as only sanitizing, not sterilizing, steps and their effectiveness depends on the techniques of the operator. Any residual contaminants on the surfaces of supply items may be transferred to the sterile gloves of an operator and may be present for possible touch contamination transfer to the preparation. This risk of contaminating a preparation will increase progressively from low-risk to high-risk preparations.

Environmental Testing

While all the elements so far mentioned, pursued with dedication, should provide a controlled environment, a testing program should be developed to verify that control is achieved and maintained. The focus of testing should be on detecting the presence

> **Key Point . . .**
>
> People are the source of the most contamination in a sterile compounding environment; so minimizing the number of people and their movements within sterile compounding areas is essential to prevent contamination of CSPs.
>
> **. . . So what?**
>
> People are social animals who enjoy interacting with others. However, sterile compounding environments are not the place to be doing so.

of microbial contaminants in the environment. Both surface testing, for the deposit of microorganisms on exposed surfaces over time, and air-volume sampling, for microorganisms suspended in the air, should be performed. In principal, baseline (minimal) microbial counts should be determined when the environment is under control. A monitoring program should then be designed to detect loss of control evidenced by increases in the microbial counts. Such increases signal the need to determine the cause and correct it. The USP has a microbiologic evaluation process for clean rooms that should be considered.[18]

Compounding Personnel

Compounding personnel in the ante and buffer areas should be limited to those adequately trained and competency-tested for aseptic technique (to be discussed later) and to the minimal number required for the planned procedures. Since the human body is constantly shedding particles, many of which are viable microorganisms, major efforts must be made to reduce the ingress of these particles into the buffer area but, particularly, into the direct compounding area. This is accomplished by good personal hygiene, thorough washing/disinfecting hands, donning garb to confine the particles as much as possible and following good aseptic technique.

Training and Evaluating Compounding Personnel

To achieve good sterile compounding practice, personnel must be adequately trained and the effectiveness of the training must be tested by written exams, observation by a trained observer, media fill testing and fingertip glove testing. Training is the most significant factor contributing the assurance of quality in sterile preparations, because personnel are recognized as the primary source of contaminants, both viable and nonviable, shed in the clean room environment. Therefore, compounding personnel must be taught to understand this natural phenomenon and how they can control particulate shedding while compounding. Considerable information regarding proper training will be found in ASHP's text and video programs on compounding sterile preparations.[19-22]

Pharmacists and technicians who compound sterile preparations must understand good compounding practice and practice excellent aseptic technique. Training should make clear that sterile preparations must have the highest level of quality and purity of all dosage forms. Trainees should be instructed in the nature of contaminants and the means for achieving the required level of purity, maintaining stability during the required beyond use dating of the preparation, and evaluating the required characteristics. Pharmacists should be sufficiently familiar with the principles of sterilization to work with technicians who perform autoclaving or hot-air sterilization of supplies or preparations. The validation of these processes for their bactericidal effect is highly critical and requires considerable expertise.

While pharmacists and technicians are not expected to be engineers, they should know the specifications for facilities and devices in which they must perform. This includes the selection of equipment (for example, an LAFW) from external suppliers or working with in-house engineers to assure proper clean air flow into the ante and buffer areas. An understanding of some engineering principles is needed to achieve required environmental standards, for example, the dynamics of air flow through a HEPA filter to achieve laminar air flow and the clean first air sweep of the direct compounding area. It is also necessary to know how to achieve the air pressure differentials to produce the cascading effect from the buffer room out through the less clean ante area.

The use of barriers to interrupt the ingress of contaminants into the direct compounding area must be understood, whether these are physical barriers such as walls or interruption barriers (e.g., removing supply items from a "dirty" cart, cleaning and disinfecting, and transferring to a "clean" cart). Another interruption barrier is the washing of hands and the donning of clean garb before entering the buffer area.

Trainees must have a basic understanding of microbiology. They need to know that microorganisms are ubiquitous and, therefore, are present in the work environment, even in the direct compounding area. They must know these organisms will multiply rapidly (doubling about every 20 minutes) when moisture, the proper temperature, and nutrients are present.

Compounding personnel should understand the principles of environmental evaluation (i.e., how to determine the effectiveness of the environmental controls used). This means knowing and selecting methods for detection of viable microorganisms in the environment, what the methods selected will detect, how samples should be gathered and incubated, proving that any viable microorganisms present will grow, and what the results signify, including when and if action is required.

Aseptic Technique

Typically, manipulations by compounding personnel are used in small-scale compounding of sterile preparations in the buffer area for low and medium-risk preparations. Medium-risk preparations may require automated compounding devices for the addition of small-volume additives to total parenteral nutrition (TPN) solutions. Compounding personnel must set up such devices, connect fresh stock containers, fill the final preparation containers, and generally monitor the operation. High-risk preparations are particularly exposed to the environment and to compounding personnel.

Garb and Behavior

Because of the inherent shedding of viable and nonviable particles from the body of compounding personnel (as many as 1 million particles of 0.3 microns and larger per minute with average arm and upper-body movement from a sitting position), serious efforts must be made to control this shedding. Means used include garbing, designed to confine most of particulate discharge within the garb; planning movements while using aseptic technique to minimize losing particles from the body; and removing human beings as far as possible from the direct compounding area. One of the advantages of using compounding aseptic isolators is the fact that the bodies of compounding personnel are physically separated from the direct compounding area.

Before entering the buffer area, compounding personnel must remove outer garments, all cosmetics (because they shed flakes and particles) and all hand, wrist, and other visible jewelry or piercings that can interfere with the effectiveness of personal protective equipment (PPE) (e.g., fit of gloves and cuffs of sleeves). The wearing of artificial nails is prohibited while working in the sterile compounding environment. Natural nails must be kept neat and trimmed.

Personnel don the following PPE in an order that proceeds from those activities considered the dirtiest to those considered the cleanest. Garbing activities considered the dirtiest include donning of dedicated shoes or shoe covers, head and facial hair covers (e.g., beard covers in addition to hair bonnets), and face masks/eye shields. Eye shields are optional unless preparing hazardous drugs. Thereafter, a hand cleansing procedure must be performed by removing debris from under fingernails using a nail cleaner under running warm water followed by vigorous hand washing. Hands and forearms are washed to the elbows for at least 30 seconds with soap and water while in the ante area. Hands and forearms to the elbows should be completely dried using either lint-free disposable towels or an electronic hand dryer. After completion of hand washing, a non-shedding gown with sleeves that fit snugly around the wrists and enclosed at the neck is donned. Gowns designated for buffer area use must be worn, and they should be disposable. If reusable gowns are worn, they should be laundered appropriately for buffer area use. Once inside the buffer area and prior to donning sterile powder-free gloves, antiseptic hand cleansing must be performed using a waterless alcohol-based surgical hand scrub with persistent activity following manufacturers' recommendations. Hands are allowed to dry thoroughly before donning sterile gloves.

Sterile gloves are the last item donned before compounding begins. Gloves become contaminated when they contact nonsterile surfaces during compounding activities. Disinfection of contaminated gloved hands may be accomplished by wiping or rubbing sterile 70% IPA to all contact surface areas of the gloves and letting the gloved hands dry thoroughly. Only use gloves that have been tested for compatibility with alcohol disinfection by the manufacturer. Routine application of sterile 70% IPA must occur throughout the compounding process and whenever nonsterile surfaces (e.g., vials, counter tops, chairs, carts) are touched. Gloves on hands must also be routinely inspected for holes, punctures, or tears and replaced immediately if such are detected. Compounding personnel must be trained and evaluated in the avoidance of touching **critical sites**. When compounding personnel exit the compounding area during a work shift, the exterior gown may be removed and retained in the compounding area if not visibly soiled, to be re-donned during that same work shift only. However, shoe covers, hair and facial hair covers, face masks/eye shields, and gloves must be replaced with new ones before re-entering the direct compounding area, and proper hand hygiene must be performed.[15]

The following lists some elements of good aseptic technique:

1. Practice good personal hygiene; be organized and calm.
2. Be healthy, without eczema or other skin rashes, and free from allergies or other conditions causing sneezing or coughing.
3. Put on garb properly, avoiding contaminating the outside of the clean/sterile gowns.
4. Replace garb or parts of garb that become contaminated while gowning or working.
5. Disinfect all interior surfaces of the LAFW (except the HEPA filter face) with sterile 70% IPA.
6. Disinfect gloves frequently while performing aseptic technique to maintain the aseptic condition of the outer surfaces.
7. Replace gloves with new sterile ones if they become punctured or torn.
8. Move with slow, smooth, gentle motions.
9. Do not talk unnecessarily.
10. Do not disrupt HEPA-filtered laminar air flow within the direct compounding area.
11. Do not interpose arms or any other nonsterile objects above a critical site in BSC or behind a critical site in horizontal laminar air flow.
12. Do no spray or splash disinfectants where the liquid might enter a preparation container or reach other preparation contact sites.
13. Do not introduce any packages into the buffer area unless they have been adequately disinfected or sterilized externally.
14. Minimize in and out movement at the LAFW, BSC or compounding isolator.

15. Disinfect gloves with sterile 70% IPA after handling any package if the outside had uncertain sterility or surfaces such as switches of mixing pumps.
16. Cooperate with other compounding personnel and mutually assist in maintaining proper aseptic technique.
17. Pass through doorways, plastic curtains, or other passageways slowly and carefully to minimize the generation of potentially contaminating air currents.
18. Do not leave open vials, tanks, or other critical sites exposed to the environment during breaks or other delays in operation.
19. Inspect all supply items before using and the finished preparation after preparation for evidence of defects.
20. Remove used supply items and clean/disinfect work area as needed.
21. Prepare and apply appropriate labels and complete documents away from the direct compounding area or, preferably, pass preparation outside so that a second person can perform the paperwork.
22. Remove used garb carefully to avoid distributing accumulated body contamination before exiting the gowning room.
23. Leave the HEPA filter blower operating at all times.

> **Key Point . . .**
>
> Competent personnel using good aseptic technique are the foundation of compounding sterile preparations made from manufacturers' sterile products.
>
> **. . . So what?**
>
> Ultimately, good sterile compounding comes down to excellent human resources management including the recruitment, training, monitoring, and coaching of employees.

Packaging and Labeling

The final container for a compounded sterile preparation needs to be sterile and maintain the sterility of the preparation to the beyond use date. It should also protect the final preparation from chemical degradation, especially if the preparation is light sensitive. The choice of package for a sterile preparation should take into account the use of the preparation. For example, ophthalmic medications need to be packaged for drops to be instilled in the eye. Irrigation solutions need to accommodate administration sets, if necessary, and ideally not be confused with intravenous drug administration containers. Plastic containers are preferred for most sterile medications to reduce cost and to prevent breakage, but a plastic container should not be used if the preparation is not compatible with plastic or if heat sterilization of the final preparation is needed.

Proper labeling is an important component of safe medication systems because it identifies the medication, quantity of medication, and beyond use date. If the preparation is patient-specific, it also associates the medication with the patient for whom it is intended and the dose that is prescribed. Labels may also include supplementary information to help assure the dose is administered properly, such as how to store the preparation, when to administer the dose, and how to prepare the dose for administration. Special techniques can be used to highlight important characteristics of drug names or doses to avoid confusion that might result from look-alike or sound-alike drug names or doses. Examples are bold letters, larger font, color, or capital letters (so-called *TALL MAN* lettering) for drug names or concentrations or doses. It is important not to include too much information on a label so that the user cannot or does not read the information.

Specific requirements for labeling compounded sterile preparations often include the following:

- Name and amounts or concentrations of ingredients
- Total volume of the compounded sterile preparation
- Beyond use date
- Appropriate route of administration
- Storage conditions (e.g., refrigerate, protect from light)
- Other information for safe use (e.g., cautionary statements, initials of responsible pharmacist, disposal instructions)

Patient specific labeling may include additional information to assure proper drug administration. This includes the following:

- Patient name and identification number
- Patient location
- Name and amount of drug(s) added and the name of the admixture solution
- Time and date of scheduled administration
- Time and date of preparation
- Administration instructions
- Initials of the persons who prepare and check the IV admixture

Verification of Compounding Accuracy and Sterility

There are two components of compounded sterile preparations that are essential—the accuracy of the content, and sterility. Manufactured products cannot be used before these two factors are assured. It is not possible to wait for the results of tests to measure content or sterility for compounded preparations because of the urgency of clinical need. Therefore, more indirect methods of quality assurance are needed.

Measures of compounding accuracy are directed toward assuring the content of the admixture matches what is ordered and printed on the label. This can be done for parenteral nutrition formulations by weighing an admixture. The expected weight of the final preparation can be calculated using specific gravity of the components. Deviations from the calculated weight would suggest that a wrong base solution or the wrong volume of one or more of the base solutions was used to compound the preparation. More commonly, the person preparing an admixture is asked to place the syringes and vial/ampuls used to compound the preparation on a tray with the final admixture for checking by a pharmacist. These supplies are checked to verify the use of the proper component(s) and volume (based on syringes drawn to the amount used) for each admixture.

Storage and Beyond Use Dating

Two important considerations in assuring the quality of pharmacy compounded sterile preparations are the conditions under which the preparation is stored and the time that elapsed between compounding and administration. These are important because of both chemical stability and sterility considerations. Chemical stability issues can be determined from the package insert, a reliable reference such as *Extended Stability for Parenteral Drugs*,[23] the *Handbook on Injectable Drugs*,[17] or other published literature.

Sterility considerations are defined in USP Chapter <797>.[15] In the absence of passing a sterility test, USP requires beyond use dating of 48 hours at controlled room temperature, 14 days at cold temperature, and 45 days in solid frozen state at -20°C or colder for low-risk level CSPs. For medium-risk CSPs, the beyond use dating is shorter: 30 hours at controlled room temperature, 9 days at cold temperature, but still 45 days frozen. For high-risk preparations, beyond use dating should not exceed 24 hours at controlled room temperature or 3 days at cold temperature and 45 days frozen unless sterility testing provides evidence to the contrary.

To protect the patient, the beyond use date should be provided on the label of the compounded sterile preparation.

Maintaining Quality after the Preparation Leaves the Pharmacy

Assurance of proper storage conditions can pose a challenge after the CSP leaves the pharmacy. Temperature limits can be exceeded during delivery to the patient or patient care area. Proper storage after the dose is received in the patient care area must be also be assured. Usually this means CSPs are stored in a refrigerator. To accomplish this, it may be desirable for the pharmacy to assume responsibility for delivery and storage of CSPs after they leave the pharmacy. If this is not possible, shorter beyond use dating can be used.

Another challenge to maintaining quality after CSPs leave the pharmacy is the reuse of the preparation for a patient other than the one for whom the original preparation was compounded. Redispensing of CSPs may avoid waste but requires oversight by pharmacy to avoid administering doses that might be contaminated or after the beyond use date. USP requires that pharmacy have the sole authority for determining whether a CSP not administered as originally intended can be used for another patient.[15] Some examples of considerations in making this decision include the following:

- CSP was maintained under continuous refrigeration
- CSP was protected from light
- No evidence of tampering
- Time remaining before originally assigned beyond use date and time

Standard Operating Procedures

USP requires that the pharmacy have written and approved standard operating procedures (SOPs) to assure the quality of the environment and operator technique used to compound sterile preparations.[15] There are specific parts to these SOPs that are recommended:

- Access to the buffer or clean area
- Decontamination of supplies in the anteroom area
- Storage of supplies not needed for scheduled operations
- Use of carts to transfer supplies and preparations
- Use of particle generating objects, such as pencils, cardboard, and paper
- Traffic flow
- Policy for cosmetics and jewelry
- Procedures for hand washing
- Policy for food items
- Procedures for cleaning surfaces in the compounding environment

- Policy for maintaining ISO class 5 direct compounding area conditions
- Handling of supplies within the direct compounding area
- Inspection and final preparation checking procedures
- Removal of preparations and supplies from the direct compounding area
- Environmental monitoring

Readers are referred to USP Chapter <797> for more detailed SOPs.[15]

Compliance with USP Chapter <797>

In the first quarter of 2009 (more than 6 months after revised USP Chapter 797 became official and enforceable), a national survey of 262 hospitals of various sizes and in various U.S. states, showed that hospital pharmacies are becoming more conversant and compliant with the standards of this chapter.[24] Only 24% of respondents to this survey reported their pharmacy meets or exceeds all requirements of Chapter 797. However, 40% said they would be fully compliant within 6 months and another 25% said it would take them 6 months to a year for full compliance.

Regulators are interested. Sixty-one percent of state board of pharmacy inspectors asked about compliance with USP Chapter 797. Sixty percent of hospital pharmacies reported that they have a cleanroom with a separate HEPA filtration system. Ninety percent of facilities clean their cleanroom on a daily basis. Sixty-nine percent of hospital pharmacies have an environmental monitoring plan (EM) in place. For those that do not, 71% plan to implement an EM plan in the near future. While 85% of hospital pharmacies train sterile compounding employees at hiring, only 68% of those facilities are conducting annual training for their compounding staff.

■ ■ ■

Key Point . . .

In compounding most sterile preparations, final sterility and accuracy testing is not possible; so having excellent policies and procedures is mandatory and compounders must use them correctly each time for consistency and uniformity of CSPs.

. . . So what?

Ultimately, the most important thing is the outcome, not the policies and procedures that result in the outcome of sterile and accurate compounding. However, it is not feasible to check every product developed, so consistent and uniform compliance with policies and procedures is used to ensure quality of sterile products.

Summary

Centralized, pharmacy IV admixture programs are an evidence-based practice for minimizing the risks of patient harm with intravenous drug therapy. This system should be in place for compounding all IV medications for routine use in the health system. There are cases where the clinical needs of the patient are too critical for the time required for a dose to be compounded in a centralized, pharmacy IV admixture area and delivered to the bedside. In these cases, doses may need to be prepared extemporaneously in patient care areas, often by nonpharmacy personnel. In these situations, greater vigilance is needed to assure the accuracy of calculations and technique used to prepare the dose. This may be done by having another caregiver double check the drug identity and dose prepared.

Alternatively and perhaps better, premixed, frozen, or point of care activated devices may be used to assure accuracy and maintenance of sterility when a dose is needed quickly. In spite of the increased safety in preparing the dose, the double check of the physician's order by a pharmacist is often bypassed with these systems. Health care professionals need to work collaboratively to choose the right system to optimize the benefits of parenteral therapy (see Chapter 15).

Suggested Reading

Buchanan EC, Cassano AT. The ASHP Discussion Guide on USP Chapter <797>. Available at: http://www.ashp.org/s_ashp/docs/files/DiscGuide797-2008.pdf Accessed Apr 21, 2009.

Buchanan EC, Schneider PJ, eds. *Compounding Sterile Preparations*. 3rd ed. Bethesda, MD: American Society of Health-System Pharmacists; 2009.

NIOSH. Preventing occupational exposures to antineoplastic and other hazardous drugs in health care settings. Available at: http://www.cdc.gov/niosh/docs/2004-165/ Accessed Apr 21, 2009.

USP Chapter <797> Pharmaceutical compounding—Sterile preparations. Revision Bulletin to USP 31-NF 26, The U.S. Pharmacopeial Convention, Rockville, MD. Official June 1, 2008.

References

1. Cohen MR. High-alert medications: safeguarding against errors. In: Cohen, MR, ed. *Medication Errors*. Washington DC: American Pharmaceutical Association; 2007.

2. Kaushaul R, Bates DW, Landrigan C, et al. Medication errors and adverse drug events in pediatric inpatients. *JAMA*. 2001;285:2114-2120.

3. Hicks RW, Cousins DD, Williams R. *Summary of information submitted to MEDMARX^SM in the year 2002. The Quest for Quality.* Rockville, MD: UPS Center for the Advancement of Patient Safety; 2003.

4. Patterson TR, Nordstrom KA. An analysis of IV additive procedures on nursing units. *Am J Hosp Pharm*. 1968;25:134-137.

5. Flack HL, Gans JA, Serlick SE, et al. The current status of parenteral hyperalimentation. *Am J Hosp Pharm*. 1971; 28:326-335.

6. Thur MP, Miller WA, Latiolais CJ. Medication errors in a nurse-controlled parenteral admixture program. *Am J Hosp Pharm*. 1972; 29:298-304.

7. O'Hare MCB, Bradley AM, Gallagher T, et al. Errors in the administration of intravenous drugs. *Br Med J*. 1995;310:1536-1537

8. Taxis, K, Barber N. Ethnographic study of incidence and severity of intravenous drug errors. *Brit Med J*. 2003;326(7391):684-687.

9. Thompson WL, Feer TD. Incomplete mixing of drugs in intravenous solutions. *Crit Care Med*. 1980;8:603-607.

10. Perlstein PH, Callison C, White M, et al. Errors in drug computations during newborn intensive care. *Am J Dis Child*. 1979; 133:376-379.

11. Pedersen CA, Schneider PJ, Scheckelhoff DJ. ASHP national survey of pharmacy practice in hospital settings: Dispensing and administration—2008. *Am J Health-Syst Pharm*. 2009:66;926-946.

12. Sanders LH, Mabadeje SA, Avis KE, et al. Evaluation of compounding accuracy and aseptic technique for intravenous admixtures. *Am J Hosp Pharm*. 1978;35:531-536.

13. Flynn EA, Pearson RE, Barker KN. Observational study of accuracy in compounding i.v. admixtures in five hospitals. *Am J Hosp Pharm*. 1997;54:904-912.

14. Trissel LA, Gentempo JA, Anderson RW, et al. Using a medium-fill simulation to evaluate the microbial

contamination rate for USP medium-risk level compounding. *Am J Health-Syst Pharm.* 2005;62:285-288.

15. Chapter <797> Pharmaceutical Compounding—Sterile Preparations. In: *United States Pharmacopeia, 31st rev./National Formulary, 26th ed.* Rockville, MD: United States Pharmacopeial Convention; 2009.

16. Turco SJ. Chap. 3 Characteristics. In: *Sterile Dosage Forms: Their Preparation and Clinical Application.* Philadelphia, PA: Lea & Febiger; 1994.

17. Trissel LA. *Handbook on Injectable Drugs.* 15th ed. Bethesda, MD: American Society of Health-System Pharmacists; 2009.

18. Chapter <1116> Microbiological evaluation of clean rooms and other controlled environments. In: *United States Pharmacopeia, 31st rev./National Formulary, 26th ed.* Rockville, MD: United States Pharmacopeial Convention; 2009.

19. Buchanan EC, Schneider PJ, eds. *Compounding Sterile Preparations.* 3rd ed. Bethesda, MD: American Society of Health-System Pharmacists; 2009.

20. Kienle PC. *Compounding Sterile Preparations: ASHP's Video Guide to Chapter <797>.* DVD & Companion Guide Workbook Package. Bethesda, MD: American Society of Health-System Pharmacists; 2009.

21. Power L, Jorgenson J. *Safe Handling of Hazardous Drugs.* DVD & Workbook. Bethesda, MD: American Society of Health-System Pharmacists; 2006.

22. Davis K, Sparks J. *Getting Started in Aseptic Compounding.* Workbook and DVD. Bethesda MD: American Society of Health-System Pharmacists; 2008.

23. Bing C, ed. *Extended Stability for Parenteral Drugs.* 4th ed. Bethesda, MD: American Society of Health-System Pharmacists; 2009.

24. Halvorsen D. The 2010 state of pharmacy compounding: Survey results: Growing confidence. *Pharmacy Purchasing and Products*, 2010 (Apr Supplement);7:1-36.

Chapter Review Questions

1. What percentage of high-alert medications might be administered through the intravenous route?
   a. 25%
   b. 50%
   c. 75%
   d. More than 75%

Answer: d. There is an excellent chapter entitled "High-Alert Medications: Safeguarding Against Errors" in the text *Medication Errors.*[1] Sixteen medications or drug categories are listed, 14 of which can or are administered by the intravenous route.

2. Enforcement of compliance with standards for compounding sterile preparations might rest with which agency?
   a. Food and Drug Administration (FDA)
   b. The Joint Commission
   c. State Boards of Pharmacy
   d. All of the above

Answer: d. Technically, the FDA is responsible for enforcing USP general chapters numbered under 1000. Realistically, the Joint Commission surveyors and/or state boards of pharmacy inspectors are more likely to ask about pharmacy compliance with USP Chapter <797>.

3. Which of the following characteristics would NOT be required for a com-

pounded sterile preparation?

a. Sterile
b. Pyrogen-free
c. Clear
d. Accurate measure of ingredients

Answer: c. While most CSPs are clear, a few are not, e.g., emulsions and suspensions.

4. **Which of the following is a primary engineering control used for compounding hazardous drugs?**

a. Horizontal laminar air flow work bench
b. Compounding aseptic containment isolator
c. Automated pump
d. Compounding aseptic isolator

Answer: b. Either a BSC or a CACI is required for the compounding of hazardous drugs both to protect the compounder from exposure and to maintain the sterility of components.

5. **Which of the following risk levels of compounding requires that the buffer area be a separate room from the ante area?**

a. Low risk
b. Medium risk
c. High risk
d. None of the above

Answer: c. High risk compounding requires an anteroom physically separated from the buffer room to provide the cleanest environment in the buffer room that surrounds the primary engineering control device.

6. **Which of the following levels of air cleanliness is required in the direct compounding area of a biological safety cabinet?**

a. ISO Class 5
b. ISO Class 6
c. ISO Class 7
d. ISO Class 8

Answer: a. ISO Class 5 (fewer than 100 particles 0.5 microns or smaller per cubic foot) is the air cleanliness required in any primary engineering control, including a BSC.

7. **Which of the following is likely to contribute the most microbial contamination to a sterile compounding work environment?**

a. Floors
b. Walls
c. Ceiling
d. Personnel

Answer: d. People generate more particles than any other source in a cleanroom.

8. **Which of the following items of garb is <u>not</u> required for sterile, non-hazardous drug compounding?**

a. Goggles
b. Gown
c. Gloves
d. Shoe covers

Answer: a. Goggles are not required unless working with a hazardous or toxic substance.

9. **Which of the following characteristics of CSPs made by a pharmacy technician must be checked by a pharmacist before the CSPs are dispensed?**
   a. Compatibility of ingredients
   b. Accuracy and completeness of labeling
   c. Appropriateness and integrity of package
   d. All of the above

   Answer: d. Pharmacists must check for compatibility of ingredients, accurate label and proper package.

10. **Which of the following laboratory tests are done for every compounded sterile preparation?**
    a. Sterility
    b. Pyrogenicity
    c. Quantitative measurement of active ingredients
    d. None of the above

    Answer: d. Low and medium risk CSPs do not require any of these tests. It is assumed that the commercially available products used in for low and medium risk CSP's are already sterile, pyrogen-free, and accurate as to labeled contents.

Chapter Discussion Questions

1. What is the evidence supporting the role of the pharmacist in compounding sterile preparations?
2. To what degree should pharmacists take responsibility for compounding sterile preparations?
3. What about medical emergencies in which compounded sterile preparations are needed?
4. Describe how to justify the cost of secondary engineering controls to an administrator.
5. How would you explain the need to remove all jewelry and cosmetics before donning sterile garb?

CHAPTER 15

Parenteral Therapy

E. Clyde Buchanan

Learning Objectives

After completing this chapter, readers should be able to:

1. Describe how parenteral drug therapy is delivered.
2. List the various devices utilized in administering parenteral therapy.
3. Explain the risks associated with parenteral therapy administration.
4. Discuss how to manage the hazards associated with administering parenteral therapies.
5. Define key terms used in talking about parenteral therapy administration.
6. List the different administration routes of parenteral therapy and their characteristics.
7. Describe national and institutional standards that influence parenteral therapy administration.

Key Terms and Definitions

- **Ampul:** A single-use container composed entirely of glass.
- **Cannula:** A tube like a needle or catheter used to infuse parenteral fluids and medications into the vascular system or other body spaces.
- **Electrolyte:** Dissolved ions that include sodium, potassium, chloride, calcium, phosphate, and others.
- **Epidural:** The space superior to the dura mater of the brain and spinal cord and inferior to the ligamentum flavum; outside the subarachnoid space where the cerebrospinal fluid flows.
- **Extravasation:** The inadvertent administration of vesicant medication or solution into the tissue surrounding an artery or vein. Extravasation is an adverse drug event.
- **Incompatibility:** Incapable of being mixed or used simultaneously without undergoing chemical or physical changes or producing undesirable effects. Undesirable effects might include loss of potency of active ingredients, formation of precipitates or toxic ingredients, color changes, etc.
- **Infiltration:** The inadvertent administration of non-vesicant medication or solution into the tissue surrounding an artery or vein. Infiltration is an adverse drug event, unless infiltration is intended (e.g., local anesthetic).
- **Intrathecal:** The space within the spinal canal.

- **Parenteral (or injectable):** Dosage form intended for injection through one or more layers of skin or other external boundary tissue, rather than through the alimentary (enteral) canal, so that the active substances they contain are administered directly into a blood vessel, organ, tissue, or lesion.
- **Sharps:** Objects in the health care setting that can be reasonably anticipated to penetrate the skin and to result in an exposure incident; including but not limited to needle devices, scalpels, lancets, broken glass, or broken capillary tubes.
- **Standard precautions:** Guidelines designed to protect workers with occupational exposure to blood borne pathogens. All blood and body fluids are treated as potentially infectious.
- **Total parenteral nutrition (TPN or hyperalimentation):** The intravenous provision of total nutritional needs for a patient who is unable to take appropriate amounts of food enterally. Typical components include carbohydrates (e.g., dextrose), proteins (e.g., amino acids), and fats (e.g., oil emulsion) as well as electrolytes, vitamins, and trace elements.
- **Vehicle:** For most parenterals, water for injection (USP) is the liquid in which active ingredients are dissolved, suspended or emulsified. Other vehicles include ethanol, and fixed, odorless, vegetable oils that are occasionally used to dissolve solutes that do not dissolve in water.
- **Vial:** A plastic or glass container with a rubber closure secured to its top by a metal ring.

■ ■ ■

Introduction

Particularly in institutional and home infusion settings, pharmacists often receive orders from physicians for drugs to be administered by a parenteral route. Because pharmacists must interpret and carry out these orders appropriately, it is their professional responsibility to understand what the physician intends and what risks are involved in the preparation and use of parenterals. See Chapter 14, which describes the compounding and quality control of sterile preparations. This chapter discusses how parenteral drug therapy is delivered, the risks associated with parenteral therapy and how to avoid those risks. Pharmacists often receive questions from nurses and other caregivers who administer parenteral medications. So pharmacists must be familiar with administration of parenteral drugs as well as preparation and dispensing.

Parenteral Drug Preparation and Dispensing

Parenteral drugs are used for a variety of diagnostic, therapeutic and palliative indications.[1] Based on the indication and information about the patient, the physician (or other licensed prescriber) develops a prescription (or medication order) for a parenteral drug. Physicians' orders require interpretation by a pharmacist for correct compounding and dispensing. Pharmacists should know the patient's age, weight, diagnoses, and allergies to fill a parenteral drug order correctly. The medication order may not give the pharmacist all the information needed to prepare doses. For example, if the order reads "ampicillin IV 1 gram every 8 hours," the pharmacist usually decides whether the dose should be given intermittently or continuously; what the diluent will be; what the concentration of ampicillin in the diluent will be; what the hours of administration will be;

the time over which the dose should be infused and how many doses to prepare. The pharmacist must determine whether the dose is in an appropriate range for the patient, whether there might be an allergic reaction and what incompatibilities to anticipate with other drugs being given by the same route. Some of these pharmacist decisions can be standardized within an institution (e.g., which diluent, what concentration, hours of administration) but other decisions are patient-specific (e.g., dose range, allergy history, incompatibilities).

Parenteral routes of administration may be prescribed for a variety of purposes, e.g., fluid and electrolyte replacement, nutrition, or as a vehicle for a prescribed drug. Parenteral drugs come in a variety of containers and sizes. Manufacturers may package parenteral drugs in ampuls, glass or plastic vials, prefilled syringes, cartridges, glass or plastic bottles, plastic bags, etc. Most injections are aqueous solutions of a drug but there are some injections in the forms of colloidal dispersions, emulsions or suspensions.

Small volume parenteral (SVP) containers may contain a single dose or multiple doses of a drug in a volume no greater than 100 mL. An example of a small volume parenteral is an IV piggy-back container (e.g., minibags or minibottles in 50 mL or 100 mL sizes) that carry a diluent for the active drug. Large volume parenterals (LVPs) are manufactured in bags or bottles up to 1000 mL. Common container sizes are 150 mL, 250 mL, 500 mL, and 1000 mL. Large volume parenterals typically contain fluids (e.g., sodium chloride 0.9%), nutrients (e.g., dextrose), and electrolytes (sodium or potassium chloride) or plasma volume expanders (e.g., albumin).

Infusion therapies fall into several categories that include the following and more:

- Antineoplastic therapy (a.k.a. cancer chemotherapy).
- Biologic therapy (e.g., active and passive immunizations, allergen extracts, monoclonal antibodies, etc.)
- Diagnostic agents (e.g., contrast media, skin tests)
- Emergency treatments (e.g., autonomic drugs, antihypertensives)
- Intravenous sedation
- Parenteral solutions (e.g., fluids and electrolytes)
- Parenteral drug therapy (e.g., antibiotics, hormones, etc.)
- Parenteral nutrition (e.g., total parenteral nutrition)
- Patient-controlled analgesia
- Radiopharmaceuticals
- Transfusions (i.e. blood and blood components)

In summary, the parenteral route of administration offers a variety of advantages[1]:

- An immediate physiological response can be achieved, which is a prime consideration in emergent clinical conditions such as cardiac arrest, or volemic shock.
- Parenterals are required for drugs that are not effective orally or that are destroyed by digestive secretions, such as vaccines, insulin or some antibiotics.
- Medications for nauseated or unconscious patients must be administered parenterally.
- When desirable, parenteral therapy gives the health care provider control of the drug, since the patient must return for continued treatment, such as situations when patients can not be relied on to take oral medication.
- Parenteral administration can result in local effects for drugs as when local anesthetics or anti-inflammatory drugs are injected at the affected site.

- When prolonged drug action is needed, parenteral dosage forms are available, including long-acting steroids injected into joints or long-acting penicillins given by deep intramuscular injection.
- Parenteral therapy provides a way of correcting serious disturbances of fluid and electrolyte balances.
- When food cannot be taken by mouth, or tube feeding, total parenteral nutrition requirements can be supplied into large veins.

■ ■ ■

Key Point . . .

Parenterals are made in a variety of sizes and containers for a variety of uses but all are injected into or beneath the skin.

. . . So what?

Once a chemical penetrates the skin barrier, the potential for an negative patient health outcome increases greatly.

Hazards of Parenteral Therapy

Regardless of the parenteral route of administration, there are disadvantages.[2] The dosage forms must be administered by trained personnel, and typically require more nursing time than those administered by other routes. Parenteral administration requires strict adherence to aseptic procedures, and can cause some pain on injection. Once a drug has been given parenterally, it becomes more difficult to reverse the physiological effects. Finally, because of manufacturing and packaging requirements, parenteral dosage forms are more expensive than similar drugs given orally.

Infusion of a parenteral product or compounded preparation into a vein can lead to phlebitis (inflammation of the vein) or thrombophlebitis (inflammation and a clot in a vein). An early sign of phlebitis is tenderness at the insertion site of the intravenous (IV) needle or cannula. As phlebitis worsens, the vein becomes red, warm and painful with edema and stiffness. In the latter stages of phlebitis, the vein appears as a palpable, tender red cord.[2] Infusion phlebitis can last for a week or more, can induce fever, and predispose the patient to sepsis. Factors associated with infusion phlebitis are the type of needle used, duration of IV therapy, chemically irritating drugs, pH of the infusion, osmolality of the IV fluid, location of the IV site, decreased blood flow and, possibly, the presence of particulate matter in the infusion.[2]

Infiltration, extravasation, or the accidental intra-arterial injection of some drugs can cause necrosis resulting in tissue damage, even loss of a limb. Caustic or vesicant drugs (e.g., chemotherapy) or vasoconstricting drugs are most often implicated in these injuries.

Particulate matter (mobile, undissolved and unintended particles other than gas bubbles) has been reported in a variety of manufactured and compounded parenterals, including large and small volume parenterals, dry-filled and lyophilized drugs, total parenteral nutrition, and others. The intravascular infusion of excessive particulate matter may clog capillary beds, contribute to phlebitis, and cause formation of granulomas or foreign body reactions. The United States Pharmacopeia (USP) has a monograph that requires manufacturers of parenteral products to limit the particulate load in their products.[3] See Table 15-1. Compounders of parenteral preparations can contribute to particulate load by any of the following errors:

- Failure to screen for incompatibilities that form precipitates, e.g., calcium phosphate complexes in total parenteral nutrition,[4]
- Failure to dissolve solutes that have precipitated, e.g., mannitol,
- Failure to filter out glass particles from opened ampuls,

- Failure to fully dissolve dry powders or lyophilized powders, e.g., antibiotics,
- Introduction of ambient particles in the compounding process.

Because of the hazards of particulate matter in compounded sterile preparations (CSPs), pharmacists checking CSPs should view the finished preparation against light and dark backgrounds to detect visible particles or cloudiness. Since some precipitates form after the CSP leaves the pharmacy (e.g., when two incompatible drugs are mixed in IV tubing), some hospitals have a policy of filtering some or all IV fluids with a 0.22 micron, 0.45 micron or 5-micron filter just before the fluids enter the administration cannula. The 0.22 and 0.45 micron filter have the disadvantages of slowing the rate of IV administration and more frequent filter blockage. This is not just inconvenient but requires more frequent manipulation of the IV line. When IV pumps are used, consideration should be given to the pounds per square inch pressure rating of the filter.[5]

Infection, the presence and growth of a pathologic microorganism, is less frequent but potentially a more serious hazard of parenteral therapy, especially IV therapy and injections into sites in joints, the eye and central nervous system, and may be life-threatening in immunocompromised patients. Intravenous infections may be infusate-related, catheter-related, or administration delivery system related.

Key Point . . .

While parenteral therapy offers advantages such as rapid onset of drug action and more reliable drug levels, medication prescribers must weigh those advantages against inherent parenteral disadvantages of pain on injection, phlebitis, extravasation, infiltration or infection.

. . . So what?

It is easy to take for granted the benefits of parenteral administration of medications and fluids. However, one must always be aware of the disadvantages of pain on injection, phlebitis, extravasation, infiltration, or infection.

Table 15-1.

USP Chapter <788> Particulate Matter in Injections

	Light Obscuration Particle Count Test Compliance*	
Large volume parenterals (over 100 mL)	Average particle count does not exceed 25 per mL equal to or greater than 10 microns	Average particle count does not exceed 3 per mL equal to or greater than 25 microns
Small volume parenterals (less than 100 mL)	Average particle count does not exceed 6000 per container equal to or greater than 10 microns	Average particle count does not exceed 600 per container equal to or greater than 25 microns

Source: United States Pharmacopeial Convention. Chapter <788> Particulate matter in injections. *US Pharmacopeia 31st ed. – National Formulary 26th ed.* Rockville, MD: United States Pharmacopeial Convention; 2008.

*The light obscuration test uses suitable apparatus based on the principle of light blockage that allows for an automatic determination of the size of particles and the number of particles according to size. When the light obscuration test method cannot be used for a parenteral product because of its particular physical characteristics (e.g., emulsions, colloids, liposomals), the microscopic particle count test may be suitable.

The hazards of incorrectly compounded and contaminated IV solutions were discussed in Chapter 14.

Administering Parenteral Medications

To prevent infection, nurses and others who administer parenteral medications must adhere strictly to hand hygiene before beginning administration.[6] Parenteral containers, syringes and needles, and IV administration set-ups must be handled with aseptic technique and standard precautions. Those using a syringe and needle to withdraw drug from a vial must be careful not to "core" a piece of rubber from the stopper with the needle. The use of extra large needles to penetrate vials' rubber closures increases the chance of coring; therefore minimum-gauge needles should be used. Ampuls can release a considerable number of glass particles into its contents when ampul necks are broken to open the ampul. Therefore, the needle that is used to enter an opened ampul should be inserted at an angle and not quite to the bottom of the ampul, but rather to one side of the ampul without touching the neck of the ampul. Alternatively, the use of a 5-micron filter needle to withdraw an ampul's contents avoids glass particles drawn up from ampuls.[7]

Site selection for vascular access must include assessment of a patient's condition, age, diagnosis, vascular condition, history of previous access devices, and type and duration of therapy. The artery or vein must accommodate the size and length of catheter required for the prescribed therapy.[8] See Table 15-2.

Parenteral Routes of Administration

Turco has described various routes of parenteral administration.[1]

- Intradermal (I.D.) administration is when the drug is injected into the superficial layer of the skin between the epidermis and the dermis. Only small volumes of solution can be given by this route and absorption is slow. Intradermal administration may be used for diagnostic skin tests and a few vaccines.
- Subcutaneous (S.C. or S.Q.) injections are given in the loose tissue beneath the skin, generally in the outer surface of the arm or thigh. Subcutaneous drug absorption is more rapid than the intradermal route. Rarely, medications can be given by continuous subcutaneous infusion (a.k.a. hypodermoclysis).[9]
- Intramuscular (I.M.) injections are made into a muscle mass, e.g., deltoid muscle of the upper arm into which as much as 2 mL can be injected in adults or the gluteal medial muscle into which up to 5 mL can be administered in adults. Drug absorption from the intramuscular route is more rapid than S.C. and much more rapid than I.D. However, I.M. dosage forms can be formulated for delayed release by manufacture

Key Point . . .

There are many routes of parenteral drug administration and all have special purposes but all require careful attention to institutional systems and procedures to avoid harm to patients.

. . . So what?

There are many different issues involved in choosing one route over another. Pharmacists should understand all of these issues if they are to help influence their appropriate use.

Table 15-2.

Typical Infusion Sites

Site Name	Infusion Site Selection
Peripheral, short	For adults, veins to be considered for peripheral cannulation are on the dorsal and ventral surfaces of the upper extremities. For neonates and pediatric patients, additional sites may include veins of the head, neck, and lower extremities. Veins of the lower extremities should not be used routinely for adults due to the risk of embolism and thrombophlebitis.
Peripheral, midline	Site selection should be routinely initiated in the region of the antecubital fossa. Veins to be considered for midline cannulation are the basilic, median cubital, cephalic, and brachial veins. For neonate and pediatric patients, additional sites may include the head, neck and lower extremities.
Peripherally inserted central catheter (PICC line)	Site selection should be routinely initiated in the region of the antecubital fossa. Prior to PICC insertion, anatomical measurements must be taken to determine the length of catheter required to ensure full advancement of the catheter with catheter tip placement in the lower third of the superior vena cava to the junction of the superior vena cava and right atrium. Veins to be considered for peripherally inserted central cannulation are the basilic, median cubital, cephalic, and brachial veins. For neonate and pediatric patients, additional sites may include the head, neck and lower extremities.
Non-tunneled and tunneled catheter and implanted ports	Site selection should be determined per manufacturer's labeled use(s) and directions for device insertion.
Arterial	Arteries that should be considered the most appropriate for percutaneous cannulation are the radial, brachial and femoral. For neonate and pediatric patients, additional site selections may include radial, post tibial and dorsalis pedalis arteries; the brachial artery is not recommended. A test should be performed when selecting the appropriate artery for cannulation, prior to device insertion, for assessment of distal arterial perfusion.

Source: Infusion Nurses Society. Standard 37 Site selection. *J Infus Nurs.* 2006 (Jan/Feb); 29 (Suppl. No. 1):S37-9.

as a sterile suspension in an aqueous or oil-based vehicle. Drugs given I.D., S.C. or I.M. may be in the dosage form of a solution, a suspension, or an emulsion.

- Intravenous (IV or i.v.) administration can deliver large or small volumes of solutions into veins. This chapter is devoted more to the IV route because it is most commonly used and poses some of the greatest risks. See previous discussions on phlebitis, infiltration, extravasation and infection. Irritating drugs can be given into large veins because of their rapid dilution with blood.
- Intra-arterial (I.A.) route is not often used. A drug administered I.A. can go directly to a targeted area which may be an organ (e.g., radiopaque dye for an arteriogram) or limb (e.g., local anesthetic for a regional block).
- Central nervous system routes; e.g., intra-spinal, an injection into the spinal column that includes epidural and intrathecal routes. Injections directly into the brain include intra-cranial and intra-ventricular.
- Other uncommon routes include: intracardiac, an injection directly into a chamber of the heart; intrasynovial, an injection into a joint fluid area; intra-articular, an injec-

tion directly into the cavity of a joint; intraosseous, an injection with a vascular access device with tip placement within the bone matrix.

Methods of Administration

Personnel administering parenterals must have a thorough knowledge of the components of administration devices. The simplest device is a sterile syringe with a sterile needle attached. With the right size syringe and the right gauge and length of needle, this set-up can be used for intradermal, subcutaneous, intramuscular or intravenous drug administration.

Infusions are usually administered with an IV set, the proximal end of which is attached to the fluid container and the distal end inserted into an IV needle (e.g., "butterfly" needle) or an IV catheter. Depending on the therapy, infusions can be administered on a continuous basis at a prescribed rate of administration or administered intermittently. See Figures 15-1 and 15-2. Continuous infusions may be given at a steady rate or the rate may be adjusted periodically depending on a patient parameter such as blood pressure, heart rate, arrhythmias etc. Periodic adjustments are often called "titrations in the rate." Rates of infusion can be measured in several units, e.g., drops per minute, mini-drops per minute, mL per hour and others.

Intermittent intravenous therapy is administered at prescribed intervals with periods of infusion cessation in order to allow patients freedom from infusions between doses.[10] The simplest intermittent therapy method is IV Push. With a syringe containing the drug solution, the caregiver inserts the needle into a port in the IV tubing and applies pressure (i.e., pushes) a bolus dose into the IV line, and then flushes the line with solution from the primary IV bag. The piggyback (Figure 15-2) method refers to a smaller secondary container (e.g., minibag or minibottle) running into a primary IV line. The

Figure 15-1. Set-up for continuous IV infusion. *Source:* Reprinted with permission from Baxter Healthcare.

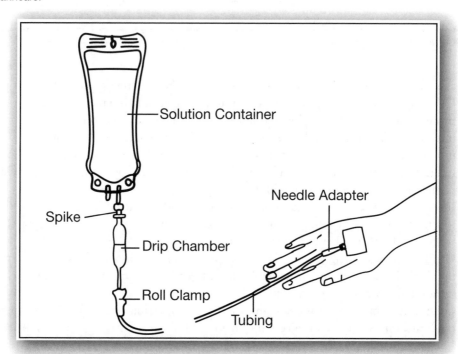

Figure 15-2. Set-up for intermittent IV infusion. *Source:* Reprinted with permission from Baxter Healthcare.

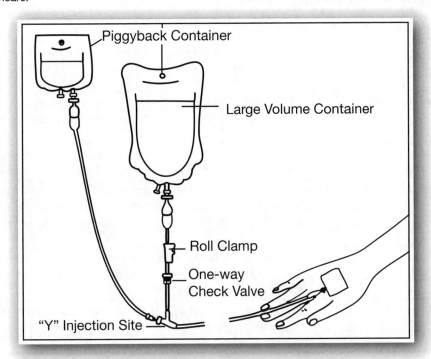

piggyback method eliminates the need for another venipuncture, achieves appropriate drug dilution and gains peak drug blood levels in a short time, e.g., 30 to 60 minutes. The piggyback method is often used to administer antibiotics.

An alternative for intermittent IV therapy method is the syringe pump. This involves slow, measured direct intravenous bolus dosing and is accomplished by a pump device that slowly injects the contents of a syringe into a Y-site in a primary IV line.

A third means for intermittent IV infusion is the burette set. This is an in-line volume measuring container made as part of the primary IV set. This method may allow a nurse to rapidly measure and administer an emergency dose of a drug. However, its use is discouraged because of the greater likelihood of a calculation or measuring error or of contaminating the primary IV line with ambient bacteria.

Intravenous fluid administration sets should be changed periodically to maintain their sterility and patency. See Table 15-3.

Infusion Pumps

To make infusion of critical drugs and fluids more accurate and uniform, flow-control devices known as infusion pumps were introduced in the 1970s. These pumps use one of several methods to accurately measure the amount of fluid being pumped into an artery or vein. There are peristaltic pumps, piston pumps, pulsatile pumps, elastomeric chambers and other methods to force fluid delivery. The type of infusion pump should suit the patient as to age, condition, prescribed infusion therapy, type of vascular access device and healthcare setting.[11]

An infusion pump should have safety features such as: audible alarms, battery life and operation indicators, anti-free flow protection, adjustable occlusion pressure levels,

Table 15-3.

Administration Set Change Intervals

Administration Set Type	Standard Administration Set Change Intervals
Primary and secondary continuous sets	Change set no more frequently than every 72 hours and immediately upon suspected contamination or when the integrity of the product or system has been compromised.
Primary intermittent sets	Change set every 24 hours and immediately upon suspected contamination or when the integrity of the product or system has been compromised.
Parenteral nutrition sets	Change every 72 hours and immediately upon suspected contamination or when the integrity of the product or system has been compromised.
Intravenous fat emulsion sets	When units of intravenous fat emulsions are administered consecutively, change set every 24 hours and immediately upon suspected contamination or when the integrity of the product or system has been compromised.
Blood and blood component sets	Administration sets and add-on filters that are used for blood and blood components must be changed after administration of each unit or at the end of 4 hours whichever comes first.
Add-on devices	Change of add-on devices such as extension sets, filters, stopcocks and needleless devices should coincide with changing of the administration set.

Source: Adapted from Anon. Chapter 48. Administration Set Change. *J Infus Nurs.* 2006; (Jan/Feb) Suppl.1 Vol. 29:S48-50.

accuracy of delivery indicator, drug dosage calculation, in-line pressure monitoring, anti-tampering mechanisms, and dose-error reductions systems.[11] Infusion pumps for vesicant drugs like chemotherapy should be capable of administering fluid under low pressure to prevent extravasation. Infusion pumps for arterial catheters must be capable of administering fluid under high pressure to overcome the back pressure of blood in arteries.[11]

Elastomeric chambers are perhaps the simplest of infusion pumps. These flow-control devices typically consist of a balloon-like chamber or fluid reservoir within a hard cylinder or shell. There is usually a pre-attached IV administration set with a flow-control clamp and a port for injection fluids and additives to the chamber. As the flow-control clamp is released, the elastic reservoir collapses, forcing fluid into the administration set. Elastomeric chambers are most commonly used for infusions of antibiotics, chemotherapy or pain medications, on either a continuous or an intermittent basis. The disadvantages of elastomeric chambers are the lack of safety features like anti-free flow protection, alarms, rate and dose indicators. Being discarded after one use, they are fairly expensive on a per dose basis; yet elastomeric chambers are often used in the home infusion setting.

IV Pumps

About 90% of hospitalized patients receive IV medications, most of which are delivered via an infusion pump.[12,13] Although conventional IV pumps improve the accuracy and continuity of IV infusions, studies estimate that these devices are involved in 35% to 60% of the 770,000 adverse drug events (ADEs) each year.[12-16] Critically ill patients are particularly susceptible to infusion pump-related ADEs because they' are more likely to receive more dangerous IV medications.[17] Most IV pump-related errors occur because a caregiver manually programs the pump with the wrong settings for the rate or dose.[16,18]

Smart Pumps

To improve the safety of IV pumps a new generation of infusion pumps called smart pumps has been introduced. By checking programmed settings against the hospital's guidelines for specific drugs and patient groups, these pumps can intercept potentially serious programming errors before they happen.[12,19] The smart pump has software that contains a drug library to alert the caregiver if programmed settings are outside of a particular medication's recommended parameters, such as dose, dosing regimen (mcg/kg/min, units/hr, etc.), or concentration.[13,15] Smart pumps record data about all such alerts, including the time, date, drug, concentration, programmed rate, and volume infused, thus providing valuable continuous quality improvement (CQI) information.[13,20] Some smart pumps can accommodate add-on syringe pump systems for small-volume IV push or bolus infusions. Others allow multiple infusions through one pump, and some are able to factor in a patient's age or clinical condition.

Before using smart pumps at the bedside, a facility programs the pumps with its own specific data sets, or "profiles." These profiles specify the infusion requirements for different patient types and care areas, such as pediatric, adult, obstetrics, oncology, anesthesia, ICU, and post-anesthesia care units. Each profile includes a drug library that contains hospital-defined drug infusion parameters, such as acceptable concentrations, infusion rates, dosing units, and maximum and minimum loading and maintenance dose, bolus limits, for 60 or more medications.[21] Pharmacists, physicians, and nurses within each institution set up and manage these profiles based on the hospital's own best practice guidelines, with on-site assistance from the pump manufacturer.[16] In 2008, 52% of hospitals reported having smart IV pumps in place and 72% of hospitals without smart pumps plan to have them within the foreseeable future.[22]

Special Purpose Infusion Devices

Special purpose infusion devices include implantable pumps and patient-controlled analgesia pumps. Implantable pumps have a catheter surgically placed into a blood vessel, body cavity or organ; the catheter is attached to a reservoir surgically implanted under the skin. The reservoir has a pumping mechanism. The purpose of an implantable pump is to provide long-term injectable access. Caregivers must be extra cautious to use aseptic technique (i.e., hand hygiene, sterile gloves, mask etc.) and small non-coring needles when adding fluids to implanted pumps.[23]

Patient-controlled analgesia (PCA) is a process in which patients can determine when and how much medication they

> ### Key Point . . .
>
> While nurses administer most IV medications, including those given by infusion pump, pharmacists must play a role in the selection, policy-making, procedure development, drug libraries and medication error monitoring associated with IV infusion devices.
>
> #### . . . So what?
>
> Pharmacists do not need to administer IV medications to influence their use. They can influence by understanding best practices, monitoring processes and outcomes associated with administration, and guide the policies and procedures used within the institution.

receive. The predominant form of PCA is a specially-designed IV pump. The pump is programmed so that the patient pushes a button, which activates a bolus dose of the analgesic. The pump may also be programmed to deliver a low-level continuous infusion of drug, for example in an opioid-tolerant patient. The pump has a bolus dose limit and a "lockout" interval that is a predetermined, programmed amount of time, for example, 10 minutes, between bolus doses and during that time additional button activation will have no effect until the designated interval has passed. Newer pumps are equipped with scanners for patient identification and double check mechanisms for the complicated programming that must be input into the device.[24,25] Patient-controlled analgesia requires not only competent caregivers but training of patients to adjust their own rate of analgesic medications. With PCA devices, patient consent, assessment, and monitoring are added to the caregiver's responsibility.[26]

Waste Disposal

All blood-contaminated and sharp items including needles, surgical blades and syringes must be discarded into nonpermeable, puncture-resistant, tamper-proof biohazard containers (a.k.a. sharps container). Sharps must not be recapped, broken or bent. Sharps containers must be replaced before they are full to avoid disposal-related injuries. All biohazardous materials, wastes and drugs must be discarded in the appropriate containers and disposed of according to local, state, and federal regulations.[27]

Infusion Therapy Documentation

Nurses and others who administer drugs must provide complete and accurate documentation regarding infusion therapy and vascular access in the patient's permanent medical record. Documentation should include at least the following[28]:

- Patient, caregiver, or legally authorized representative's participation in and validated understanding of therapy and care procedures.
- Type, brand, length, and size of vascular access device.
- Date and time of insertion, number and location of attempts, type of catheter stabilization and dressing, patient's response to the insertion, and identification of the person inserting the device.
- Identification of the insertion site by anatomical descriptors, landmarks, or appropriately marked drawings.
- Infusion site condition and appearance using standard assessment scales for phlebitis, infiltration, and extravasation.

Parenteral Medication Safety

As mentioned in Chapter 14, the USP reported that "the intravenous route of administration often results in the most serious medication error outcomes" based on reports submitted to USP's MEDMARX[SM].[29] A summit on preventing patient harm and death from IV medication errors was convened on July 2008, by the American Society of Health-System Pharmacists (ASHP), ASHP Research and Education Foundation, Institute for Safe Medication Practices, USP, Infusion Nurses Society, The Joint Commission, and National Patient Safety Foundation. USP's MEDMARX[SM] data on parenteral medication errors from more than 1 million error reports from 850 hospitals between 2002 and 2006 were presented at the summit. Parenteral medication errors were nearly three times as likely to cause harm or death (3.0%) compared with other errors reported to MEDMARX[SM] (1.2%). The majority (79%) of harmful or fatal parenteral errors involved the IV route of administration (other errors involved the subcutaneous, epidural, intravascular, or intrathecal routes), and 58% of parenteral medication errors originated during the administration step of the medication-use process. The therapeutic categories most commonly associated with harmful or fatal parenteral medication errors were insulin, opioid analgesics, and blood coagulation modifiers: all "high-alert" medications.[30]

Who is to blame for parenteral medication errors? Smetzer pointed out that simply holding healthcare practitioners accountable for giving the right drug to the right patient in the right dose by the right route at the right time fails to ensure medication safety. Adding a sixth, seventh, eighth, or ninth right (e.g., right reason, right formulation, right line attachment, timely and accurate documentation) is not the answer either.[31] The "rights" are merely broadly stated goals or desired outcomes of safe medication practices that offer no procedural guidance on how to achieve these goals and they fail to acknowledge that human factors and system weaknesses contribute to errors, and that the focus of the "rights" on individual performance does little to reflect that safe medication practices are a combination of both interdisciplinary efforts of many individuals and reliable systems. Health caregivers can only be held accountable for following the processes that their organizations have designed as the best way to verify the "rights." For example, nurses and pharmacists cannot really verify that the right drug is provided in a given vial, or that it contains the right dose/strength. But they can be held accountable for reading the label, requesting an independent double check if required, questioning orders for drugs/doses that are illegible or appear unsafe, using bar code technology if functional, and so on. These are procedural steps the organization has deemed sufficient to verify the right drug and the right dose. If the procedural rules cannot be followed because of system issues, health caregivers also have a duty to report the problem so it can be remedied.[31]

With the systems approach in mind, the aforementioned multidisciplinary summit meeting stated optimum IV system characteristics. See Table 15-4. Another multidisciplinary group looked specifically at the safety of intravenous drug delivery systems.[32] Table 15-5 summarizes some of the benefits and problems associated with each delivery system that were identified by this group. Note that centralized pharmacy admixture programs rank fourth in relative safety among the four IV drug delivery systems, being safer only than when a direct care giver admixes doses on the floor. Commercial manufactured, ready-to-use products were clearly viewed as the safest in terms of potential and actual risk of harm to patients, e.g., administration of wrong medication, infections, phlebitis etc.

Pharmacist Cynthia Dusik makes the point that IV safety for pediatric patients requires extra precautions in healthcare institutions.[33] Here are her dozen safety maneuvers to minimize IV medication risk for pediatric patients:

- Ensure that all staff members are educated and competent to work on behalf of neonates, infants, children, and adolescents.
- Mandate that the patient's weight and allergy status be included on all physician medication orders. Allow only metric units for weight and height (kg and cm) to avoid confusion and potential dosing errors.
- Provide medications in the most ready-to-use format, preferably in unit-of-use packaging.

Table 15-4.

Priority IV Medication Safety Practices

Step in Medication-use Process	Priority IV Medication Safety Practices
Formulary management and medication-use policy	▪ Implement standardized infusion concentrations (dose, rate, units) based on local and national practices that are appropriate for most practice settings and allow exceptions, if needed
	▪ Use commercially available ready-to-administer IV medications if available (except parenteral nutrient solutions)
	▪ Limit available concentrations of parenteral medications on the formulary
	▪ Implement hospital-wide standardized processes for high-alert medications
	▪ Prohibit use of patients' own parenteral medications or establish strict criteria for exceptions
	▪ Establish comprehensive IV medication administration policies, with standardized administration times, upper and lower dosage limits, and administration rates (especially for IV push and adjusted medications); policies for special patient populations; and policies that specify any required monitoring, special equipment, or unique competencies for administration
	▪ Establish communication procedures for product shortages, recalls, and safety advisories, including recommendations for alternative agents
Prescribing and ordering	▪ Use standardized IV medication orders (paper or electronic format)
	▪ Prescribe standardized infusion diluents, concentrations, and units (preferably commercially available products)
	▪ Limit use of nonstandardized infusions to clinical indications in which benefits outweigh potential risks
	▪ Use hospital-wide standardized dosing protocols for emergency drugs and high-alert medications (e.g., heparin, insulin)
	▪ Differentiate look-alike medications when ordering
	▪ Use clinical decision support at the point of care (e.g., drug allergy and drug interaction alerts, dosage calculators)
Storage	▪ Stock commercially available ready-to-administer infusions for emergency use in patient care areas where possible
	▪ Differentiate look-alike medications, including separate storage locations
	▪ Prohibit or impose tight security precautions on stocking concentrated injectable products and more than one concentration of an IV medication on patient care units
	▪ Designate storage locations of authorized medications on patient care units (i.e., minimize variability in storage locations)
	▪ Adopt ISMP guidelines on interdisciplinary safe use of automated dispensing cabinets (ADCs)

(continued)

Table 15-4. (continued)

Priority IV Medication Safety Practices

Step in Medication-use Process	Priority IV Medication Safety Practices
Preparation and dispensing	▦ Dispense IV medications and admixtures in ready-to-administer form (i.e., a form that requires no manipulation prior to administration)
	▦ Standardize process for compounding sterile preparations, with procedures to minimize unnecessary interruptions and distractions, trace and verify the accuracy of compounding, and provide for pharmacist checking of compounding accuracy
	▦ Label IV admixtures using standard format with information needed by staff who will administer admixtures prominently displayed
	▦ Ensure competency of pharmacists and technicians who prepare IV medications
	▦ Use best practices for preparation of IV admixtures in addition to practices for assuring stability and sterility in USP Chapter <797>
	▦ Use machine-readable codes to verify accuracy of medication dispensing and filling of automated dispensing cabinets (ADCs)
Administering	▦ Require independent double checks and documentation of administration of selected high-alert medications, including pump settings
	▦ Standardize IV medication administration, with provisions to (1) minimize unnecessary interruptions and distractions, (2) focus on one patient at a time, (3) refer to an accurate medication administration record at the bedside, (4) engage the patient or parent and family members in medication administration process, (5) use two patient identifiers, (6) trace tubing to the body before administering medication into tubing, and (7) label distal and proximal infusion sites when using pumps with multiple channels or multiple pumps (e.g., for epidural medications, enteral nutrition)
	▦ Ensure competency of staff who prepare and administer IV medications
	▦ Involve patients and families in IV medication safety and provide written scripts to guide interactions between health care providers and parents
	▦ Use clinical tools customized for high-risk patient populations (e.g., dose calculators for pediatric patients or patients with renal insufficiency)
	▦ Limit the preparation of IV admixtures by nursing staff to life-threatening emergencies and preparations with limited stability
	▦ Use intelligent infusion devices (e.g., smart pumps) with dose-limiting feature enabled
Monitoring medication use and medication use processes	▦ Have antidotes, supportive medications, dosing and administration information, and resuscitation equipment immediately available in patient care areas
	▦ Establish baseline and ongoing monitoring procedures for selected parenteral, high-alert medications (e.g., anticoagulants, insulin, vasopressors, oncologic agents) so that medication ordering is linked with appropriate laboratory test results

(continued)

Table 15-4. (continued)
Priority IV Medication Safety Practices

Step in Medication-use Process	Priority IV Medication Safety Practices
Monitoring medication use and medication use processes	▨ Establish standard operating procedures for communication at the time of patient transition from one care setting to another to provide for continuity of care and medication reconciliation
	▨ Establish standard operating procedures for communicating about and responding to actual or suspected medication errors
	▨ Use data from intelligent infusion devices and information systems to improve medication-use processes

Source: Modified from Table 1 in Proceedings of a summit on preventing harm and death from IV medication errors. *Am J Health-Syst Pharm.* 2008; 65:2367-2379.

Table 15-5.
Issues Associated with IV Drug Delivery Systems

Product Type	Benefits	Problems	Safety Rank
Manufacturer ready-to-use	Low risk for contamination, ease of use and dispensing, maximum available expiration dating	Products not available for special populations, pharmacoeconomic data lacking, frozen products may require thawing	1
Outsourced ready-to-use	Can customize dose for each patient, low risk for contamination	Cost analysis suggested, requires advance planning and storage	3
Point of care activated	Works well with automated cabinets, maximum available expiration dates	Products not available for special populations, cost analysis suggested, risk of inactivation errors	2
Pharmacy compounded	Can customize dose for each patient, significant quality control, labeled in accordance with hospital standards	Risk of contamination, significant operational requirements related to USP Chapter <797>	4
Non-pharmacy compounded at point of care	Can customize dose for each patient, immediate availability	High potential for error, low compliance with regulatory requirements, labeling typically handwritten or absent, risk of contamination	5

Source: Modified from Table 2 in Sanborn MD, Moody ML, Harder KA et al. Second consensus development conference on the safety of intravenous drug delivery systems—2008. *Am J Health-Syst Pharm.* 2009; 66:185-192.

- Use appropriate measuring devices to deliver pediatric doses.
- Have a formulary process in place that includes drug evaluation, selection, therapeutic use, potential risk, and any other issues to maximize safe medication use.
- Limit the number of concentration and dosage strengths available within the organization to minimize the risk of selecting the wrong concentration. Do not make concentrated electrolyte solutions available as floor stock in patient care areas.
- Standardize concentrations of medications that are delivered via continuous infusion. Eliminate the use of "rule-of-six" to calculate continuous infusions.
- Prior to dispensing and administration of medication, ensure that a pharmacist reviews all orders for appropriate indication, dosing regimen, potential allergies, and potential drug and/or food interactions.
- Limit the availability of medications on override in automated dispensing cabinets (ADCs) to those that are needed in emergent situations. Discourage removal of medications prior to a pharmacist's review. Regularly review override reports to identify trends.
- Use bar code technology when refilling ADCs and at the point of patient care to minimize wrong drug/concentration filling errors and administration errors. If bar code technology is not available, establish procedures of multiple checks when restocking ADCs to minimize wrong drug/concentration filling errors. In institutions not utilizing ADCs, establish multiple checks when unit stock is replaced.
- Even the most thorough implementation of smart pumps does not guarantee compliance with their intended and appropriate use. Establish a practice of regular data review to determine compliance with drug library use and to determine if adjustments to dosing limits are warranted.
- Establish an ongoing method to review medication processes throughout the institution. Involve all disciplines to evaluate medication use processes and apply continuous quality improvement principles to identify and eliminate problematic practices.

Just as pediatric age group patients require special precautions for parenteral therapy, so do other susceptible patient groups like cancer patients, geriatric and transplant patients.

Key Point . . .

Special populations such as pediatric, cancer, geriatric, transplant patients require special precautions for parenteral therapy.

. . . So what

Interventions targeting patient populations at greatest risk of adverse outcomes of parenteral therapy can be more cost-effective than treating everyone the same.

Summary

Parenteral drug therapy can be highly beneficial for patients but can be riskier than other routes of administration. Health caregivers must be highly trained and conscientious in carrying out institutional procedures to minimize the risks of parenteral drug therapy. The complexity of modern parenteral therapy, for example with automated pumps, toxic drugs and risky administration sites, make training health care personnel and holding them accountable to procedures all the more important. Leaders in health care institutions in which parenteral drug therapy is employed are responsible for the policies, procedures and competency of their personnel. Leaders in health care institutions that serve pediatric, cancer or geriatric patients must make extra precautions in developing policies, procedures and personnel competency measures.

Suggested Reading

Alexander M, Corrigan A, Gorski L, et al. *Infusion Nursing: An Evidence-Based Approach.* Norwood, MA: Infusion Nursing Society; 2009.

Anon. Safe practices for parenteral nutrition. *J Parenter Enteral Nutr.* 2004;28:S39-S70.

ASHP Reports. Proceedings of a summit on preventing patient harm and death from IV medication errors. *Am J Health-Syst Pharm.* 2008;65:2367-79.

Breland BD, Michienzi KA. Advancing patient safety with intelligent infusion technology. *Pharm Purchas Prod.* 2009 (Mar);Suppl:1-13.

Hankin CS, Schein J, Clark JA, et al. Adverse events involving intravenous patient-controlled analgesia. *Am J Health-Syst Pharm.* 2007;64:1492-1499.

Sanborn MD, Moody ML, Harder KA, et al. Second consensus development conference on the safety of intravenous drug delivery systems—2008. *Am J Health-Syst Pharm.* 2009;66:185-192.

Schneider PJ, Buchanan EC. Chapter 14. Sterile preparations and admixture programs. In: Introduction to Institutional Pharmacy Practice. Bethesda, MD: American Society of Health-System Pharmacists; 2010.

References

1. Turco S. Chap. 1 Introduction. In: Turco S, ed. *Sterile Dosage Forms.* Philadelphia PA, Lea & Febiger, 1994:1-10.

2. Turco S. Appendix 4. Hazards associated with parenteral therapy. In: Turco S, ed. *Sterile Dosage Forms.* Philadelphia: Lea & Febiger; 1994:405-437.

3. United States Pharmacopeial Convention. Chapter <788> Particulate matter in injections. In: *United States Pharmacopeia 31st Ed./National Formulary 26th Ed.* Rockville, MD: United States Pharmacopeia; 2008.

4. Food and Drug Administration. Safety alert: hazards of precipitation associated with parenteral nutrition. *Am J Hosp Pharm.* 1994;51:1427-1428.

5. Infusion Nurses Society. Standard 32 Filters. *J Infus Nurs.* 2006(Jan/Feb);29(No. 1S):S33-34.

6. Centers for Disease Control and Prevention. Guidelines for hand hygiene in healthcare settings. *Morbid Mortal Weekly Rep.* 2002(Oct 25);51:1-45.

7. Consentino F. Chap. 6 Handling and administration. In: Turco S, ed. *Sterile Dosage Forms.* Philadelphia: Lea & Febiger; 1994:79-96.

8. Infusion Nurses Society. Standard 37 Site selection. *J Infus Nurs.* 2006(Jan/Feb);29(No. 1S):S37-39.

9. Infusion Nurses Society. Standard 64 Continuous subcutaneous access devices. *J Infus Nurs.* 2006(Jan/Feb);29 (No. 1S):S68-69.

10. Turco S. Chap. 8 Large volume sterile solutions. In: Turco S, ed. *Sterile Dosage Forms.* Philadelphia: Lea & Febiger; 1994:115-195.

11. Infusion Nurses Society. Standard 33 Flow control devices. *J Infus Nurs.* 2006 (Jan/Feb);29 (No. 1S):S34-35.

12. Husch M, Sullivan C, et al. Insights from the sharp end of intravenous medication errors: Implications for infusion pump technology. *Qual Saf Health Care.* 2005;14(2):80.

13. Vanderveen T. Averting highest-risk errors is first priority. Available at: www.psqh.com/mayjun05/averting.html. Accessed Jun 8, 2009.

14. Reeves JG. "Smart pump" technology reduces errors. Available at: www.apsf.org/resource_center/news-letter/2003/spring/smartpump.htm . Accessed Jun 8, 2009.

15. Eskeu JA, Jacobi J, et al. Using innovative technologies to new safety standards for the infusion of intravenous medications. *Hospital Pharm.* 2002;37(11):1179.

16. Rosenthal, K. Smart pumps help crack the safety code. *Nurs Manage.* 2004;35(5):49.

17. Rothschild JM, Keohane CA, et al. Intelligent intravenous infusion pumps to improve medication administration safety. *AMIA Annu Symp Proc.* 2003:992.

18. Adachi W, Lodolce AE. Use of failure mode and effects analysis in improving the safety of IV drug administration. *Am J Health Syst Pharm.* 2005;62(9):917-920.

19. Rothschild JM, Keohane, CA, et al. A controlled trial of smart infusion pumps to improve medication safety in critically ill patients. *Crit Care Med.* 2005;33(3):533.

20. Wilson, K and Sullivan, M. Preventing medication errors with smart infusion technology. *Am J Health Syst Pharm.* 2004;61(2), 177-183.

21. Beattie S. Technology today: Smart IV pumps. RNWeb. Dec 1, 2005. Available at: http://rn.modernmedicine.com/rnweb/article/articleDetail.jsp?id=254828) Accessed May 8, 2009.

22. Halverson D. The state of pharmacy automation. Pharm Purchas & Prod. 2008 (Aug). Available at: www.pppmag.com/pp-p-state-of-pharmacy-automation-2008/sopa-survey-results-taking-technology-for-gr.html. Accessed May 8, 2009.

23. Infusion Nurses Society. Standard 45 Implanted ports and pumps. *J Infus Nursing.* 2006 (Jan/Feb);29(No. 1S):S45-46.

24. Viscusi ER, Schechter LN. Patient-controlled analgesia: Finding a balance between cost and comfort. *Am J Health-Syst Pharm.* 2006;63(Suppl.1):S3-13.

25. Steinfass SK. Beyond pumps: Smarter infusion systems. *Nurs Manage.* 2004;35(Suppl. 5):10.

26. Infusion Nurses Society. Standard 67. Patient-controlled analgesia. *J Infus Nurs.* 2006 (Jan/Feb);29 (No. 1S):S73-74.

27. Infusion Nurses Society. Standard 25. Disposal of sharps, hazardous materials, and hazardous wastes. *J Infus Nurs.* 2006 (Jan/Feb);29 (No. 1S):S30.

28. Infusion Nurses Society. Standard 14 Documentation. *J Infus Nurs.* 2006 (Jan/Feb);29 (No. 1S):S22-23.

29. Hicks RW, Cousins DD, Williams R. *Summary of information submitted to MEDMARX[SM] in the year 2002. The Quest for Quality.* Rockville, MD: USP Center for the Advancement of Patient Safety; 2003.

30. ASHP Reports. Proceedings of a summit on preventing patient harm and death from IV medication errors. *Am J Health-Syst Pharm.* 2008;65:2367-2379.

31. Smetzer J. The five rights: A destination without a map. ISMP Newsletter 2007 (Jan 25). Available at: http://www.ismp.org/newsletters/acutecare/articles/20070125.asp?ptr=y Accessed April 29, 2009.

32. Sanborn MD, Moody ML, Harder KA et al. Second consensus development conference on the safety of intravenous drug delivery systems – 2008. *Am J Health Syst Pharm.* 2009;66:185-192.

33. Dusik CM. Best practices for IV safety in pediatrics. *Pharm Pur & Prod.* 2009 (Apr);6:12-15.

Chapter Review Questions

1. **Which of the following would be considered parenteral routes of administration?**
    a. Intradermal
    b. Intravenous
    c. Epidural
    d. All of the above

    Answer: d. Any injectable route that is administered through the skin is considered parenteral.

2. In their orders, physicians must specify all the information necessary to compound a parenteral drug.
a. True
b. False

Answer: b. For parenteral drugs, physicians often just order the active ingredient, dose, route and regimen without specifying the diluent, concentration or rate of administration.

3. Which of the following nutrients can be given parenterally?
a. Carbohydrates
b. Proteins
c. Fats
d. All of the above

Answer: d. Carbohydrates, proteins and fats are administered together with electrolytes, vitamins and trace minerals for total parenteral nutrition.

4. Which of the following is the most commonly used parenteral route?
a. Intravenous
b. Intramuscular
c. Subcutaneous
d. Intrathecal

Answer: a. The intravenous route is most commonly used because veins accommodate a larger volume of injection, a wider variety of active ingredients and more predictable blood levels.

5. Which of the following is NOT an intermittent method of intravenous drug administration?
a. Elastomeric chambers
b. Smart pumps
c. Patches
d. Syringe and needle

Answer: c. Elastomeric chambers, smart pumps and syringes can all be used to give intermittent doses of drugs. A patch is applied to the skin surface to provide a continuous drug action.

6. Which of the following requires special precautions to prevent glass particulates from entering a compounded sterile preparation?
a. Syringe
b. Cartridge
c. Ampul
d. Vial

Answer: c. When ampuls are broken at the neck for opening, many small glass particles fall into the solution. Special placement of needles with the ampul or a filter needle is required to avoid withdrawal of glass particles that can be injected into a compounded sterile preparation.

7. **What makes a "smart pump" smart?**
   a. Internal programmable drug library
   b. Patient group specific dosing and rate limits
   c. Recording of administration data, such as which patient received what drug and when
   d. All of the above

   Answer: d. Smart pumps are capable of all these safety features and more.

8. **During what part of the medication-use process do most parenteral medication errors take place?**
   a. Prescribing
   b. Administering
   c. Compounding
   d. Dispensing

   Answer: b. According to MEDMARX^{SM} data from 2002 to 2006, 58% of parenteral medication errors originated during the administration step of the medication-use process.

9. **According to the systems approach, for which of the following "rights" should a nurse be held more accountable?**
   a. Right drug
   b. Right dose
   c. Right route
   d. None of the above

   Answer: d. Health care institution leaders must develop operating processes and procedures (e.g., double checks, proper labels, fail-safe connections, etc.) that lead to right medication use. Nurses should only be held accountable for following the recognized processes and procedures of the institution in which they work.

10. **What is required before a patient is given responsibility for a PCA pump?**
    a. Pump programming
    b. Patient training
    c. Patient monitoring
    d. All of the above

    Answer: d. For patient-controlled analgesia to be safe, caregivers are responsible for all these actions plus more before patients can be given responsibility for self-administering strong pain killers by vein.

Chapter Discussion Questions

1. What makes parenteral therapy so complex?
2. What makes parenteral therapy dangerous?
3. Name and discuss some procedures, devices and systems that make parenteral therapy safer.
4. Discuss the pharmacist's role in developing safe and effective parenteral therapy.
5. Why do different patient populations (e.g., pediatric patients, elderly patients) need customized procedures to maintain their safety during parenteral therapy?

CHAPTER 16

Leadership and Management

David A. Holdford

■ ■ ■

Learning Objectives

After completing this chapter, readers should be able to:

1. Define leadership and contrast it with management.
2. Discuss what it takes to be a leader.
3. Identify ways to develop leadership skills.
4. Describe six common leadership styles.
5. Identify situational characteristics that might require different leadership styles.

Key Terms and Definitions

■ **Attitude theory:** A theory stating that the beliefs leaders hold about people greatly influences both the manager's behavior and the followers' responses. The theory divides leaders into two categories; Theory X Leaders and Theory Y Leaders.

■ **Behavioral theories:** A group of leadership theories that argue that the greatest predictors of leadership effectiveness are the behaviors and abilities that people learn over time. They all revolve around the degree to which leaders are task-oriented or follower-orientated.

■ **Big L leaders:** This is a label used to describe individuals in formal positions of authority.

■ **Emotional intelligence:** A group of soft skills critical for productive interactions with others. It is comprised of self-awareness, self-regulation, motivation, empathy, and social skills. These qualities help confer the ability to apply different leadership styles to different situations.

■ **Follower-oriented leaders:** They express greater concern for the follower than the task at hand. These leaders demonstrate supportive behavior.

■ **Laissez-faire leadership:** This describes a hands-off approach to leadership. It is not really considered a leadership style in this chapter because true leadership requires active attempts to influence.

■ **Leadership:** It is the process through which an individual attempts to intentionally influence another individual or group in order to accomplish a goal.

- **Leader:** A term used to describe individuals who influence by setting direction for others, communicating a common vision, and motivating and inspiring followers. Considered different but closely related to the term manager.

- **Little L leaders:** This is a label that describes people with influence who do not possess a formal position of authority.

- **Manager:** A term used to describe people who influence by providing order and consistency through the activities of planning, budgeting, organizing, staffing, controlling, and problem solving. Considered different but closely related to the term leader.

- **Power:** Ability to influence. Consists of six commonly recognized types: formal, reward, punishment, expert, charismatic, and informational.

- **Situational theories:** These are a group of theories that attempt to understand, explain, and predict the role of context in effective leadership. According to these theories, the greatest predictor of leadership effectiveness and success is the situation faced by leaders and how leaders react to those situations.

- **Structure:** The degree to which a leader frames responsibilities and goals for achieving tasks. It consists of setting goals, providing training, defining expectations, setting limits on behavior, and establishing rules and procedures to be followed.

- **Supportive behavior:** The degree to which a leader indicates respect and concern for followers. Treats them as human beings, watches out for their welfare, and expresses appreciation for their contributions.

- **Task-oriented leaders:** They focus on accomplishing the assigned job with much less concern about the followers who accomplish the job. Task-oriented leaders concentrate on providing the necessary structure followers need to complete their work.

- **Trait theories:** Describes a group of theories that argue that the greatest predictors of leadership effectiveness and success are the traits and dispositions with which people are endowed at birth or develop early in life.

■ ■ ■

Introduction

The concept of leadership is widely discussed as critical to the future of institutional pharmacy practice, but serious concerns have been raised about a looming leadership shortage[1,2] It has been estimated that up to 5,000 new health-system pharmacy leaders will be needed in the next decade.[3] At the same time, students and pharmacists are less willing to seek leadership positions for a broad range of personal and professional reasons.[3]

It has been suggested that leadership should be seen as an everyday activity of all pharmacists and pharmacy students. Nurturing the "everyday leader" should be a goal where all pharmacists show leadership in effectively influencing the behavior of physicians, nurses, pharmacy technicians, interns, and others.[4] To achieve this goal, pharmacists and pharmacy students must understand their leadership responsibilities and their capacity to lead. Leadership skills must be well understood and nurtured in the profession to build everyday pharmacy leaders.

Despite an extensive number of leadership papers written in pharmacy, most discussions deal with the topic in abstract, personal ways. The typical leadership article presents lessons learned from the personal experience of a leader. Common themes in these papers are exhortations for pharmacists to develop a vision, be a servant to others, and to influence change, but they rarely present easily applicable lessons for individuals with little leadership or life experience. Although these papers may inspire, they tend to lack an evidence-based discussion of the subject.

This chapter presents a description of major leadership concepts in the literature. It distills the extensive leadership literature into a limited number of pages geared to individuals with no previous leadership training or education. By necessity, it emphasizes explanation over comprehensiveness. Still, it is evidence-based because it is based upon an extensive understanding of leadership theory and research. The goal is to offer pharmacists and students lessons which can increase leadership effectiveness.

What is leadership?

There are numerous definitions for the term "leadership." One of the most concise and useful definitions defines **leadership** as "the process through which an individual attempts to intentionally influence another individual or group in order to accomplish a goal."[5] This definition calls attention to the following key issues associated with leadership:

- *Leadership is a process.* It is a series of actions exerted by individuals to accomplish goals. As with any good process, leadership should effectively accomplish goals, efficiently use people and resources, and be respectful of individuals involved in or affected by the process.
- *Leadership is intentional.* Leadership does not just happen. It requires deliberate effort on the part of a leader who must willingly accept responsibility and take action. In fact, "**Laissez-faire leadership**" is a misnomer because, by definition, this so-called style of leadership uses a hands-off approach to people and events. Thus, laissez-faire indicates an abdication of any leadership role.
- *Leadership requires exerting influence.* Influence can be accomplished in a multitude of ways, from the transactional (e.g., Do this, and I will give you that) to the inspirational (e.g., Here is our purpose. Let's achieve it!).
- *Leadership centers on people (i.e., leaders and followers) and the relationships between them.* Good leadership accomplishes its goals in a way that develops

> **Key Point . . .**
>
> Leadership is a process that should effectively accomplish goals, efficiently use people and resources, and be respectful of individuals involved in or affected by the process.
>
> **. . . So what?**
>
> Leadership is not a person or an outcome. It is a process. It is practiced by individuals to achieve an outcome and relies on others to achieve those outcomes. Leaders should be judged both on the process used and the outcomes achieved. A good process respect the human beings involved, because it helps establish and maintain commitment toward a leader's vision. Also, disrespect for individuals is contrary to the common good.

and strengthens long-term relationships. Strong relationships based upon trust help establish and build follower commitment to goals.

- *Leadership is goal-directed.* The ultimate purpose of leadership is to achieve desired goals. In health care, leadership demands the balancing of multiple goals, to the organization's mission, the people in the organization, and the individuals served.
- *Leadership should be for the common good.* Good leaders maximize utility to society. This means that tyrants and despots like the highly influential Adolf Hitler can be deemed poor leaders because they damage the common good.

Sources of Leadership Power

A fundamental element of leadership is the willingness and ability to use **power**, defined as the ability to influence. Leaders influence others by exerting different sources of power available to them, and individuals become leaders through their willingness and ability to wield that power. Indeed, the more power one has, the more potential influence and ability to lead.

However, the ability to influence is not enough. Some people choose not to use their power to influence change. In pharmacy settings, many managers and pharmacists refuse to use the power available to them to improve the profession and help their patients. Instead, they conclude that they are powerless to affect the world around them.

The power to lead others comes from many sources. Within an organization, there are six commonly recognized types of power: formal, reward, punishment, expert, charismatic, and informational.[6,7]

Formal power: Formal power (also called legitimate power) is the power bestowed on a person in the form of positional authority. For example, when a pharmacist is made director of pharmacy, the organization gives him or her authority to hire and fire, make budgetary decisions, and set policy within the department. This power is used to accomplish organizational goals. In the hierarchy of a health system, a pharmacy director has more formal power than a staff pharmacist, and a staff pharmacist has more formal power than a technician.

Reward power: Reward power refers to one's ability to reward others who act in a desired manner. People with formal power in organizations often have the authority to reward the behaviors of individuals with pay raises, promotions, and praise. Although often associated with formal positions of authority, anyone can reward others. A subordinate who compliments a leader for gaining a pay raise for employees rewards that behavior, and that compliment can cause the leader to fight harder for employee pay raises in the future.

Reward power depends greatly on how a reward is valued by the individual being influenced—a pharmacist whose financial situation is precarious is more subject to influence by monetary rewards than one who is more financially secure. If a leader cannot provide a desired reward to a follower, reward power is minimal.

Punishment power: The power to punish (also called coercive power), like reward power, usually accompanies formal authority in organizations. Punishments exercised by managers range from mild warnings to job termination. Punishment power is used to discourage undesired behaviors.

Although subordinates cannot formally punish a manager, they can punish a manager informally by withholding information, avoiding interactions with the manager, spreading rumors or negative stories, and even reprimanding the manager. For example, a subordinate may confront a manager regarding excessive criticism and lack of accessibility or support.

Expert power: Expert power derives from the expertise of a person who has special knowledge, skills, and experience. Expertise can be traded for influence. Individuals with computer expertise often wield tremendous power within health care organizations because of the reliance on information systems. Pharmacists use expert power within health care systems through their knowledge of drugs and drug therapy.

Charismatic power: Charismatic power (also called referent power) is an individual's ability to influence another by force of character or charisma. People who are admired by others are able to exert influence through a desire of followers to emulate or please them. Charismatic power is another source of power that is not exclusive to managers. Mahatma Gandhi was one of the great leaders of the 20th century, but he never held a formal leadership position.

Information power: Information power comes from the possession of critical information needed by others. It differs from expert power, which deals with abilities and expertise. In this information age, a person who controls information can exert considerable power. For instance, savvy pharmacists and managers cultivate information sources in organizations who can inform them about organizational politics and upcoming events. This information is often critical to the success of pharmacy initiatives.

Leadership Without Formal Authority

Individuals in formal positions of authority have greater potential to influence others. White[4] refers to these individuals as **"big L" leaders**. Big L leaders typically have more power because they have additional resources available to them—greater access to information, more contact with other influential people, and the like. However, formal authority does not necessarily make one an effective leader.

A title only gives more opportunities to influence. If the power available to formal leaders is misused, no one will follow. Indeed, followers may even actively oppose individuals in formal positions of authority. In the short run, people may be able to get away with abusing their formal positions by taking credit for the work of subordinates, showing favoritism, disrespecting the humanity of workers, or doing any other number of things. But over time, abuse of formal power will reduce a leader's effectiveness.

In the end, leadership cannot be awarded or assigned by a formal position of authority. It must be earned. People who are placed in a position of authority, such as director of pharmacy or supervisor, have very little power to influence others if they do not effectively utilize the various forms of power available to them. The ability to lead is based upon the perceptions of others. If people believe that a leader has power, they will choose to follow. A title cannot make one a leader, neither can a person declare himself or herself to be a leader. Only followers can decide who will lead them. Maxwell said it best when he said, "The only thing a title can buy is a little time, either to increase your level of influence with others or to erase it."[8]

In a similar vein, people do not have to possess a formal managerial position to lead. Without a managerial title, staff pharmacists can still use reward, punishment, expert, charismatic, and information power to influence change in organizations. White[4] calls these individuals **"little L" leaders**. In many pharmacy organizations, informal leaders wield substantial power—leading change from the bottom up. In fact, effective pharmacy leaders rely on these "little L" leaders—from developing initiatives to enhance clinical services on the nursing units to new ways of running the pharmacy. Indeed, front-line pharmacists are now expected to be leaders in their everyday responsibilities.[9]

Contrasting Leadership and Management

Leadership and management are two distinct but related activities. The concepts are often confused because they both seek to bring about change in organizations by influencing behavior. In truth, the distinction may be irrelevant because organizations need individuals who are both good leaders *and* managers. Nevertheless, the distinction can highlight different strategies employed in influencing individuals.

According to Kotter,[10] **managers** exert influence by providing order and consistency. This is accomplished through the activities of planning, budgeting, organizing, staffing, controlling, and problem solving. Each is critical to day-to-day operations, especially when conditions are calm and change is unnecessary. However, managerial tasks and the order and consistency associated with them are less useful in turbulent and changing circumstances, because adaptability is more important in responding to fluid circumstances.

Adaptability is typically the role of leaders. **Leaders** excel at coping with change, setting direction for others, communicating a common vision, and mo-

■ ■ ■

Key Point . . .

"The only thing a title can buy is a little time—either to increase your level of influence with others or to erase it."

. . . So what?

A title gives formal power to a leader and the ability to reward and punish, and it also provides access to information unavailable to those without titles (e.g., personnel files). However, the ability to reward and punish is limited because it is constrained by an organizations policies and culture. Heavy-handed use of rewards and punishment to manipulate followers is typically discouraged in organizations. Information power is also tempered because a formal title causes followers to withhold information for fear of being punished or not receiving a reward. A title simply provides an opportunity for a leader to establish the trust and commitment of followers to pursue a common vision for the pharmacy. If that trust and commitment is lost, followers may ignore, even resist, the leader.

tivating and inspiring followers.[10] Leaders exert influence by relinquishing much of the **structure** and order of managerial tasks and encourage followers to take responsibility for their work and work settings. Leaders provide vision and direction to organizations, and they attempt to inspire followers to work independently, without much direction.

Thus, the distinction is that *leaders focus on getting people to commit to a common goal, while managers concentrate on getting people to take action toward that goal.* Accordingly, the difference between leaders and managers lies in the degree of commitment expected from followers.

For managers, commitment is less important than compliance. Managers want people to do what they are told. They are less interested in their reasons for doing so. In fact, a manager may care little whether people want to do something—only that they do it.

On the other hand, leaders seek commitment over compliance. They are interested not only in behavior but also in feelings, motivations, thoughts, and perceptions associated with behaviors. Since mental processes are so integral to behavior, they are necessary to bring about maximum effort in workers. If leaders can capture the hearts of workers, greater commitment to goals and tasks will result.

Figure 16-1 illustrates the fundamental differences between management and leadership. Pharmacy managers push the staff to complete tasks by providing an organized framework of rules and controls to guide them. This framework is backed up by a system of rewards and punishments for acceptably completing the tasks. The problem is that systems based upon rewards and punishments may encourage action but they rarely encourage high levels of commitment needed to rise to the challenge of extraordinary or changing conditions.[11]

For example, budget cuts and staff shortages may require significantly greater effort by the staff with no increase in pay and deteriorating working conditions. Stress, uncertainty, anxiety, and conflict can complicate the situation. Responding under these conditions often takes more commitment to the pharmacy organization than is generally inspired by a manager.

Commitment is better "fired up" by leaders who have gained the trust and respect of followers. Leaders pull followers toward a shared vision (e.g., patient health). The steps for achieving this vision are left largely to the followers.

Although there is value in differentiating leaders and managers, the dichotomy may be trivial in the end because pharmacy leaders must be able to effectively employ push and pull strategies depending on the circumstances. Even the most motivated followers need to be pushed sometimes. Both management and leadership are essential to the success of organizations and neither is necessarily more important than the other. Actually,

Figure 16-1. Contrasting leadership and management.

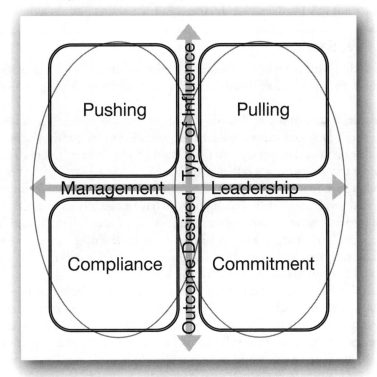

the dichotomy may really be illustrating different styles of leadership rather than two separate concepts. Therefore, the remainder of this chapter will view leaders and managers to be essentially the same thing and use the terms interchangeably.

Leadership Theories

Leadership theories can help pharmacists understand and explain problems faced in influencing change. Theories supplement pharmacists' common sense and intuition when deciding which courses to choose in various situations. They allow pharmacists to apply the best evidence available about what is known about influencing individuals and groups.

Theories assist in exploring why some leaders are effective and others are ineffective. They help in assessing the reasons some leaders act the way they do and can aid in developing strategies that enhance the impact of leaders. Theories make it easier to identify leadership characteristics, behaviors, and responses to situations that need to be monitored.

The challenge is to understand the basics of theories and to determine how well a particular theory applies to a situation. A basic understanding of leadership theories assists in recognizing common leadership problems and potential solutions. No single theory explains every situation. Nor can they provide cookbook answers to complex problems. Instead, they offer insight that can be used to develop nuanced solutions to leadership dilemmas.

Leadership theories can help answer the following questions: (1) What should be looked for in selecting an effective leader? (2) What characteristics and behaviors are associated with good leaders? (3) Under what conditions do different leadership behaviors work best? (4) How can pharmacists improve their own leadership effectiveness?

Most leadership theories can be categorized as relating to the nature of leaders, the general behaviors in which they engage, and their responses to changing situations (Figure 16-2). The categories overlap because the major variables—leader, behaviors, and situation—are not independent of each other.

Nature of Leaders

Theories that deal with the nature of leaders attempt to identify what characteristics are associated with effective leaders. They can be used to select good leaders or be developed over time.

Trait theories are a group of theories that argue that the greatest predictors of leadership effectiveness and success are the traits and dispositions with which people are endowed at birth or develop early in life.[12] By the time a person reaches a leadership position, these characteristics are difficult to obtain or to change.

Not so long ago, people believed that leadership capabilities were hereditary. If individuals had royal blood, they were thought to have a capacity to lead. Over time, however, objective observers noticed that royal bloodlines bore little relationship to the ability to lead. In fact, an argument can be made that leadership positions awarded upon the basis of heredity can lead to the inbreeding of genes and ideas, both of which can hinder the ability of an individual to effectively lead others.

Many studies have attempted to identify specific traits in people that might be predictive of leadership capability. It was believed that if these traits were identified, they could be used to screen for good leaders. For example, leaders might be selected on the basis of intelligence quotient (IQ), if IQ could be shown to consistently predict good leadership ability. Thousands of studies have explored physical, social, personality, and

Figure 16-2. Variables influencing effectiveness of leaders.

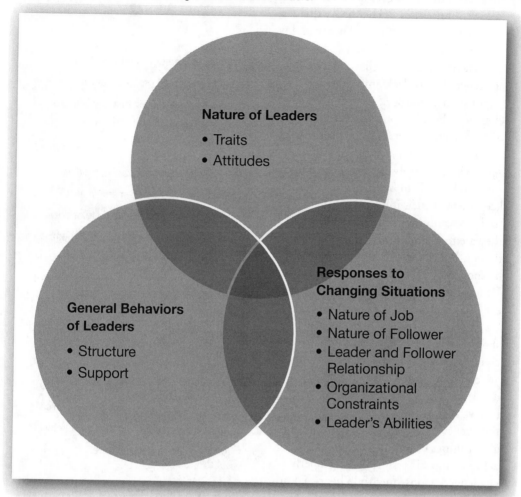

Nature of Leaders
- Traits
- Attitudes

General Behaviors of Leaders
- Structure
- Support

Responses to Changing Situations
- Nature of Job
- Nature of Follower
- Leader and Follower Relationship
- Organizational Constraints
- Leader's Abilities

task-related traits in leaders. The traits studied include physical traits, such as height, age, and attractiveness; social traits, such as charisma, charm, tact, and popularity; personality traits, such as adaptability, assertiveness, and emotional stability; and task related traits, such as the drives to excel, accept responsibility, and take initiative. Reviews of the literature suggest that the most desirable traits in leaders are drive, motivation, integrity, self-confidence, intelligence, and knowledge.[12,13]

However, the relationship between these traits and good leadership has not been found to be strongly predictive. Lord et al.[14] observed that the relationship between these traits and leadership capabilities is weak and inconsistent at best, making many traits poor predictors of good leaders. Intelligence, for instance, may be seen in many good leaders because a sharp mind is needed for many of the technical demands of leaders (e.g., complex problem solving, understanding complex systems). However, there are also many intelligent people who are terrible leaders because they lack self control, interpersonal skills, or any other equally important capabilities needed by effective leaders.

A different theory dealing with the nature of leaders considers their attitudes toward followers. **Attitude theory** states that the beliefs leaders hold about people greatly influences both the manager's behavior and the followers' responses.[15] The theory divides leaders into two categories; Theory X Leaders and Theory Y Leaders.

Theory X leaders believe that people are generally lazy, lack ambition, avoid responsibility, and seek security instead of challenge. Based upon this attitude, Theory X leaders believe that the people they lead must be carefully watched and managed. Tight controls must be placed upon them to keep them busy. The best way to keep them at their job is to tell them what to do, reward them when they do what they are told, and punish them when they do not. Phrases which might commonly be spoken by a Theory X manager include, "If I don't keep after them, they will slack off." "They don't care about this place." "Why should I compliment them? They should be lucky to have a job!" Thus, coercive and controlling leadership methods are common with Theory X leaders.

In contrast, Theory Y leaders generally believe that people are not lazy. Instead, they believe that people are ambitious about things of importance and will achieve fantastic results when properly challenged. Consequently, Theory Y leaders act quite differently toward followers than Theory X leaders. Theory Y leaders treat followers with respect and ask as much from followers as they ask of themselves. They challenge followers to achieve and assume that followers will succeed. Phrases which might commonly be spoken by a Theory Y manager might include, "When I give my employees the right conditions and tools to do a job, they always impress me." "How do you think we should handle this problem? I value your judgment." Consequently, democratic, coaching, and supportive leadership techniques are preferred by these managers.

The take-home lesson from attitude theory is that a leader's attitudes towards followers can act as a self-fulfilling prophecy. If a leader perceives followers to be lazy and inept, he/she will treat them that way. And when followers are treated as lazy and inept, they will act that way. On the other hand, if a leader perceives and treats followers as respected professionals, they will reward his/her faith in them by acting as professionals.

> **Key Point . . .**
>
> If a leader perceives and treats followers as respected professionals, they will reward his/her faith in them by acting as professionals.
>
> **. . . So what?**
>
> The social science literature, including education and management, indicates that human beings tend to live up to or down to other people's expectations of them. Yet, personal and culture factors often lead us to develop negative perceptions of our fellow man or woman. This can cause leaders to expect the worst in followers. Low expectations can push leaders to micromanage, continually question, and act in a bossy manner toward followers. This typically leads to a vicious cycle in which followers respond by acting up, thereby justifying the leader's attitude.

General Behaviors of Leaders

Behavioral theories recognize that knowing the nature of leaders only provides a foundation for understanding leadership. It is really the knowledge of the behaviors associated with good leaders that can help in identifying and training them. Behavioral theories argue that the greatest predictors of leadership effectiveness are the behaviors and abilities that people learn over time.[5] Behavioral theories attempt to answer the question, "What leadership behaviors are most effective?" A variety of behavioral theories have been proposed,[16-19] but they all revolve around two primary dimensions of behavioral orientation adopted by leaders, task- and follower-orientations.

Task-oriented leaders focus on accomplishing the assigned job, while concerns about the followers involved in the job take a back seat. Task-oriented leaders concentrate on the important work of providing the necessary **structure** (defined as setting goals, providing training, defining expectation and limits on behavior, and establishing rules and procedures) followers need to complete their work.

Some task orientation in leaders is essential because followers need some structure to complete most tasks. However, there is a point where structure is no longer useful and becomes restrictive—even irritating. For example, a pharmacist typically needs to provide technicians general procedures and expected outcomes for tasks and later check up to see if the tasks have been accomplished. However, if the pharmacist continually checks up on the technician every few minutes and frequently interrupts the task with unsolicited advice or suggestions, the technician will probably find the guidance overbearing and unhelpful.

Follower-oriented leaders focus less on the job at hand and express greater concern for the follower in words and actions. Such leaders actively support followers by treating them as human beings—not cogs in a machine attempting to achieve some task. These leaders demonstrate **supportive behavior** by showing respect, gaining trust, demonstrating consideration, and being friendly and approachable.

Both orientations are necessary in organizations, but taken to the extreme either orientation can be problematic. Too much focus on the task may cause followers to chafe at the restrictions. It can lead followers to label the leader as a "micromanager" or "slave driver" and will cause followers to feel abused and taken advantage of. On the other hand, too much emphasis on the followers will result in failure to meet deadlines and goals. Most leaders try to balance a task orientation with a follower orientation. The appropriate behavior to use depends on the situation faced by the leader.

Responses of Leaders

Situational theories are a group of theories that attempt to understand, explain, and predict the role of context in effective leadership. According to these theories, the greatest predictor of leadership effectiveness and success is the situation faced by leaders and how leaders react to those situations.[5] Traits, abilities, and behaviors are important, but they are seen as situation-specific. In one circumstance, certain traits and behaviors serve a leader well, while in another they may be disastrous. An understanding of the role of context can help leaders adapt to the dynamics of a leadership situation.

Although individual situational theories vary in content and emphasis,[20-23] they generally agree that the appropriate leadership style depends on the job, the followers, the relationship between the leader and the led, organizational constraints, and the leader's abilities (Figure 16-3).

■ *The nature of the job.* Jobs can be classified as (1) routine and non-routine or (2) structured and unstructured. Leading people in routine, structured tasks requires different strategies than non-routine, unstructured tasks. For instance, simple tasks such as counting, lifting, and reading instructions require different oversight than more complex professional tasks like designing therapeutic plans or evaluating the source of a medication error.

Figure 16-3. Influences on leadership situations.

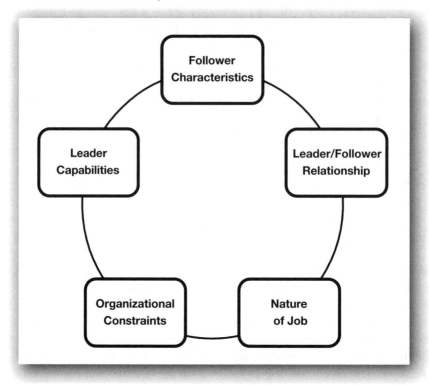

- *Follower characteristics.* Some followers are highly motivated, energetic, willing to accept responsibility, and competent. These individuals may need little direction and structure in their jobs, while unmotivated and less capable people require close oversight and direction.
- *Relationship between leader and followers.* A strong relationship based upon mutual trust and respect gives leaders the ability to collaborate and cooperate as a team. A bad relationship leads to suspicion, second guessing each other's motives, and adversarial interactions.
- *Organizational constraints.* Leaders are often constrained by organizational policies and procedures, corporate culture, and lack of time and resources. Thus, leaders are often hindered in their ability to communicate with, hire, fire, discipline, and reward staff members.
- *The leader's abilities.* Some leaders are more capable and experienced in dealing with leadership situations than oth-

> **Key Point . . .**
>
> Leadership success depends more on the leader's ability to adapt to a situation than the ability to change it.
>
> **. . . So what?**
>
> In the short term, it is difficult for pharmacists to change the nature of their jobs, followers, or organizational constraints. Therefore, they must adapt to circumstances in how they relate to followers and the leadership actions they take.

ers. A leader's ability to adapt to changing situations helps to adjust to different tasks, followers, and organizational constraints.

Leaders have little control over many factors influencing leadership situations. For the most part, leaders cannot substantially change the nature of the job, the characteristics of the followers, or the organizational constraints. Most pharmacy leaders "inherit" their workers and are given tasks that must be accomplished within the constraints of the organization. According to situational theory, leadership success depends more on the leader's ability to adapt to a situation than the ability to change it.

Styles of Leadership

Six basic leadership styles that can be applied to changing work situations have been identified: the coercive, transformational, affiliative, democratic, pacesetting, and coaching styles.[24]

The coercive style. A coercive (or directive) leadership style uses rewards and punishments to influence behavior.[21] This type of leader is very task oriented and controlling of others. Of all leadership styles, the coercive style appears to be the least effective in the most situations when used as the primary form of leadership.[24] Coercive leaders tend to create an "us-versus-them" environment in which followers feel manipulated and disrespected. Followers become frightened or resentful. They avoid enthusiastic participation in new initiatives or programs because of a fear of making mistakes or a perception that their input is not appreciated. Instead, they wait for the leader to tell them what to do and are likely to say, "I just do what I'm told."

Although often considered ineffective when used as the primary leadership style, coercive leadership is essential as a supplement to other styles. Coercion is sometimes necessary to have individuals assume undesirable but necessary responsibilities. It is also indispensible for dealing with difficult individuals who can damage the productivity of the team. Coercion can be critical in crises, such as when a business is failing and people need to be frightened into changing their work practices. Fear can be a potent motivator in getting people to change entrenched behaviors. For some employees, a threat of suspension or termination may be the only way to change poor work habits. Nevertheless, even under these conditions, coercive leadership should be used sparingly and for limited periods.[24]

The transformational style. The transformational style mobilizes people toward a vision articulated by a leader.[25] Transformational leaders rely on charismatic power, not rewards and punishments, to influence others. They influence others because followers identify with them and their message. Martin Luther King is an example of a transformational leader. King had a dream of what society could be like in America, and through actions and words he inspired millions to make that dream their own.

Of the six leadership styles, the transformational style has been found to be most effective in the greatest number of situations.[24] Transformational leaders can inspire people by clearly defining how their work fits into a larger vision for the organization. This, in turn, maximizes the commitment of followers to the vision and energizes them to seek the best path for achieving it. Feedback from the leader focuses less on the process of achieving goals and more on the outcomes, encouraging individuals to innovate and take risks.

The transformational style can fail when the leader is unable to articulate a clear vision. Not every leader is good at doing this. When done poorly, attempts at inspirational leadership may be seen as pompous or out of touch. Such a leader will not be able to inspire others.

The affiliative style. The affiliative style of leadership revolves around meeting the emotional needs of followers. It focuses on people, whereas coercive leadership focuses on the task.[21] Affiliative leaders seek happiness, harmony, and, ultimately, mutual loyalty between leaders and followers. They attempt to build trust by demonstrating respect to others and communicating openly. They offer positive feedback for good work in order to build confidence and self-esteem. When they are critical, it is provided with the greatest care and concern for an individual's feelings. Some pharmacy managers mistakenly assume that positive feedback will cause employees to slack off in their work, so they offer only criticism. In reality, positive feedback can enhance productivity by enhancing communication, loyalty, trust, and innovation.

At the same time, overreliance on the affiliative style can have negative effects. Followers who hear only praise will not know when they need to improve their behavior. Poor performance can go uncorrected if followers feel that mediocrity is acceptable. It can also lead to a sense of entitlement.[26,27] Concerns have been voiced that recent generations of workers have received so much praise from their parents, teachers, and sports coaches that they expect "kudos for just showing up."[27] It has been stated that overreliance on kudos has turned some young adults "into narcissistic praise-junkies"[27] who become insecure in the absence of regular compliments.

Whether this is true or not, all workers—young and old—need structure to do their jobs. Therefore, affiliative leaders need to supplement supportive behaviors with styles that offer more structure.

The democratic style. Leaders who practice the democratic style give followers a say in decisions that affect their work lives. They solicit input from followers and attain their buy-in for major decisions and initiatives. This approach generates a sense of ownership by the staff in an organization's goals, nurtures the generation of ideas by including more individuals in the process, and helps build mutual trust and respect.

On the other hand, democracy can be frustratingly inefficient. It often leads people to debate trivial issues and haggle over decisions rather than take action. Another pitfall is that reaching consensus leads to compromises that produce less than optimal results. This is a real problem under the pressure of deadlines or when individuals lack the qualifications to help with the decision. Finally, some leaders use the democratic style to avoid making difficult decisions (i.e., those that might have a negative impact on a leader's career). Instead, they attempt to shift responsibility—and potential blame—to followers.

The key is to choose those situations where democratic leadership works well and does not work well. The democratic style works optimally when there is sufficient time for the democratic process to unfold, the best course is uncertain, and followers are sufficiently competent to contribute. When these conditions are in place, the democratic leadership style can be very successful.

The pacesetting style. Pacesetting leaders set extremely high performance standards for both followers and themselves.[21] Pacesetters lead by example—demonstrating effort and sacrifice and asking the same of others. If the pacesetter puts in long hours or gives up weekends for work-related projects, everyone else is expected to do the same. In essence, the pacesetter says, "Do as I do." Followers who cannot keep up with the leader are replaced by others who will.

Pacesetting leaders are often praised as admirable, and the pacesetting style is adopted by many pharmacy leaders. It is a common style adopted by people who have been in the military or participated in competitive athletics. When applied appropriately, a pacesetters leadership style often builds credibility with followers by setting a good example.

The problem is that the pacesetting style can have an unintended negative impact on morale and performance.[24] A pacesetter's demands for total job commitment can seem unreasonable and overwhelming to many followers. Not everyone has the same dedication to the job as the pacesetter, especially if the leader has not inspired the followers toward a shared vision.

Another problem is that some pacesetters are not clear in what performance they expect of others, because the meaning of actions can be ambiguous. For instance, a leader may try to communicate through his actions the message, "If we all work as hard, we are going to be the best pharmacy in town." But the follower may misinterpret the leader's message as, "If you do not work as hard as I do, you aren't good enough." When pacesetting leaders do not supplement actions with clear statements of expectations, followers are left to guess the leader's intentions. When they are not made explicit, perceived expectations of performance boil down to "be as good as me."

Nevertheless, the pacesetting style can be effective when done well. It is effective in situations with self-motivated and highly competent followers who need little direction to complete tasks such as professional sports and medicine. It also works well when used in combination with other styles that supplement the pacesetter's actions with explicit written and spoken communication. Finally, it succeeds when pacesetters use the style humbly, in a way that does not appear arrogant or narcissistic.

The coaching style. Coaching leaders strive to develop the abilities of their followers so they can work more independently and effectively toward organizational goals. They help workers to set goals and achieve them through career development, training, and skill development. Coaches work cooperatively with the staff to improve productivity and performance, and they provide them with the tools necessary to attain success. They challenge followers and delegate tasks to them that help develop their skills.

Key Point . . .

When pacesetting leaders do not supplement actions with clear statements of expectations, followers are left to guess the leader's intentions.

. . . So what?

It is hard to argue with the idea of leading by example. The problem lies in the implementation. Actions may speak louder than words, but the message they send can be unintentional. Facial expressions, body language, tone and volume of voice, and other things that accompany a leader's words can be easily misinterpreted, especially in emotional situations. Words *and* actions are necessary to communicate what is expected of followers without misunderstandings.

Coaching can be a very effective leadership style, but it is often underutilized because managerial demands often do not permit leaders sufficient time for the slow and laborious work involved.[24] In many cases, it is easier for leaders to do a task themselves than teach others to do it. However, when subordinates learn a new skill, it can free leaders for other commitments. People who are taught to do something can take over the responsibility for it. They may even do a better job than the coach.

Coaches do better with followers who are motivated to improve their performance and mature enough to accept feedback. Coaching does not work as well when followers resist change or new ideas. It can also be ineffective in a crisis, when quick actions are necessary.

Leaders Need Many Styles

The more leadership styles a person masters, the better he or she can adapt to changing leadership situations. Leaders who have mastered four or more styles—especially the transformational, democratic, affiliative, and coaching styles—tend to establish and maintain the best working environment and show better business performance.[24] Equally important to mastery of the style is the ability to switch among them as the situation demands.

Some leaders adapt to their leadership deficiencies by finding environments that match their styles and abilities. For example, a coercive leader might try to find a situation in which the staff prefers lots of structure and the tasks are routine and standardized. Or a democratic leader might seek followers who are participative and circumstances where democracy can thrive. The problem is that situations constantly change. Several famous wartime leaders, including Ulysses S. Grant, Winston Churchill, and George S. Patton, failed as peacetime leaders because they were unable to adapt their leadership to the new environment.

Other leaders adapt by working with others who are willing and able to cover up their leadership weaknesses. This requires leaders to understand their own weaknesses, identify individuals who have skills they lack, and be willing to delegate key responsibilities to those individuals with the requisite skills. For instance, a leader who is not a "people person" may try to delegate sensitive personnel issues to subordinates with good interpersonal skills. The major problem with this solution is that it forces leaders to rely on others to do key aspects of their job. When key subordinates are not available or they leave for other jobs, the leader is left in a difficult position. The leader can also lose credibility with followers if too many responsibilities are delegated because the leader cannot or will not handle them.

A better solution may be to develop the ability to apply multiple leadership styles to different situations. This requires the leader to expand his or her repertoire of leadership styles as much as possible. It also requires the leader to learn to identify effective styles for various leadership situations.

Developing Leadership Abilities

It is widely accepted that individuals can learn to increase their capacity to lead. According to Maxwell,[8] as people develop their leadership skills, they pass through four phases. In phase 1, "unaware and ineffective," individuals have underdeveloped leadership skills. They may have strong opinions and be quick to offer advice, but they have done very little leading themselves and have modest understanding of what it takes to lead others. These people have marginal impact on what goes on around them. Unless they develop their leadership skills, they will continue to be unaware and ineffective.

In phase 2, "aware and ineffective," people have accepted leadership roles and found out how hard it is to be a good leader. They make many mistakes and are relatively ineffective. At this point, some individuals get frustrated and choose to avoid further leadership roles. Luckily, others decide to develop their leadership skills, and over time, become increasingly effective at influencing others.

People in phase 3, "aware and effective," must work hard to apply their leadership skills, but doing so makes them steadily more effective. In this third phase, Individuals consciously apply what they have learned about leading others. They make mistakes, but they learn from them. By systematically identifying and changing ineffective behaviors, they continually improve their ability to lead.

In phase 4, "unaware and effective," leadership is less a conscious act and more a part of a person's life. Leadership becomes automatic, but the impact is tremendous. In this phase, leaders no longer consciously think while they influence others. They just do it, because it is a natural extension of who they are and what they want to achieve. They may still consciously assess their leadership performance and make appropriate adjustments, but for the most part, the behaviors become internalized as part of a leader's individual persona.

Role of Emotional Intelligence

Researchers have identified **emotional intelligence** (EI) as critical to leadership.[28] EI comprises self-awareness, self-regulation, motivation, empathy, and social skills. These qualities help confer the ability to apply different leadership styles to different situations. The greater the EI, the larger the number of leadership styles that can be appropriately applied. Leaders who are deficient in certain components of EI are likely to be less effective in applying particular styles. For example, a leader who lacks empathy will have difficulty using the affiliative style, while one who has poor social skills may not effectively use the coaching or transformational styles.

Improving leadership requires identifying which EI components are lacking and developing strategies for improving them. A leader who lacks the ability to use the affiliative style might attempt to improve empathetic listening skills or do a better job at relationship building. Of course, that is easier said than done, but it is possible to cultivate greater EI and consequently improve leadership. In fact, many chief executive officers of large corporations employ personal coaches to enhance their EI.[29]

The following are some suggestions how pharmacists can increase their E.I. and ability to lead.

- Identify and work with a mentor during the early stages of one's career. Since leadership is an art as well as a skill, it is essential to have continual and intensive coaching from an experienced leader.
- Become a thoughtful student of leadership. Observe others who are good leaders and reflect on what makes them so. Read up and study the topic of leadership. There are many excellent books on leadership available in bookstores and libraries where pharmacists can learn from the published experiences of others.
- Never stop trying to understand yourself. One way of doing so is through self-administered questionnaires such as with Meyers-Briggs Personality or E.I. tests. Another way is to ask for feedback from others such as your boss, coworkers, or subordinates.
- Identify the skill sets necessary for leaders in health-systems pharmacy. Leadership is multidimensional requiring a mix of hard technical and soft people skills. ASHP has developed a list of competencies needed for individuals seeking to move up the institutional pharmacy leadership ladder (Table 16-1).
- Practice leadership. The only way to truly learn how to lead is through personal experience. Take on leadership positions which force you to do things that stretch your capabilities. Get into the habit of replaying and analyzing your leadership experiences—both successes and failures. Analyze the causes of successes or failures and think about

Table 16-1.

Competencies Needed for Leaders in Health-System Pharmacy[30]

Technical Capabilities	People Skills
▨ Medication-use system management	▨ Human resources management
▨ Pharmacy operations management	▨ Leadership and vision
▨ Financial management	▨ Self-development and teachability
▨ Information/technology management	▨ Self-awareness and self-management
▨ Planning and organizational skills	▨ Empathy and social skills
▨ Problem solving and critical thinking	▨ Communication skills
	▨ Integrity
	▨ Commitment (initiative and persistence)
	▨ Responsibility (selfless accountability for actions)
	▨ Caring about others

how outcomes might have changed under different conditions or actions. For example, if you challenge a technician to be more productive, ask yourself "Did I get the desired result with my action?" If not ask, "Why?" and "What other action could I have taken which might result in a different outcome?"

Barriers to Developing Leaders in Health Systems

"At present, leadership opportunities within the profession are too often impeded instead of fostered."[9] This occurs for many reasons. One is that many students and pharmacists do not consider leadership development to be important, desirable, and/or relevant to their lives. Some avoid leadership responsibilities to maintain an ideal balance between work and life. Others prefer to focus on clinical practice instead. Still others feel that the additional pay for formal leadership positions may not be seen as worth the extra time, effort, and stress.

The educational system is part of the problem because leadership training of students is inadequate and inconsistent.[9] Leadership training in pharmacy schools is rarely a priority. Insufficient didactic and experiential education on the topic has led to a lack of awareness about the basics of leadership and the practical application of leadership skills.

▨ ■ ▨

Key Point . . .

The only way to truly learn how to lead is through personal experience.

. . . So what?

Leadership is a not a spectator sport. Unless you have taken on responsibility for leading others, you have never had your leadership skills tested. You may have conceptual knowledge about human motivation and influence, but knowing and doing are two separate things. If you want things to change in your practice setting, do not sit on the sidelines. Jump in and lead.

This problem is compounded because many clinical faculty members do not understand or appreciate the importance of leadership training. Thus, when teaching and mentoring students, they focus on the clinical to the exclusion of other topics.[9]

Leadership training after graduation is also haphazard in many pharmacy work settings.[9] One reason is that the immediate day-to-day demands of practice can absorb the entire work day leaving little time for leadership training. Another reason is that many pharmacists in formal positions of authority are ineffective mentors and teachers. Many have received no formal training themselves, often receiving the appointment for their clinical skills or their willingness (but not readiness) to accept a formal leadership role. Indeed, bad leadership can be self-perpetuating—meaning that ineffective leaders are more likely to do a poor job developing future leaders. They will make unwise choices in selecting future leaders, provide ineffective feedback and guidance, and discourage potential leaders from pursuing formal management positions.

The American Society of Health-System Pharmacists is actively addressing these barriers. One of the most important initiatives is its Section of Pharmacy Practice Managers, an interest group within the society that seeks to help members become more effective advocates and leaders. The section plans continuing education programs at major society meetings, sponsors special conferences that connect establish leadership experts with new and potential pharmacy leaders, provides teaching materials on leadership and management, develops standards and guidelines for best practices, and offers practice tools on pharmacy management and leadership-related topics. The section has a website link at ASHP's website located at www.ashp.org.

Summary

This chapter provides an overview of current leadership theories and recommendations for pharmacists. It condenses extensive leadership literature into a relatively limited number of pages. As a result some ideas are simplified for the reader and others are left out. For example, the chapter does not address emerging leadership theories such as Servant Leadership.[31] Nevertheless, the chapter summarizes most key concepts pharmacists need to know about leading others.

Therefore, the only thing left is for pharmacists to start their leadership journey. Every pharmacist in an organization can be a leader. Each of us has many sources of power which can be used to improve the quality of health care. Many problems faced by the profession could be improved if more pharmacists would exercise leadership at different levels of pharmacy organizations. Any leadership deficiencies can be overcome by developing leadership capabilities over time.

Suggested Reading

Bartolome F. Nobody Trusts the Boss Completely: Now What? *Harv Bus Rev.* 1989;67:135-142.

Collins JC. *Good to Great: Why Some Companies Make the Leap ... and Others Don't.* New York: HarperBusiness; 2001.

Goffee R, Jones G. Why should anyone be led by you? *Harv Bus Rev.* 2000;78:62-70, 198.

Kouzes JM, Posner BZ. *Credibility: How Leaders Gain and Lose It, Why People Demand It.* 2nd ed. San Francisco: Jossey-Bass; 2003.

Maxwell JC. *The 21 Irrefutable Laws of Leadership.* Nashville, TN: Thomas Nelson, Inc.; 1998.

Pollard SR, Clark JS. Survey of health-system pharmacy leadership pathways. *Am J Health-Syst Pharm.* 2009;66:947-952.

Rickert DR, Smith RE, Worthen DB. The seven habits: building pharmacist leaders. *Am Pharm.* 1992;NS32:48-52.

References

1. ASHP Reports. Proceedings of a leadership retreat conducted by the ASHP Foundation and the John W. Webb Visiting Professor Program: Boston Massachusetts October 24, 2004. *Am J Health-Syst Pharm.* 2005 April;62:856-863.

2. Ashby DM, Mannasse HR. ASHP Reports: 2004 Leadership report on strategic direction: Creating a unique vision for the profession. *Am J Health-Syst Pharm.* 2004 September;61:1825-1932.

3. White SJ. ASHP Reports: Will there be a leadership crisis? An ASHP Foundation Scholar-in-Residence report. *Am J Health-Syst Pharm.* 2005 April;62:845-855.

4. White SJ. Leadership: Successful Alchemy. Harvey A.K. Whitney Lecture. *Am J Health-Syst Pharm.* 2006;63:1497-1503.

5. Pointer DD, Sanchez JP. Leadership: A framework for thinking and acting. In: Shortell SM, Kaluzny AD, eds. *Health Care Management: Organizational Design and Behavior.* 3rd ed. Albany, NY: Delmar Publishers; 1994:85-112.

6. French JRP, Raven B. The bases of social power. In: Cartwright D, Zander AF, eds. *Group Dynamics.* Evanston, IL: Row Peterson; 1960:607-623.

7. Lee B. *The Power Principle.* New York: Simon and Schuster; 1997.

8. Maxwell JC. *The 21 Irrefutable Laws of Leadership.* Nashville, TN: Thomas Nelson, Inc.; 1998.

9. Student New Practitioner Leadership Task Force. Addressing the Pharmacy Leadership Gap: Leadership as a Professional Obligation. Bethesda, MD: American Society of Health-System Pharmacists Foundation; 2008 Jun 27.

10. Kotter JP. What leaders really do. *Harv Bus Rev.* 1990;(May-June):103-111.

11. Herzberg F. One More Time: How Do You Motivate Employees? *Harv Bus Rev.* 1987 September;65(5):109.

12. Donnelly JH, Gibson JL, Ivancevich JM. Leading people in organizations. *Fundamentals of Management.* Ninth ed. Chicago: Irwin Publishing; 1995:377-411.

13. Kirkpatrick SA, Locke EA. Leadership: Do traits matter? *Acad Manage Exe.* 1991;(May):48-60.

14. Lord RG, DeVader CL, Allinger GM. A meta-analysis of the relation between personality trait and leadership: An application of validity generalization procedures. *J Appl Psych.* 1986;71(3):402-410.

15. MacGregor D. *The Human Side of Enterprise.* New York: McGraw-Hill; 1960.

16. Tannebaum R, Schmidt WH. How to choose a leadership pattern. *Harv Bus Rev.* 1973;(May-June):162-180.

17. Likert R. From production- and employee-centeredness to systems 1-4. *J Manage.* 1979;5(2):147-156.

18. Blake RR, McCanse AA. *Leadership Dilemmas—Grid Solutions.* Houston, TX: Gulf Publishing; 1991.

19. Schreisheim CA, Bird BJ. Contributions of the Ohio State studies to the field of leadership. *J Manage.* 1979;(Fall):135-145.

20. Fiedler FE, Garcia JE. *New Approaches to Effective Leadership: Cognitive Resources and Organizational Performance.* New York: John Wiley; 1987.

21. House RJ, Mitchell RR. Path-Goal theory of leadership. *J Contemp Bus.* 1974;(Autumn):81-97.

22. Vroom V, Yetton P. *Leadership and decision making.* Pittsburgh, PA: University of Pittsburgh Press; 1973.

23. Hersey P, Blanchard KH. *Management of Organizational Behavior.* Englewood Cliffs, NJ: Prentice Hall; 1993.

24. Goleman D. Leadership that gets results. *Harv Bus Rev.* 2000;(March-April):78-90.

25. Bass BM. From transitional to transformational leadership: Learning to share the vision. *Organ Dyn.* 1990;(Winter):140-148.

26. Zaslow J. Blame it on Mr. Rogers: why young adults feel so entitled. Wall Street Journal Online. 2007 Jul 5;B5.

27. Zaslow J. The most praised generation goes to work. Wall Street Journal Online. 2007 Apr 20;W1.

28. Goleman D. What makes a leader? *Harv Bus Rev.* 1998;(Nov-Dec.):93-102.

29. Morris B. So You're a Player. Do You Need a Coach? The hottest thing in management is the executive coach: part boss, part consultant, part therapist. Who are these people? And what are they doing in your company? *Fortune.* 2000;141[4]:141-147.

30. ASHP Director of Pharmacy and Leadership Assessment Form. *American Society of Health-System Pharmacists;* 2009. Available at: www.ashp.org/DocLibrary/LeadershipAssessmentTool.aspx. Accessed March 11, 2009.

31. Greenleaf RK. *Servant Leadership: A Journey into the Nature of Legitimate Power and Greatness.* Mahwah, NJ: Paulist Press; 1977.

Chapter Review Questions

1. **Leaders are born, not made.**
   a. True
   b. False

   Answer: b. False. Theories of leadership which argue that that leadership is genetic have been generally found to unsupported. Instead, it has been shown that leadership can be developed over time.

2. **Leaders who do not have formal leadership positions are called _____ leaders.**

   Answer: "Little L" leaders. These are individuals with sources of non-formal power who lead change in pharmacy settings from the bottom up.

3. **A leader who believes that followers have "bad attitudes" is likely to encourage "bad attitudes" and unproductive behaviors in those followers.**
   a. True
   b. False

   Answer: a. True. The leader above is likely to fall into the category of a Theory X leader. Leadership attitude theory states that the bad attitudes of Theory X leaders toward followers will encourage followers to match the leader's bad opinions.

4. **Leaders exert influence by their willingness and ability to exert _____.**

   Answer: Power. Leadership is about influencing change and power is the ability to influence.

5. **Which of the following is LEAST EFFECTIVE in most situations when used as the primary leadership style?**
   a. Coercive
   b. Affiliative
   c. Coaching
   d. Pace-setting
   e. Transformational

Answer: a. Coercive. Coercive leadership uses a push strategy that, when used excessively, can cause followers to push back either covertly or overtly. Pull strategies are more effective in gaining follower commitment.

6. **Task-oriented leaders are more likely to provide support to followers than follower-oriented leaders.**
   a. True
   b. False

   Answer: b. False. Task-oriented leaders provide more structure than support.

7. **What form of power is most associated with transformational leaders?**

   Answer: charismatic power. Charisma is the ability to inspire enthusiasm. Transformational leaders inspire enthusiasm in followers by providing a vision of what is possible.

8. **Effective leadership can be done without conscious effort.**
   a. True
   b. False

   Answer: a. True. The highest phase of leadership abilities occurs when a leader is "unaware but effective." In this phase, leadership becomes automatic.

9. **How can a pacesetting leadership style be ineffective?**

   Answer: When expectations of performance are not clear to followers, when demands are deemed to be unreasonable or overwhelming, or when the pacesetter is perceived to be arrogant or narcissistic.

10. **A leader can be very successful in a dynamic environment with a single leadership style.**
    a. True
    b. False

    Answer: b. False. A dynamic environment requires the ability to apply multiple leadership styles to changing circumstances. The more styles available to leaders, the more likely the leader will be able to adapt.

Chapter Discussion Questions

1. Describe how a good leadership process can lead to bad results, and bad leadership processes can lead to good outcomes. What implications does this have for how leaders learn from experience.
2. What leadership styles are likely to be most effective in hospital pharmacy settings? What leadership styles have you observed in hospitals?
3. John was a pharmacist leader who was a strong believer in leading by example. He was a highly competent, hard working Director of Pharmacy at a hospital. He worked long hours and did not have much of a life outside of work. John was never satisfied with the productivity of the pharmacists and technicians he supervised. He criticized them for not meeting his productivity standards and continually pressured

them to work after their shift ended. He thought nothing of calling departmental meetings on weekends or after hours. What is the likely consequence? What recommendations would you give to John?

4. What types of power are available to pharmacy technicians in a pharmacy? Give examples.

CHAPTER 17

Recruiting, Selecting, and Managing Pharmacy Personnel

David A. Holdford

Learning Objectives

After completing this chapter, readers should be able to:

1. Explain the role of human resources management in providing high quality pharmacist services.
2. Identify critical steps in the recruitment and selection of employees.
3. Discuss strategies for retaining and motivating pharmacy employees.
4. Describe the principles and practices of employee performance feedback.

Key Terms and Definitions

- **Behavioral interviews:** Behavioral interviews ask applicants to provide examples about past events and what the applicant did during those events. Behavioral interviewing is based upon the assumption that past behavior best predicts future behavior.
- **Equal Opportunity Employment Commission (EEOC):** The Equal Employment Opportunity Commission (EEOC) is charged with enforcing laws associated with the Federal Civil Rights Act.
- **Federal Civil Rights Act of 1964:** The law and its amendments prohibit discrimination in employment hiring, promotion, compensation, and treatment based upon gender, race, age, religion, and other characteristics.
- **Performance standards:** Performance standards are clearly written, objective expectations of how well employees must do their jobs. They tell employees what to do, how well to do it, and how fast.
- **Position (or job) descriptions:** These contain detailed information on training, experience, knowledge, and skills necessary for minimally acceptable employees. They establish an employee's responsibilities and necessary qualifications for a position.
- **Progressive discipline:** Progressive discipline is a series of managerial actions that escalate incrementally when unacceptable performance does not improve within a specified time period.

The usual steps are a verbal warning, a written warning, a suspension, and termination.

■ **Situation (or role play) interviews:** Situation interviews ask candidates to describe what they would do if faced with a difficult imaginary situation. Situation questions assess applicants' imaginations and their ability to think up quick solutions to problems, although they do not necessarily reveal how a candidate will actually act in real life.

■ **Stress interviews:** Stress interviews deliberately attempt to unnerve candidates by asking blunt, even rude questions. The questions might be delivered in an unfriendly, forceful manner and accompanied by interruptions and persistent pursuit of specific topics. Stress interviews attempt to distinguish a candidate's preparation for the interview and ability to handle stress.

■ **Traditional interviews:** Traditional interviews gather general information about candidates by engaging them in a general conversation about themselves. Common questions are "Tell me a little about yourself?" and "Why do you want to work at our institution?"

■ ■ ■

Introduction

One of the most important issues in pharmacy practice is something for which most pharmacists are least prepared and trained to deal with: personnel management. Indeed, ask pharmacists in institutional settings their greatest aggravation at work, and they will likely answer with some type of complaint about dealing with people, coworkers, other professionals, and supervisors. Successful management of people can make the difference between a smooth running pharmacy and a dysfunctional, unsuccessful one.[1]

Personnel management in institutional pharmacy practice is integral to the provision of patient-centered pharmaceutical care. Managing a patient-centered institutional pharmacy depends on the clear communication of expectations to staff and timely feedback about performance. This helps minimize unproductive conflict in interpersonal relationships and builds strong professional relationships. Pharmacists in well-run and managed pharmacies are likely to make fewer medication errors and have more time and desire to effectively deal with drug-related problems. They will be less distracted, more focused, better organized, and more engaged in their work.

On the other hand, badly run pharmacies can impede patient-centered care. It is not too strong to make the statement, "Poor management of people in pharmacies kills patients." Bad management can kill by hindering professionals' ability to provide safe and effective care. Unengaged, inefficient, and unfocused employees make errors—and errors can be deadly in hospitals and other health care settings. Problem employees can also hurt teamwork by causing conflicts and disrupting the workflow. They can increase workplace tension and generally make the pharmacy a miserable place to work. On top of that, problem employees tie up managers in conflict management, counseling, and supervision—time that can be better spent on other important tasks. Recruiting and retaining good employees is arguably the most important job of pharmacy managers.

Laws and Regulations Affecting Human Resources Management

Most actions in the management of pharmacy personnel are influenced by laws and regulations passed by local, state, and federal governments intended to protect workers from unfair employer practices and biases toward individuals.[1] The most important piece of legislation affecting personnel management is the **Federal Civil Rights Act of 1964** and subsequent amendments to the Act. The original purpose of the Act was to outlaw racial segregation in employment and public settings. It has since been expanded to prohibit discrimination in employment hiring, promotion, compensation, and treatment of protected employee groups—those who might be discriminated against based upon their gender, race, age, religion, sexual preference, height, weight, arrest record, national origin, financial status, military record, or disability.

The **Equal Employment Opportunity Commission (EEOC)** is charged with enforcing laws associated with the Federal Civil Rights Act. Although some actions of the EEOC are considered controversial (e.g., affirmative action), the EEOC can help ensure a smooth running of pharmacy by enforcing what any good manager should already be doing, developing and implementing fair and explicit human relations management.[1] The EEOC prohibits discrimination in any of the following[2]:

- hiring and firing
- compensation and benefits, assignment, or classification of employees
- transfer, promotion, layoff, or recall
- job advertisements
- recruitment
- testing
- use of company facilities
- training and apprenticeship programs
- and other terms and conditions of employment

> ■ ■ ■
>
> **Key Point . . .**
>
> Poor management of people in pharmacies kills patients.
>
> **. . . So what?**
>
> Few people think about ineffective managers and management practices this way. Most realize that poor management can make the workplace intolerable or that it can waste a lot of time and resources. But few think about how it can kill patients. But if you look at the root cause of any fatal medical error, you will see that poor management is a contributing factor. For instance, the people involved might not have been given the necessary training, tools, or feedback, or a disorganized work setting may have distracted an employee. Pharmacists in well-run and managed pharmacies are likely to make fewer medication errors and have the time and desire to provide better service to patients and deal with their drug-related problems.

In addition, EEOC prohibits practices such as harassment of protected employee groups or retaliation against individuals for exercising their rights under EEOC rules.[2] Clashing with the EEOC can cause legal problems for a pharmacy and hinder efforts to recruit and retain excellent employees. Therefore, pharmacy managers need to familiarize themselves with Federal and state laws associated with hiring and firing and consult with their human relations department throughout any sensitive personnel management cases. The department of human relations can review and advise manager actions on appropriate procedures to be followed and adequate documentation.

The Employment Life-Cycle

Employment in an institution can be likened to a life-cycle (Figure 17-1), where an employee's life at an institution begins when hired, the employee grows and matures as training and experience is gained, and the end comes when the employee terminates employment.

Figure 17-1. The employment life cycle.

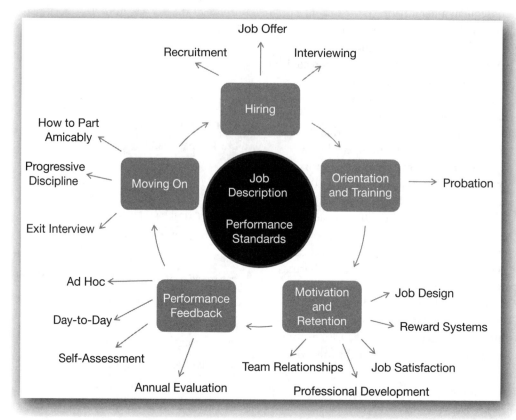

Each phase of the life-cycle builds upon the other in the growth of a good employee. Successful recruitment and hiring make all of the other steps easier by starting with a good foundation. Good training and development, job design, and feedback increase job satisfaction and employee productivity. And when the time comes for an employee to leave a position, it will likely be for good reasons (e.g., a promotion or retirement after a long and successful career) if all of the other steps have been well done.

Hiring

The pharmacy department's shares hiring and other managerial tasks with the department of human relations (also called the personnel department). Human resources departments typically advertise positions, manage applications and paperwork, screen candidates, advise about legal and policy questions, check references, and extend job offers.[1] Their expertise and efforts are invaluable in freeing pharmacy managers and staff to focus on the selection process.

Presence of a human resources department does not mean that pharmacists should surrender their responsibility in recruiting and choosing new employees.[1] At minimum, pharmacists need to supervise the process because human resources personnel do not understand the needs of pharmacy practice as well as pharmacists. Furthermore, human resources personnel do not suffer the same consequences of a bad pharmacy employee choice as individuals in the pharmacy department. Human resources will not be reminded daily about a poor employee choice, but the staff in the pharmacy department will.

Hence, pharmacists should seek to maintain as much control as necessary over the recruiting and selection process.

Ideally, the recruiting process should be inclusive and allow all employees to contribute. Employees should be encouraged to recommend the position to qualified friends and professional acquaintances. They should also help review position descriptions to ensure that the descriptions are accurate and up-to-date. Employees should be involved in interviewing candidates, especially if they are going to being working with the individuals eventually hired. Including staff in the process will broaden the potential for insights into candidates and increase the chance of selecting good individuals.

The Recruiting Process

There are numerous activities associated with recruiting qualified candidates. Job descriptions and performance standards are their center (Figure 17-1). **Position (or job) descriptions** are the foundation of human relations management because they describe an employee's purpose. Clearly written and conceptualized job descriptions are essential for communicating expectations of employees. They are used in setting salaries, communicating performance expectations, and writing up annual performance evaluations. They are also crucial in helping screen out unqualified candidates and encouraging qualified candidates to apply.

Job descriptions contain detailed information on training, experience, knowledge, and skills necessary for a minimally acceptable candidate. They establish the candidate's responsibilities and necessary qualifications for the position. The following information may be included in a position description[3]:

- Position title and classification
- Duties, essential job functions, and responsibilities of the position
- Education, training, experience, and licensure required
- Knowledge, skills, and abilities needed to perform the assigned duties
- Reporting and coordinating relationships
- Scope of authority (i.e., the degree to which decisions can be made without consulting a superior)
- Pay grade and salary range (optional)
- Education and training required to maintain competence
- Other specifications of the position required by law or the organization

Key Point . . .

Employment can be likened to a life-cycle, where an employee's life at an institution begins when hired, the employee grows and matures as training and experience is gained, and the end comes when the employee terminates employment.

. . . So what?

Employees have different needs depending on where they are in their employment life-cycle. At the beginning, they need a good foundation for later success. This includes an orientation to the organization's culture and developing skills needed to accomplish their jobs. As an employee progresses through the life-cycle, their needs and desires change. Managers who align employee interests to the needs of the organization will be more likely to have a satisfied and productive staff.

Performance Standards

Performance standards utilize information from the job description to establish benchmarks for employee behaviors and accomplishments. **Performance standards** are clearly written, objective expectations of how well employees must do their jobs. They tell employees what to do, how well to do it, and how fast. They are used in orientation, training, performance appraisal, coaching, counseling, disciplining, and almost any other personnel management task.

Performance standards can help reduce managerial bias in interactions with employees, because they are explicit and objective expectations of performance. The employee is held accountable for unambiguous benchmarks of acceptable and unacceptable performance rather than the subjective perceptions of the manager. This benefits both the employee by clarifying job expectations and the manager by providing a yardstick upon which to judge employee performance. That yardstick is useful in reducing employee claims against unfair treatment—it is harder to argue against objective measures of performance—and can head off charges of discrimination and bias.

Figure 17-2 provides an example of a performance standard for a pharmacist for the act of dispensing. Expected performance is detailed and quantifiable. A pharmacist who has more than two justified complaints in the process of reviewing medication orders, addressing drug related problems, and related communications does not meet minimally expected performance. Two complaints or less meet minimal performance expectations.

> **Key Point . . .**
>
> Performance standards tell employees what to do, how well to do it, and how fast. They are used in orientation, training, performance appraisal, coaching, counseling, disciplining, and almost any other personnel management task.
>
> **. . . So what?**
>
> It is surprising how many pharmacy employees do not know or contribute input to the performance standards to which they are held accountable. This can be problematic when attempting to justify their contributions to the pharmacy or in responding to criticism about one's work. When managers and employees understand and agree on standards of performance, strategies for improving output can be developed and conflict over expectations reduced.

Most standards consist of more than just two levels of performance. Other levels might be added such as "meets expectations but needs improvement," "exceeds expectations," and "significantly exceeds expectations." Clear descriptions of these performance levels need to be developed and communicated to employees, so they can know exactly what accomplishments are needed to achieve a desired rating.

Since expectations of pharmacy personnel are multidimensional, standards are typically developed for various types of performance.[4] Compliance standards require obedience to established policies and procedures such as expectations of employee attendance, showing up to work on time, and compliance with department dress code. Other standards might deal with an employee's temperament and ability to work with others including quality of communication, initiative and ability to work independently, and ability to

Figure 17-2. Performance standard for dispensing.

> **Performance description:** Dispenses medications in accordance with state and federal laws, all regulatory agencies, and departmental policies.
>
> **Minimally expected performance:** No more than two justified complaints received during the year regarding serious medication errors or routine dispensing functions. This includes but is not limited to:
>
> - Reviewing all orders prior to dispensing
> - Maintaining and regularly reviewing patient medication records for potential drug related problems
> - Contacting physicians, nursing staff, and others as needed to resolve questions regarding medication orders
> - Documenting actions in the electronic medical record

work as part of a team. Standards are also set for the primary tasks of a position including the quality of work, the quantity of output, and the timeliness of completing tasks.

The following characteristics are associated with good performance standards[4]:

- They must be explicit about what determines unacceptable, acceptable, and superior performance.
- They must be specific, objective, and measureable.
- Standards should be challenging but attainable. This means that expectations should not be so high that an employee does even try to meet the standards, but not so low that little effort is needed to achieve them.
- Performance must be under an employee's control. Therefore, employees should not be judged on performance failures or successes related to the system or other uncontrollable factors.
- Standards should be accepted by both the employer and employees. Disagreements over standards of performance need to be resolved. If not, conflicts over performance feedback and evaluations will likely result.

Recruitment Strategies

Recruitment strategies should be individualized to the type of position being filled. As a general rule, the more important the position (e.g., department chair), the more effort and time needed. Systematic recruitment planning is recommended due to the potential cost of making a bad hire. Planning should consider what has worked or not worked in past recruiting efforts. Many institutions recruit continuously even when no job openings are available, so a ready list of individuals is available when an opening does occur.[1,3]

Recruiting individuals from within the department or from other departments has advantages over recruiting from outside of the institution. One advantage is a better understanding of the capabilities and performance of candidates. Another advantage is that it shows commitment to the development of employees. Hiring from within confirms that employees are respected by the management. Internal recruitment can be less expensive by precluding the need to advertise positions, pay for housing and transportation for out-of-town candidates, and pay recruiters to find qualified candidates, In addition, scheduling interviews is easier for internal candidates thereby reducing the disruption of daily work.

Internal recruitment begins very early in the employment life-cycle. Indeed, even before hiring an employee, interviews should ascertain an employee's career aspirations and interests in promotion within an organization. After being hired, employees should be offered training opportunities and tasks to prepare for future roles within the institution.

Nevertheless, recruitment from outside of an institution has advantages too. The primary advantage is the potential for recruiting from a larger number of qualified candidates. Another advantage is that external candidates can inject new perspectives and ideas into the pharmacy. Without introducing outside talent into an institution, organizations can become insular and narrow-minded in their practices. To recruit individuals outside of the organization, the following common methods are used[3]:

- Advertisements in professional journals, newspapers, state professional society newsletters, and electronic bulletin boards.
- Personnel placement services provided by national or state professional societies.
- Oral and written recommendations from colleagues.
- Offering a finder's fee for hires that result from an employee referral.
- Personal discussions or correspondence with potential candidates.
- Recruitment visits to colleges of pharmacy or to facilities that conduct technician-training programs.
- Using professional recruiting firms, which typically charge the organization a percentage of the position's annual salary. In addition, recruitment advertising companies offer access to a list of job seekers for a fee.
- Familiarizing students with the organization by offering summer jobs or participating in college of pharmacy experiential rotations.
- Offering tuition assistance programs for students in exchange for future work commitments.
- Maintaining a "prospect list" of individuals applying for previous job openings, which can often be supplied by the human resources department.
- Attending community job fairs and local or state welfare-to-work programs, and organization-sponsored events such as continuing education sessions, award presentations, or community outreach programs.

Being an employer of choice in a region makes recruiting easier. Employers of choice have a reputation for being the most desirable place to work. They can pick and choose among the best candidates for positions. Managers can help an institution become the employer of choice by earning the respect of employees, making the pharmacy a better place to work, and providing opportunities for professional growth. Managers can also lobby for adequate compensation programs for employees (including salary, fringe benefits, and raise structure).

Applications and Screening

The interview process typically starts when a candidate fills out a job application. The job application and any related correspondence (e.g., resume, letters of recommendation) are stored in the candidates file.

After submitted a job application, candidates are screened for their suitability for the position. Screening is done to weed out unqualified applicants from the pool of potential candidates. Common screening criteria include lack of job qualifications (e.g., license, degree, residency, experience), poorly completed applications (e.g., misspelling, missing information, sloppy writing), and negative applicant history (e.g., felony conviction, lying on the application, frequent changes in employment).[1]

After screening the candidate applications, a screening interview is commonly conducted. The purpose of the screening interview is to provide a quick assessment of the appropriateness of a potential candidate for a position. Screening interviews are usually conducted by the human resources department or the direct supervisor for the position.[3] The interview may be conducted at the institution, by telephone, or at professional gatherings such as the ASHP Annual Midyear meeting. Notes from the screening interview should be placed into an applicant's file.

The Interview Process

Interviews are scheduled after identifying qualified candidates for a position. If multiple applicants are qualified, candidates are typically ranked according to their desirability. The top ranked candidates receive initial invitations to interview, while the less qualified candidates are commonly left in a reserve pool of backup individuals who will only be invited to interview if none of the top candidates are acceptable.

Preparation for an interview is as important for the interviewer as it is for the candidate.[15] Preparations should take into account the schedules of individuals who will be involved in interviewing and use realistic estimates of the time needed in planning and interviewing. Table 17-1 provides a suggested list of interview preparation steps.[1,3]

Table 17-1.
Steps to Prepare for an Interview

1. All interviewees should be sent information about the position including the job description and standards for performance, the institution, local information about the city and state (if an out-of-town candidate), travel directions, and clarification about reimbursement for expenses incurred during the interview. This helps candidates prepare for the interview.

2. Objectives for the interview should be established. Objectives may vary depending on the immediate needs of the organization. If the pharmacy has acute, immediate needs, only those candidates who are immediately available might be considered. In other situations, the pharmacy may be willing to wait for an excellent candidate to graduate from pharmacy school or complete a commitment made to another employer.

3. The position description and performance standards should be reviewed. These documents will form the basis of many interview questions.

4. Applications, letters, and resumes should be explored for accomplishments and credentials upon which to question the candidate. Key concerns should also be noted including frequent job changes, gaps in employment, demotions, inconsistencies in history, or incomplete information on references.

5. A list of interview questions should then be developed that attempt to assess the candidate's ability to achieve job requirements specified in the performance standards. Examples of questions can be found in a variety of sources.[3,11-13] Human resources departments are also helpful in crafting questions.

6. It is often desirable to ask a core group of standard questions of all candidates to allow interviewers to compare candidate responses. Those standard questions should then be supplemented with questions specific to the candidates' responses and unique qualifications for the position.

7. A quiet, uninterrupted interview time and place should be scheduled.

8. Coworkers should be scheduled to meet and interview the candidate.

Source: Reference 1.

Most interviews follow a predictable number of steps. The first step consists of introductory small talk designed to put the candidate at ease. Rather than jumping immediately into the questioning, a few minutes of small talk attempts to establish some rapport with the candidate. After the small talk, interview questions are posed of the candidate.

Interviews questions can be posed using different interviewing techniques.[1] **Traditional interviews** engage candidates in a general conversation about themselves. Common questions are "Tell me a little about yourself?" and "Why do you want to work at our institution?" This line of questioning is useful in gathering general information about the candidate. **Situation (or role play) interviews** ask candidates to describe what they would do if faced with a difficult imaginary situation. For example, "You are a pharmacist, and a technician has just told you that another pharmacist just covered up a dispensing error. What would you do?" Situation questions assess applicants' imaginations and their ability to think up quick solutions to problems, although they do not necessarily reveal how a candidate will actually act in real life. **Stress interviews** deliberately attempt to unnerve candidates by asking blunt, even rude questions such as "We were looking for someone with more experience for this position. What makes you think that you are good enough to fill this position?" The questions might be delivered in an unfriendly, forceful manner and accompanied by interruptions and persistent pursuit of specific topics. Stress interviews attempt to distinguish a candidate's preparation for the interview and ability to handle stress. The downside is that qualified candidates might be insulted and go to other employers. In addition, stress interviews may not effectively discriminate between successful and unsuccessful individuals. **Behavioral interviews** seek examples of an applicant's past behavior under the assumption that past behavior is likely to predict future behavior. Specific questions are asked about past events and the applicant's involvement in the events. Applicants are asked questions that start with "Describe a situation when you had to…." or "Tell us about your worst experience…" Behavioral interviewing is based upon the assumption that past behavior best predicts future behavior. It is common for interviewers to employ several interview styles.

After the questioning phase is finished, candidates are usually encouraged to ask questions of the interviewers. Managers should be prepared to describe relevant facts about the job including opportunities for professional growth, descriptions of employee benefits, the initial salary and salary range for the position, and the employee's work schedule. Non-managers should expect questions about the daily work, general morale of employees, and the like. Interviewers should give the candidate a realistic view of the position, including both favorable and unfavorable information to avoid overselling the position.[3] At the end of the interview, applicants either meet with other interviewers or are given a tour of the facilities. If the candidate is from out of town, a tour of the area should be given too.

After the interview, the candidate should be updated on progress with interviews. At minimum, a follow-up letter should be sent after the interview expressing thanks for the candidate's interest and explaining when a decision will be made about the position. A friendly phone call to the candidate might be made to express continued interest in the candidate and answer any additional questions.

The final choice of an employee typically comes down to how well a candidate can address the following questions of the interviewers.[1]

■ "Can this person do the basic job?" Job openings occur because of an organization's need. The better the candidate can craft an argument that he or she is the best one for solving this need, the more likely he or she will be hired.

- "Will the candidate make my job easier?" The interview process is conducted by human beings who have personal interests in how the position will be filled. The candidate who makes the best case that an interviewer will benefit by hiring the candidate will have a jump on the competition.
- "Would I want to work with this person?" Applicants who are likeable and able to develop rapport with interviewers enhance their chance of being selected for a position.

Before a final offer can be extended to a candidate, a background verification check should be completed. The check verifies information provided by a candidate and is typically completed by the human resources department. Information about the candidate and the candidate's responses may be checked against the following sources[3]:

- Personal letters of reference provided by the applicant
- Letters of reference provided by previous employers or preceptors (with the applicant's permission)
- State board of pharmacy records
- Academic records
- Legal background searches (when permitted by law and/or by the applicant)

■ ■ ■

Key Point . . .

The person who gets a position is typically determined by how well the candidate addresses the questions: "Can this person do the basic job?" "Will the candidate make my job easier?" "Would I want to work with this person?"

. . . So what?

The smartest, more technically competent person is often not the person chosen for a job. Interpersonal skills and the ability to do the basic job are sometimes more important. For example, a pleasant work environment commonly has people who get along with each other, who contribute their fair share, and who do not cause problems for employers. A candidate's chances are improved if he or she can get an interviewer to think, "I want to work with this person."

After a candidate passes the background verification check, a compensation package is put together and an offer extended. Job offers should be extended as soon as a hiring decision is made to prevent a candidate from accepting another position. The offer is typically made by phone because the phone is expedient and more personal than other forms of electronic communication like e-mail. If the offer is not accepted or rejected immediately, a deadline for responding is usually negotiated between the candidate and the employer. Once an offer is accepted, a starting date is negotiated and the employee works with the human relations department to complete necessary paperwork and other requirements of new employees.

Retention

The issue of retaining pharmacists and other employees hired by a pharmacy is a major concern of institutional pharmacy managers. Indeed, the costs of pharmacist turnover has been estimated to range from more than 20 thousand dollars to almost 90 thousand dollars.[5] The issue of employee retention is linked to all parts of the employment life-cycle and failure at any point of the hiring, training, or performance feedback stages can lead to the loss of a pharmacist. Table 17-2 summarizes a checklist that can identify areas that need improvement for retaining pharmacists and other pharmacy employees.

Table 17-2.
Pharmacist Retention Checklist

Salaries

- Our salaries and benefits are competitive to other hospitals in our region.
- Our salaries and benefits are competitive to other non-hospital pharmacist employers in our region.
- We regularly monitor, track and adjust pharmacist salaries (e.g., quarterly).

Employee Development

- We provide annual opportunities for our staff to obtain additional training or attend professional meetings at hospital expense.
- We provide opportunities for pharmacists to progress into areas of greater responsibility based on experience and skills.
- We promote and reward professional development growth in our performance appraisal system.
- We actively mentor new, inexperienced practitioners.

Lifestyle

- We offer preferred shifts and schedules whenever possible. We shift non-time sensitive work to fit the preferred shifts.
- We offer significant incentives to those who work non-preferred shifts.
- We meet with our staff at least annually to discuss quality of life issues and adjust our work environment where possible.
- We offer flexible/creative schedules when possible to meet special needs.

Practice

- Staff have the necessary tools to do their jobs-adequate references and electronic information sources, hand held computers, space, access to computers.
- Most of our pharmacists practice in an environment that is professionally challenging and rewarding with patient contact.
- We use automation and technicians to perform duties that do not require pharmacist knowledge and expertise.
- Our pharmacists are in a position to positively affect patient care and outcomes.

Environment

- Our staff have regular communication from management.
- Our staff have regular opportunities to communicate issues to management.
- Our management staff and other staff members are enjoyable to work with.
- Our technician staff is well trained and work collaboratively with our pharmacist staff.
- Our relationship with other professionals-such as physicians and nurses is positive, constructive and collaborative.

Source: Reference 14.

Motivating Performance

Once an employee is hired, a major role of a manager is to encourage superior performance and or at least avoid discouraging it. This role can be accomplished when human relations management is accomplished by individuals who can apply principles of human motivation to facilitate employee performance. Ideas about human motivation are controversial, and no single theory answers all questions a manager might have about how to motivate people. However, research does provide some general rules-of-thumb for pharmacists and managers.[6-9]

- Communicate what is expected of employees in speech, writing (e.g., policies and procedures), and action. Be consistent in all communications.
- Perceptions matter. In many cases, doing the right thing may not matter if employees perceive things differently. Therefore, managers should try to understand issues from the employees' viewpoints.
- Systems for measuring employee performance need to accurately and fairly distribute rewards.
- The more a manager knows about the needs of the people with whom he or she interacts, the better the manager will be able to identify what issues are most important and likely to motivate an employee. For instance, an employee who values free time may not be motivated to take on additional challenges with monetary bonuses. On the other hand, giving additional time off in exchange may work.
- Provide positive feedback often and provide it much more than negative feedback.
- Employees who feel threatened are often less productive. Threats of job loss or excessive criticism by managers, no matter how well deserved, can cause unintended consequences in employee behavior. Threats can cause anxiety, fear, and resentment and distract employees from their work. Therefore, negative feedback should be used thoughtfully and sparingly. When used, negative feedback should provide explicit actions for employees to improve performance and be accompanied by supportive comments to take the sting out of the criticism.
- Include employees in decisions that affect their lives. Participation can help them gain ownership of the processes under which they work and are assessed. It can help them better understand and accept how rewards are distributed and the behaviors required to receive those rewards.
- Focus on encouraging feelings of accomplishment and pride in one's work. Help them find the joy in their current job or help them develop their skills for a better job.
- Try to pay people a fair, reasonable amount and then do everything

> **Key Point . . .**
>
> Perceptions matter. In many cases, doing the right thing may not matter if employees perceive things differently.
>
> **. . . So what?**
>
> To a great extent, management is about influencing perceptions. Perceptions are reality. If employees perceive that a manager is being unfair in the treatment of employees, the reality of the situation is irrelevant to how they are going to react. Therefore, managers not only need to do the right thing, they need to be perceived as doing the right thing.

possible to encourage them to forget about their pay. A preoccupation with money distracts everyone, employers and employees, from issues that really matter.

■ Help employees realize that most reward systems are unfair to someone, in some way, and at some time. Try to be seen as doing the best you can for employees given the current flawed reward system.

■ Set an example for others by demonstrating pleasure in what you do.

Performance Feedback

Managers are judged on how well the team performs, and effective performance feedback is essential for productive and well functioning teams. Performance feedback attempts to communicate how well employees are achieving the objectives in their job description and performance standards. It also suggests ways that performance can be improved.

Performance feedback can occur any time a manager interacts with an employee. Indeed, feedback is continually provided from a manager's words, voice, body language, and behaviors. For that reason, managers need to be continually aware of the messages they send to employees in day-to-day interactions. Awareness needs to be accompanied by self control too, because a misplaced comment or a poorly articulated criticism can cause unnecessary tension or communicate an unintended message.[10]

Day-to-day discussions are the most effective form of performance feedback because they are immediate and frequent. Behavior is more likely to change in day-to-day feedback because it can occur shortly after that behavior occurs. For that reason, managers often try to look for a situation that illustrates problem behavior to be discouraged or a positive behavior to be reinforced. This process can be improved if employees are encouraged to provide his or her view of the situation. This encourages employees to analyze their behaviors and engages them in the change process. If there is disagreement about the problem behavior, the manager should speak in terms of his or her perception of situation. Rather than saying, "This is what you did," it is better to say "Correct me if I am wrong. This is what I observed." Focusing on perceptions is less confrontational but still very effective in addressing behavioral issues. Once an agreement is reached on the need to change, the employee should be encouraged to come up with a strategy to improve. Once agreed upon, the manager should periodically check to see if employee performance improves.

Annual (or semi-annual) performance reviews are another form of feedback to employees. Annual performance reviews are sometimes dreaded by both employees and managers because they take a lot of time and effort, can be stressful, compete with other priorities, and can be seen as a bureaucratic chore.[4] Nevertheless, performance reviews are important because they require managers and employees to step back and think about progress throughout the year and make plans for the future. Annual performance reviews augment and summarize feedback provided by managers in day-to-day feedback.[1]

Ideally, the performance review should be an exchange of information and ideas— not a report card of the worthiness of an employee.[4] Certainly, reviews will have an evaluative component of employee performance. But equally important, they serve as a planning session for long-term employee and departmental goals.

Effective reviews should attempt to achieve several goals.[4] They should summarize information provided to the employee in day-to-day feedback. If daily feedback has been effective, then nothing in the performance review should be a surprise to the employee. Reviews should encourage self-appraisal by the employee and offer an opportunity for the employee to communicate accomplishments that might have been overlooked by the manager. Employee performance should be recognized, and performance deficiencies should be addressed through a collaborative, dual problem solving process. Discussion should emphasize the future instead of past performance because the past cannot be changed. Good reviews should attempt to positively affect an employee's self-esteem and improve the relationship between employees and managers.

A typical performance evaluation consists of the following steps:

- Performance standards are reviewed and any issues associated with the standards are clarified.
- Objectives from previous evaluations are examined.
- The manager evaluates past performance with the employee and expresses appreciation for any accomplishments.
- The manager discusses causes for any performance deficiencies and mutually develops strategies with the employee for improvement.
- Any long-term career goals are discussed and strategies for achieving them are developed.
- Relevant points discussed in the interview recorded and both the employee and manager sign the performance review document.

Efforts should be made to avoid common appraisal problems.[4] One problem is biased assessment of employees. Biased assessments may result when the reviewer bases judgments primarily on recent job performances of employees (called the recency effect) instead of on performance over the whole evaluation time period. Another bias is the halo effect, where evaluators judge individuals based on general perceptions of the person and not objective, quantified measures of behavior. Another appraisal problem is trying to be nice rather than objective about an individual's performance. Other assessment problems include rating everyone the same, not taking the process seriously, using the review primarily to assign salaries instead of improving performance, having insufficient or superficial knowledge of an employee's performance, emphasizing the negatives during the review, and blindsiding individuals with unexpected issues that had never been brought up before in day-to-day feedback.

Reviews should be conducting with the understanding that they may eventually be challenged in institutional grievance proceedings or in legal settings. Therefore, reviews need to be procedurally and legally justifiable.[4] This means that all statements should be factual and based upon measurable performance. For instance, an employee should not be described as having a "bad attitude." More precise criticism

> **Key Point . . .**
>
> Progressive discipline consists of a series of managerial action that escalate incrementally when unacceptable performance does not improve within a specified time period.
>
> **. . . So what?**
>
> Progressive discipline seeks to protect employees and managers by employing a structured process to managerial feedback and discipline. Employees are protected because they are provided with detailed feedback about unacceptable performance and given opportunities to improve it. Managers are protected because they are given a process of disciplinary actions that is legally defensible against charges of bias.

should be offered, such as the number of complaints from nurses and co-workers about the individual's behavior. Reviews should also be based on an employee's job responsibilities and performance objectives. Thus, if an employee's dress or hairstyle is not relevant to expectations of performance, it should not be discussed. Finally, reviews should be consistent across employees so those of similar job descriptions are held to similar standards of performance.

Progressive Discipline

Progressive discipline is a form of feedback designed to improve *unacceptable* employee performance such as absenteeism, tardiness, unprofessional behavior, violation of rules, and unsatisfactory work performance. **Progressive discipline** consists of a series of managerial action that escalate incrementally when unacceptable performance does not improve within a specified time period.

The usual steps in progressive discipline are a verbal warning, a written warning, a suspension, and termination. Verbal warnings are formal oral reprimands about poor performance and what will occur if performance does not improve. A chronically tardy technician might receive a verbal warning that he or she is not meeting performance standards and must show up to work on time to avoid further disciplinary action. A note should be made by the manager about the time and place of the reprimand and what was discussed. If behavior does not improve, a written warning follows. A written warning is a formal document of disciplinary action that should clearly describe the unacceptable behavior, previous warnings, specific expectations of future behavior to be achieved by a precise deadline, and the consequences of not meeting expectations.[1] For example, a formal warning might state, "You were verbally warned about tardiness on January 16 of this year. You have continued to be tardy at a rate above that specified in your performance standards. If you are late for work more than twice within the next month, you will be suspended for one day without pay." The written warning makes explicit to the employee that if behavior does not improve, the next step in progressive discipline occurs: suspension. Suspensions are disciplinary actions that force employees to take unpaid leave for a specified time period. They are designed to jolt the employee into taking action and demonstrate the seriousness of a situation. They act as a final warning that current behavior is unacceptable. The written documentation is similar to that of a written warning except that the consequences of further unacceptable behavior are more severe (i.e., termination of employment).

Termination of Employees

Hopefully, termination will be a rare event for individuals in a pharmacy because it is a difficult experience for everybody involved. In truth, it reflects a failure of the human resources management system.

Termination of an employee means that the system failed to choose the right person for the job and/or give the employee what was needed to succeed. For the terminated employee, it can negatively impact self-esteem and damage financial security. For the manager, the termination is an unpleasant confrontation at best, and at worst, a potential lawsuit for wrongful dismissal.

The repercussions of termination can be minimized if institutional termination policies and procedures are followed and the human resources department is consulted and involved throughout the process. Policies and procedures protect both the employee and the manager, and the human resources department can prevent common errors from occurring. In all cases, termination should be done with compassion and in a manner that seeks to maintain the employee's dignity and self-respect. The process should be well documented and witnessed.

Summary

By necessity, a single chapter can only provide a quick overview of recruiting, selecting, and managing pharmacy personnel. The subject is complex and can require years of experience before one gains sufficient expertise. This chapter can only begin to highlight key issues of managing pharmacy personnel which are so critical for serving the patient. Hiring, training, performance feedback, and other key elements of managing people are interrelated such that all must be done well to get the most out of pharmacy personnel. Individuals who are well managed are more likely to be productive and enjoy their jobs. Competent, productive employees in a pharmacy are better able to provide pharmaceutical care and achieve better health outcomes for patients.

Suggested Reading

ASHP technical assistance bulletin on the recruitment, selection, and retention of pharmacy personnel. *Am J Health-Syst Pharm*. 1994;51:1811-1815.

Desselle S. Performance appraisal systems. In: Desselle SP, Zgarrick DP, eds. Pharmacy Management. New York: McGraw-Hill/Appleton & Lange; 2004:185-202.

Donnelly JH, Gibson JL, Ivancevich JM. Human Resource Management. Fundamentals of Management. 9th ed. Chicago: Irwin Publishing; 1995:444-479.

Murawski MM. Introduction to personnel management: training your support team for clinical practice. *Drug Topics*. 1996;140[Jun 10]:170-179.

Pierpaoli PG. Three challenges: redefining production, embracing pharmaceutical care, and empowering staff. *Am J Hosp Pharm*. 1990;47:321-323.

Smith JE. Integrating human resources and program-planning strategies. *Am J Health-Syst Pharm*. 1989;46:1153-1161.

Thomas KS. Intrinsic Motivation at Work. San Francisco: Berrett-Koehler Publishers, Inc.; 2002.

Umiker W. Management skills for the new health care supervisor. 3rd ed. Gaithersburg, MD: Aspen Publishers, Inc.; 1998.

Vermeulen LC, Rough SS, Thielke TS, et al. Strategic approach for improving the medication-use process in health systems: The high-performance pharmacy practice framework. *Am J Health-Syst Pharm*. 2007;64:1699-1710.

White SJ. Human resource management in patient-centered pharmaceutical care. *Top Hosp Pharm Manage*. 1994;14:46-52.

White SJ, Generali JA. Motivating pharmacy employees. *Am J Hosp Pharm*. 1984;41:1361-1366.

References

1. Holdford DA. Human Resources Management Functions. In: Desselle SP, Zgarrick DP, eds. *Pharmacy Management*. New York: McGraw-Hill/Appleton & Lange; 2004:171-183.

2. Federal Laws Prohibiting Job Discrimination Questions and Answers. The U.S. Equal Employment Opportunity Commission. 2009. Available at: http://www.eeoc.gov/facts/qanda.html. Accessed May 2010.

3. ASHP technical assistance bulletin on the recruitment, selection, and retention of pharmacy personnel. *Am J Hosp Pharm.* 1994;51:1811-1815.

4. Umiker W. Performance Feedback. *Management Skills for the New Health Care Supervisor.* 3rd ed. Gaithersburg, MD: Aspen Publishers, Inc.; 1998.

5. Cost of Pharmacist Turnover. ASHP Member Center on Staffing, HR Resources, & Pharmacy Workforce . 2009. American Society of Health-Systems Pharmacists. Available at: http://www.ashp.org/s_ashp/docs/files/turnovercost.pdf. Accessed May 2010.

6. Donnelly JH, Gibson JL, Ivanevich JM. Motivation. *Fundamentals of Management.* 9th ed. Chicago: Irwin Publishing; 1995:302-341.

7. Hiam A. *Motivating and Rewarding Employees.* Holbrook, MA: Adams Media Corp.; 1999.

8. Kohn A. Why incentive plans cannot work. *Harv Bus Rev.* 1993;74:54.

9. Fournies FF. *Why Employees Don't Do What They're Supposed To Do and What To Do About It.* 2nd ed. New York: McGraw Hill; 1999.

10. Holdford DA. Managing Yourself. *J Am Pharm Assn.* 2009;15:45-54.

11. Reinders TP. *The Pharmacy Professional's Guide to Résumés, CVs, & Interviewing.* 2nd ed. Washington, DC: American Pharmacists Association Publications; 2005.

12. Medley HA. *Sweaty Palms. The Neglected Art of Being Interviewed.* 2nd ed. Berkley, California: Ten Speed Press; 1984.

13. Nimmo CM. *Human Resources Management: ACCRUE level II.* Bethesda, MD: American Society of Hospital Pharmacists; 1991.

14. Pharmacist Retention Checklist. ASHP Member Center Staffing, HR Resources, & Pharmacy Workforce. 2009. American Society of Health-Systems Pharmacists.

Chapter Review Questions

1. The following is a good performance standard: "All employees should try not to be late for work."
   a. True
   b. False

Answer: False. The above standard is neither specific in the expected behavior (trying to not be late for work is a vague expectation) nor quantitative (it is not clear how many times being late for work is unacceptable).

2. The purpose of screening job applicants is to identify the best candidate for the position.
   a. True
   b. False

Answer: False. The purpose of screening is to eliminate all applicants deemed unqualified for the job.

3. Interview questions should be based upon:
   a. Position descriptions
   b. Performance standards
   c. The interviewer's personal interests
   d. Details about the candidate's resume and application

Answer: a, b, c, and d. Any of the above can and should inform the interview. Answer "c" might be controversial based on the argument that questions based upon personal interests might lead to bias. However, the process is conducted by human beings and personal interests cannot and should not be excluded from the interview.

4. _____ interview questions are based upon the assumption that what people have done in the past is predictive of what they will do in the future.
   a. Stress
   b. Behavioral
   c. Situational
   d. Traditional

   Answer b. Behavioral. Behavioral interview questions ask candidates to provide examples of previous accomplishments or behaviors assuming that they are more predictive of future performance than questions answered under stress, based upon made-up situations, or general discussions about oneself.

5. Perceptions matter more in interactions between managers and employees than the truth.
   a. True
   b. False

   Answer: True. Perceptions are reality in dealing with human beings. For example, a manager's actions that are perceived as unfair by employees, even if judged fair by objective observers and standards, will suffer the same consequences of a manager who is truly unfair.

6. Employees should be included in all managerial decisions.
   a. True
   b. False

   Answer: False. Employees should only be included in managerial decisions that affect their lives. Selection of coworkers is an example of a decision that affects employees' lives, so they need to be involved as much as possible.

7. Which of the following methods of performance feedback are most effective, on average, in influencing employee behavior?
   a. Day-to-day feedback
   b. Annual performance evaluations
   c. Progressive discipline

   Answer: a. Day-to-day feedback. Day-to-day feedback immediately and frequently reinforces desired behavior and discourages undesired behavior. Annual performance evaluations occur too rarely to have long-lasting impact on daily performance. Progressive discipline is not typically used for the average employee and therefore is unlikely to have much influence on the behaviors of most employees.

8. Greater pay motivates better performance in employees.
   a. True
   b. False

   Answer: Maybe. Many might argue that the answer is "True" because the answer is simply common sense and the foundation of our economic system where those who produce more should receive greater rewards. Others might say "False" by responding that not everyone is motivated to receive greater pay or that better performance is often not rewarded with more pay. However, the question is much more complex than one might see at first glance. The answer to this question probably can never be definitively answered because of the complexity of human behavior and the convoluted way that humans respond to incentives. For one thing, the statement above does not define how much pay, how the pay is linked to good performance, how well performance measures distinguish good performance from not so good performance, how motivated employees are to put in the additional effort needed to achieve the pay, or the host of other variables affecting motivation. Therefore, pay-for-performance systems in personnel management need to be supported by good leadership and management.

9. **Which of the following actions might indicate an ineffective performance review?**
   a. The manager emphasizes the award of a pay raise during the review.
   b. The manager focuses on all of the negative behaviors of the employee through-out the evaluation period.
   c. The employee and manager engage in mutual problem solving on identified performance weaknesses of the employee.
   d. The manager links performance assessment to the employee's performance standards.

Answer: a and b are associated with ineffective performance reviews. Discussions about pay increases may be important to the employee, but they can distract from the real purpose of performance reviews, to assess past performance and plan for ways of improving performance in the future. Focusing on the negative during performance evaluations will leave employees demoralized and overshadow any achievements made during the year. Performance evaluations should be mutual problem solving sessions between employees and managers. Evaluations should assess performance against established standards of performance and result in mutually agreeable strategies for improving future performance.

10. **The primary purpose of progressive discipline is which of the following?**
   a. Improve minimally acceptable employee behavior to behavior that is superior.
   b. Get rid of employees who are not contributing members of the team.
   c. Encourage employees to change from unacceptable performance to acceptable performance.
   d. Document employee punishments to avoid being sued.

Answer: c. The purpose of progressive discipline is to motivate employees to move from unacceptable to acceptable performance. It is not meant for employees who are at least minimally acceptable. Its primary purpose is not to get rid of employees either, although that may be the end consequence of the process. And the primary purpose of progressive discipline is not to provide cover to managers to avoid being sued. If avoiding lawsuits is a goal, one could probably achieve that goal by doing nothing to address poor employee performance.

Chapter Discussion Questions

1. What should go into a clinical pharmacist's performance standards?
2. Do you think the EEOC hinders or helps pharmacists serve their patients? Why?
3. Do think that your annual reviews have always been fair? Explain.
4. Provide an example from your life that supports or refutes one of the motivational rules-of thumb described in the section *Motivating Performance.*
5. Do you think that progressive discipline is used more to mend the behaviors of problem employees or to get rid of problem employees? Why?

CHAPTER 18

Training for Careers in Hospitals and Health Systems

Thomas P. Reinders and David A. Holdford

■ ■ ■

Learning Objectives

After completing this chapter, readers should be able to:

1. Identify what training and skills are necessary to succeed in hospital and health-system pharmacy practice
2. Compare the various training and educational options for hospital and health-system pharmacy practice
3. Contrast graduate education with residencies and other forms of experiential training

Key Terms and Definitions

■ **American Pharmacist Association's (APhA) Pathway Evaluation Program:** Provides a process for exploring pharmacy careers and provides resources for making informed career decisions.

■ **American Society of Health-System Pharmacy Midyear Clinical Meeting and Exhibition:** A national annual meeting in December where individuals interested in post-graduate training can attend the Residency Showcase.

■ **Curriculum vitae (CV):** Provides detailed information about an individual's qualifications and experiences. It differs from a resume because it is typically longer and more detailed (more than two pages).

■ **Internship:** On-the-job training experience for students enrolled in pharmacy school.

■ **Porfolio:** A collection of information about an individual designed to provide a comprehensive picture of experience, accomplishments, and training. It typically contains actual work completed, for example, a written project or poster presentation, that can showcase one's capabilities.

■ **Resume:** Document summarizing relevant education, training, and job experience. It differs from a CV because it short (one or two pages).

Introduction

Congratulations! You have decided to be a pharmacist. Now your next step is to answer the question, "What kind of pharmacist do I want to be?" The answer to this question lies greatly in the type of practice setting you choose to work after graduation.

Determining a career path in pharmacy can be a challenging task due to the variety of options available within the profession. Students can practice in independent community pharmacies, super markets, corporate chains, mass merchandisers, mail order pharmacies, specialty pharmacies, hospitals, long-term care facilities, government institutions, managed care, and many other locations. The career choices within each of these locations (e.g., clinical pharmacist, manager, specialist) make the task even more challenging.

Successful student pharmacists begin by taking an early and active role in shaping who they will become as a pharmacist. Since there are many choices, it is best to explore options before making a final decision on your career path. Too often, students are admitted to a school or college of pharmacy after being exposed to one particular facet of pharmacy practice—typically community pharmacy. Then, they declare a preference for this type of practice throughout their pharmacy education without exploring the other options available to them. This preference is often intensified by community pharmacy chains, mass merchandisers, and other employers of pharmacists who approach students early in their careers as students and offer tuition assistance packages and part-time jobs. Appealing to student concerns about paying off tuition and choice of career, these employers encourage students to lock onto one career path by signing commitments to work for them after graduation.

The downside of choosing a career path without adequately exploring other alternatives is that opportunities can be missed. Realization of the missed opportunities occurs typically when students reach the experiential phase of their pharmacy education. Through their exposure to dynamic pharmacist role models who actually practice pharmacy in team-based

Key Point . . .

Your ability to identify and compete for hospital and health-system practice positions is influenced by steps you take in pharmacy school.

. . . So what?

If you have no idea what you want to do with your life at graduation time, you may be at a serious disadvantage in regard to your career. Many of your classmates and colleagues at other schools have been taking steps to prepare for a career in hospital and health-system pharmacy practice. They have chosen their coursework and practice experiences to teach them concepts and skills that will prepare them to practice. They have built a resume of experiences and accomplishments that differentiate themselves from other potential job candidates. They have interviewed for residencies and other jobs in hospital and health-system practice and probably have offers in hand. However, if you are still at least a year or two from graduation, you still have time to take the steps that can help you obtain a career in hospital and health-system pharmacy practice.

surroundings (just like the professors say in pharmacy school), they ask themselves, "Why didn't I know about this earlier?" This realization then leads to regret about not exploring more career options while progressing through the curriculum.

The concern over potential regret causes another problem—putting off any career moves until tomorrow. Many students delay making any decision about what they want to do with their career for perfectly good reasons including:

- "I don't know enough about my options."
- "I am afraid of making the wrong choice."
- "I might miss out on good opportunities if I narrow my focus."

The problem with delaying any action is that your ability to identify and compete for hospital and health-system practice positions is influenced by steps you take in pharmacy school. To compete for residencies and the best entry level positions, you need to compile a portfolio of experiences that demonstrates you are able to succeed after graduation.

We recommend exploring career opportunities but not locking in on any specific one. Head in a general career direction that interests you, but do not close yourself off to any option. Do not say, "I do not need to know about X, because I am going to be practicing Y." Take advantage of all of the options your education provides you, within the classroom and outside of it. Learn as much as you can, stay focused on your studies, network, join organizations, and have fun. No matter where you practice in pharmacy, you will be able to build a challenging and satisfying career.

Key Point . . .

Take advantage of all of the options your education provides you—within the classroom and outside of it. Learn as much as you can, stay focused on your studies, network, join organizations, and have fun.

. . . So what?

It is hard for pharmacy students to develop a good resume if they confine themselves to the classroom and study areas. Well-rounded resumes demonstrate a life outside of the classroom in addition to academic accomplishment. In addition, the relationships made in pharmacy school can continue long after graduation. The pharmacy profession can be a small world, and the quality of relationships developed during the years at school can pay off in the future.

Planning a Career Path

So how do you know which career paths might be right for you? The steps are relatively straightforward:

1. Assess your personal strengths and weaknesses
2. Develop an understanding about yourself and the kind of life you want to live
3. Think about how you make decisions
4. Reflect on the types of decisions you will make as a student pharmacist
5. Begin to prepare a plan for your future

Throughout your tenure as a student pharmacist, you will need to be diligent in taking advantage of opportunities to learn about every aspect of the profession. Each year of study will lead to an expansion of your knowledge and skills. Table 18-1 lays out a series of activities you can complete during your four years of pharmacy school. It also suggests which years are optimal for completing these tasks.

A valuable tool to assist you is the **American Pharmacist Association's (APhA) Pathway Evaluation Program**. You can access the program from the career tab on the APhA Academy of Student Pharmacists website (www.aphanet.org). Many pharmacy schools require their students to complete exercises in the Pathway Evaluation Program, so many students are already familiar with it. These students would probably be well served by reviewing their findings periodically to clarify their own career preferences. If you have never completed the program, you can explore it on your own by going to the website. You will benefit from the time taken to complete the survey and examine the exercises.

The Pathway Evaluation Program offers individuals the opportunity to assess which career options best suit their personal interests and strengths. A unique feature of the program is the opportunity to compare one's rating of 48 critical factors common to pharmacy practice (e.g., work schedule, job security, prestige and opportunities for advancement) with the ratings of actual pharmacists in a variety of practice settings. Table 18-2 lists critical job factors that were highly rated by staff pharmacists, clinical specialists and pharmacist managers practicing in health-system settings including hospitals, home health care, and long term care. The table also provides a short assessment of the

Table 18-1.
Career Planning Activities During Your Years at Pharmacy School

Activities	P-1 Year	P-2 Year	P-3 Year	P-4 Year
Introductory pharmacy practice experiences	X	X	X	
Advanced pharmacy practice experiences				X
Elective courses related to your future practice goals		X	X	
Talk with mentors	X	X	X	X
Acquire internship experience	X	X	X	X
Shadow practicing pharmacists	X	X	X	
Become active in student organizations	X	X	X	X
Attend local, state, national pharmacy meetings	X	X	X	X
Review state and national pharmacy websites	X	X	X	X
Prepare and update career statement, resume, curriculum vitae, and electronic portfolio	X	X	X	X
Review pharmacy residency programs		X	X	X
Review post-graduate programs		X	X	X
Prepare residency or post-graduate study application				X

presence of these factors in hospital and health-system pharmacy practice. Findings from the pathway program indicate that pharmacists in hospital and health-system practice, on average, are intellectually challenged by the work itself and the individuals with whom they work. They have a chance to apply what they learned in pharmacy school, and they enjoy competitive compensation, good working conditions, and the opportunity for professional development. If these are things you desire in your career, the opportunities in health-system settings might be right for you.

Table 18-2.

Important Critical Factors for Health-System Pharmacists

Critical Factor	Assessment
Collaboration with other professionals	Pharmacists spend a significant amount of time during their daily activities in working with other health professionals, especially physicians and nurses. Since the health professionals are usually within the same facility and have access to a patient's health record, there is constant written and verbal communication concerning the drug therapy of patients. Collaboration in this setting is important since the success of any health system depends on its ability to function as a collaborative unit.
Variety of daily activities	Pharmacists have a great variety of tasks and duties during a routine day. The health-system setting spans a wide range from ambulatory care to critical care. The medication-related needs of patients for this continuum of care creates variability. While some activities can be repetitive, there is always a balance between routine and challenging tasks and duties.
Multiple task handling	The health-system setting is a dynamic environment where pharmacists are not always able to work on a single task until it is completed. The setting, by its very nature of promptly dealing with the acute needs of patients, often requires the pharmacist to handle multiple tasks.
Applying medical knowledge	Pharmacists in the health system setting have an opportunity to apply their medical and scientific knowledge on a daily basis. There is a constant need for accurate and reliable drug information related to the medication needs of patients in this setting.
Job security	Job security and stability is apparent since there is a continuous need for pharmacists in the health-system setting. Pharmacists with specialized knowledge and skills are provided even more security.
Income	Compensation is important to pharmacists. During the past decade the salaries for pharmacists in this setting have increased so that they are often equivalent to salaries offered in the community setting. Pharmacists with additional credentials and management responsibilities usually receive additional compensation.
Benefits (vacation, health, retirement)	Benefit packages are important to pharmacists seeking employment. Overall, the health-system setting provides generous benefit packages. Some benefits (e.g., additional vacation, travel funds, child care, fewer weekend shifts) are a major reason that some pharmacists have been attracted to this setting.
Professional involvement	Professional involvement is important to pharmacists in this setting. Pharmacists are concerned about the respect for their work and seek to share ideas and knowledge among peers. Opportunities are provided to attend meetings and events related to the profession. Health-system employers generally encourage and reward professional involvement.

(continued)

Table 18-2. (continued)

Important Critical Factors for Health-System Pharmacists

Critical Factor	Assessment
Autonomy	Pharmacists in this setting like their ability to make independent decisions about their practice activities. Pharmacists are viewed as a medication use expert and their opinions about medications are trusted by other health care professionals. While independent decision making is evident, pharmacists in this setting favor the ability to provide their recommendations while functioning as a healthcare team member.
Self-worth	Satisfaction based upon recognition and feedback is important to pharmacists in this setting. Likewise, it is important to have a high level of confidence in the quality of their work and to fulfill personal and professional goals.
Additional training	Health-system settings are known to encourage and promote additional training for their employees due to the number of disease conditions and treatments, advances in technology and trends in this setting. This provides the opportunity for professional growth which can enhance career satisfaction and lead to additional compensation. Many health-system employers will provide some or all of the expense associated with position-related education and training.
Interaction with colleagues	There is a high level of interaction among colleagues within the health-system setting. This involves interaction with staff within the pharmacy as well as all other health professionals providing patient care.

Source: Reprinted with permission from reference 1.

Gaining Experience

IPPEs and APPEs

Recent changes in the accreditation standards for schools and colleges of pharmacy offer all students a chance to learn about health-system pharmacy. Schools now require exposure to practice settings during the initial years of a pharmacy student's education —through **Introductory Pharmacy Practice Experiences (IPPEs)**. This requirement affords an opportunity for all students to explore pharmacy practice in a health-system setting. Also required in the latter part of the curriculum, students complete an advanced pharmacy practice experience in health-system pharmacy practice—**Advanced Pharmacy Practice Experiences (APPEs)**. APPEs in health-system pharmacy provide more in-depth observations about practice in this setting and require students to demonstrate common practice competencies such as the preparation of intravenous drug products and responding to drug information requests from physicians.

Even if students have no intention of practicing in hospital and health-system settings, they need to pay attention during these rotations because many of the skills can be useful in non-hospital and health-system settings. For instance, some independent pharmacists prepare intravenous infusions for small hospitals and home health care companies, and chain pharmacies now employ clinical pharmacists in specialty pharmacy settings. General knowledge about hospital and health-system pharmacy practice can also be useful to non-hospital and health-system pharmacists in handoffs of patients between practice settings (e.g., medication reconciliation when moving from hospital to community locations).

Student Organizations

Involvement in student pharmacist organizations offers opportunities to learn more about hospital and health-system pharmacy practice. Some organizations, such as the Academy of Student Pharmacists, represent all facets of professional practice, while others represent specialized practice, such as student chapters of the American Society of Health-System Pharmacists (ASHP). Joining either type of organization can provide a starting point for learning more about the practice of the profession in a health system. Taking leadership roles within professional organizations can help in developing leadership skills and offer better professional networking opportunities. Some student ASHP chapters offer shadowing experiences with health-system pharmacists, similar to the exposure provided during introductory practice experiences.

Didactic Curriculum

Students gain information about health-system practice as part of their didactic curriculum. Formal lectures and required readings offer an entry point for exploring health-system practice. Some schools and colleges provide required and elective courses revolving around health-system practice. These courses offer readings from the health-system pharmacy literature, presentations from invited hospital and health-system pharmacist lecturers, and field trips to health-system pharmacies. The clinical pharmacy curriculum also presents information about hospital and health-system practice in both required and elective courses (e.g., cardiology, critical care, and oncology).

Some schools and colleges offer specialized educational tracks for students who wish to practice in health systems and/or to pursue a residency. If your school does not offer one of these tracks, you can always work with your faculty and administrators to develop your own personal track, arranging a portfolio of practice experiences that will allow you to be competitive when seeking a residency.

Internships

Internships in a health system provide a basic understanding of hospital and health-system practice. This can be especially helpful when pursuing a pharmacy residency upon graduation because it provides a sound introduction to the basics of practice and training in relevant skills. Residency candidates with additional experience in health-system practice may have an advantage over those with limited hospital and health-system practice experience.

Key Point . . .

Even if you have no intention of practicing in an hospital and health-system setting, pay attention during health-system IPPEs and APPEs because many of the skills learned in these rotations can be useful in non-hospital and health-system settings.

. . . So what?

Many faculty members at schools of pharmacy are aware of the exasperating declaration made by students, "I don't need to know X because I am going to be practicing in Y." In truth, no one really knows what the future holds for them or what they really need to know. However, many conditions once treated only in hospitals now are handled in ambulatory or long-term care settings. That trend is likely to continue. Therefore, many of the skills learned during health-system IPPEs and APPEs may come in handy in the future for almost any pharmacy practice setting.

Mentors

Mentors can be an invaluable source of support and encouragement for student pharmacists or new graduates. Ask them about their career path and what they would recommend to someone who is just starting out in the profession. Just be aware that they will likely be passionate about their chosen area of practice and may advocate for this path over other practice areas. Talk with many mentors and peers, listen to what they say, and make your own choice.

Professional Meetings

Consider attending local, state and national meetings to learn more about the profession and begin building a network of colleagues. Attending the **American Society of Health-System Pharmacists Midyear Clinical Meeting** is valuable for students seeking a residency. Most residency program directors participate in a residency showcase program during the meeting. The event is structured to allow you to meet program directors, staff and current residents. The residency showcase is an important first step in learning about the variety of programs and to begin preparing a list of questions related to pursuing a residency.

Key Point . . .

You can always work with your faculty and administrators to develop your own personal track, arranging a portfolio of practice experiences that will allow you to be competitive when seeking a residency.

. . . So what?

Do not wait for others to give you what you need to compete for a residency. Take control by making your own arrangements. In fact, a candidate who shows enough drive to build his or her own portfolio of practice experiences may be looked at more favorably than one who simply follows a pathway established by others.

Internet

Do not forget the Internet. Pharmacy organizations provide a wealth of information for you to explore by visiting their websites. Many have included a special section devoted to student interests. For example, the American Society of Health-System Pharmacists website provides information about career planning and preparation, professional and leadership development and other education resources for students.

Developing a Career Plan

No matter what you plan to do after graduation, career planning should consider the acquisition of skills common to hospital and health-system practice, because many of these skills are transferrable to other jobs. Training in health-systems provides many chances to develop clinical pharmacy skills—expertise that is transferable to any arena of pharmacy practice including long-term care, ambulatory pharmacy, and managed care. Training in sterile product preparation and admixtures can be useful in home health care and hospice settings. Other skills learned in hospital and health-system settings include the ability to work with teams of professionals, managing technicians, managing medication distribution systems, and electronic data management.

At some point, you will need to decide on a specific area of interest within the pharmacy profession. If you choose to pursue a career in health-system practice, remember that you can change your mind in the future. In truth, many individuals who started in hospitals and other health-system settings now work for pharmacy benefits managers, pharmaceutical companies, state and federal agencies, and more.

When you finally make a commitment, you can better craft a message about your career intentions. This increases your chances for success.

One way of communicating your commitment is to put it at the beginning of your resume or curriculum vitae in the form of a "career objective." A few examples of career objectives include: (1) To obtain a pharmacy intern position; (2) To obtain a pharmacy practice residency position; (3) To obtain a pharmacist position in a health-system practice setting; and (4) To obtain a clinical pharmacist specialist position.

You may consider expanding your career intentions with a "personal statement." You are most likely to be asked for a personal statement if you apply to a residency program, a fellowship program, or a graduate program. Frequently, programs will ask you to respond to an open-ended question such as, "What led you to choose a career in pharmacy?" or "How will this program help you reach your professional goals?" Your statement should be original and sincere. You can reflect on how your education and practice experiences have contributed to your personal and professional growth. Don't fail to mention specific strengths such as leadership or communication skills and offer a few specific examples or anecdotes that support your points. Finally, avoid repeating information that is readily available in your **resume**, **curriculum vitae**, or electronic **portfolio**.

> ### Key Point . . .
>
> Many individuals who started in hospitals and other health-system settings now work for pharmacy benefits managers, pharmaceutical companies, state and federal agencies, and more.
>
> #### . . . So what?
>
> The skills developed by hospital pharmacists can be transferred to a lot of other settings. New pharmacists who start work in health-system settings have many different alternative career paths open to them as experience is gained.

As you develop your personal career plan, seek the advice of others but take all recommendations with a grain of salt. Obtaining advice from experienced individuals can be invaluable, but listen to it with a critical ear because many well-meaning individuals give bad advice. And even when the advice is good, it may not be right for your circumstances. Only you can determine the right career path for you.

Students who express an interest in pursuing a health-system practice position upon graduation, are often told that they *must* complete a pharmacy residency to become a successful pharmacist. But such firm advice fails to recognize that there are many paths to success and many forms of success. Pharmacy graduates are prepared for entry level positions, and those positions in health-systems do not necessarily require advanced training. A residency experience may significantly enhance your knowledge and skills by providing opportunities to which a staff pharmacy may not be exposed. It also provides an accelerated path to skill development and training that would take many more years to achieve without a residency. On the other hand, an entry level non-residency position may allow you to build your career at your own pace instead of a residency's fast pace. Many institutions have career ladders that provide a series of skill development tasks and new responsibilities that groom and can be followed for pharmacists seeking promotion.

Obviously, the choice of whether to pursue a residency depends on the availability of residencies, the type of hospital and health-system practice setting where you want to work, and the opportunities available to you as a staff pharmacist. Upward promotion in some facilities may be hindered without a residency, especially if one is required or preferred for employment. However, personal commitment is needed for any residency or post-graduate training. Some students may find that they cannot dedicate themselves to an additional year or two of residency. Personal factors such as limitations in geographic location, debt burden, weak academic performance, and limited practice experience may also serve as deterrents.

Graduate Education

Graduate education is an alternative career option that does not receive as much attention as the residency path. A graduate degree provides unique training and development of skills not typically acquired in residencies. Indeed, some residencies are combined with Masters Degree programs to address some of the didactic deficiencies of residencies. Table 18-3 provides a comparison of the residency with common graduate degree options available to pharmacists.

Many pharmacists pursue graduate degrees on a part-time basis after graduating, often with financial assistance from their employer. Others pursue graduate certificates that provide additional expertise (e.g., board certification in pharmacotherapy, graduate certificate in gerontology).

Key Point . . .

Seek the advice of others but take all career recommendations from others with a grain of salt. Obtaining advice from experienced individuals can be invaluable, but listen to it with a critical ear because many well-meaning individuals give bad advice. And even when the advice is good, it may not be right for your circumstances.

. . . So what?

When talking to almost any successful pharmacist about how they chose their career path, the pharmacist will likely describe a conversation or series of conversations with an individual who gave some guidance. The successful pharmacist probably also received a lot of advice which was not heeded. Indeed, sometimes success is determined not only by the advice which is taken but also by the advice which is ignored.

Summary

The steps you took to become a successful student pharmacist will be similar to those needed to become a successful pharmacist. You should expect that your career goals will change throughout your career. Continue to document your professional activities and achievements by routinely updating your resume, curriculum vitae or electronic portfolio. Continue to reassess your career goals and determine if your current career path is allowing you to achieve what you want. Make a commitment to lifelong learning and seek to enhance your knowledge and skills as you progress throughout your career.

Table 18-3.
Advanced Training Opportunities for Pharmacists

	Description	Average Time to Complete	Career Opportunities
Pharm.D.	Professional degree that prepares individuals to obtain a pharmacy license to practice pharmacy.	2 to 4 years of pre-pharmacy; 4 years pharmacy	Staff pharmacist positions in hospital, community, long-term care, mail order, and managed care settings. People with Pharm.D. degrees can gain supervisor and pharmacy management positions with practice experience. This prepares students for 80% of current jobs available in pharmacy. Staff pharmacists may be excluded from many managerial, clinical, and academic opportunities without advanced training.
Residency	Practical training experience that permits resident to attain high levels of professional and clinical expertise.	1 to 2 years beyond Pharm.D.	Prepares pharmacists for advanced practice pharmacist positions in hospital, community, long-term care, mail order, and managed care settings. Often a requirement for managerial and clinical positions in health care systems and a prerequisite for most fellowships.
Fellowship	Research training experience that also provides advanced clinical and teaching experience. Typically specializes in a therapeutic area of focus.	2 years beyond residency	Prepare individuals to work in education (often in a tenure line position), industry (clinical liaison or researcher), or government (FDA). In comparison to the Pharm.D./M.S. program, the fellowship offers greater depth of research and training in a specialty area, but less course work, and no graduate degree.
Master of Science M.S.	Graduate degree program that trains students to attain advanced knowledge and research expertise.	2 years beyond Pharm.D.	This degree prepares students to conduct basic research (e.g., clinical trial, practice intervention, database study). The skills learned in attaining this degree prepares individuals for pharmaceutical industry, health system management, governmental positions (e.g., FDA), managed care, and some academic positions.

(continued)

Table 18-3. (continued)

Advanced Training Opportunities for Pharmacists

	Description	Average Time to Complete	Career Opportunities
Masters in Business Administration (M.B.A.)	Professional managerial degree that trains individuals in finance, accounting, marketing, management, and other fields of business.	2 years beyond Pharm.D.	Prepares individuals for managerial positions in any business including pharmacy and health care. Careers include director of pharmacy, health system management, corporate chain pharmacy management, entrepreneurial business opportunities, pharmaceutical industry management, and governmental positions.
Masters in Public Health (M.P.H.)	Graduate degree that trains individuals to develop, manage, and evaluate health programs for patient populations.	2 years beyond Pharm.D.	The MPH program provides students with the skills for employment in leadership roles in a broad range of local, state and national public health agencies as well as health systems and managed care.
Ph.D.	This is a research degree and is the highest educational degree possible. Graduates attain high levels of research and analysis capabilities.	4 years beyond Pharm.D.	Prepares individuals for any opportunity they wish to pursue. Many of the highest level officials in government, academia, consulting, and industry have Ph.D.s. The degree has significant prestige and the skills associated with it are highly sought out by employers. Career opportunities are global.
Certificates (e.g., gerontology)	A program of coursework for individuals with a Ph.D., Masters, or Bachelor's degree in a defined topic area.	varies	Provides individuals with additional training and credentials in a specific area of practice.

Suggested Reading

Andrusia D, Haskins R. *Brand Yourself: How to Create an Identity for a Brilliant Career.* New York: Ballantine Books; 2000.

American Society of Health-System Pharmacists. Survival strategies for your new career. Washington, DC: American Society of Health-System Pharmacists; 2007.

Bolles RN. *What Color is Your Parachute?* Berkeley, CA: Ten Speed Press; 2009.

Holdford DA. Managing yourself: an essential skill for managing others. *J Am Pharm Assoc.* 2009;49(3):436-445.

Reinders TP. *The Pharmacy Professionals Guide to Resumes, CVs, and Interviewing.* 2nd ed. Washington, DC: American Pharmacists Association; 2005.

Reference

1. APhA Career Pathway Evaluation Program for Pharmacy Professionals. Washington, DC: American Pharmacists Association; 2007.

Chapter Review Questions

1. **A pharmacy graduate needs a residency to become a health-system pharmacist.**
    a. True
    b. False

    Answer: b. False. A residency is not an absolute requirement to become a health-system pharmacist, but it provides an important advantage. All things equal, the candidate with a residency will be preferred over a candidate without residency experience. And the candidate with a residency may have better choice of positions. Nevertheless, many new graduates get jobs in health-systems without residency training. Many factors go into the hiring of pharmacists and residency training is just one.

2. **I am about to graduate from a Doctor of Pharmacy program. I really want to work as a hospital pharmacist, but I was thinking of working for a community pharmacy chain first until I pay off my student loans. Then I would look for a hospital job. Is this a good idea?**
    a. Yes
    b. No
    c. Maybe
    d. Probably not

    Answer: d. Probably not, for at least two good reasons. One is that postponing what you really want to do, for whatever reason, might lead you to put off your plans forever. If you want to be a hospital pharmacist, be a hospital pharmacist. Another reason to start your career as a hospital pharmacist is that the skills and training that prepare a person to succeed in chain pharmacy practice are different from the skills and training needed for hospital pharmacy. Therefore, it might be harder to switch to hospital pharmacy than you might think.

3. **I do not know what I want to do with my life. Should I get a Masters of Business Administration (MBA)?**
    a. Yes
    b. No
    c. Maybe
    d. Probably not

    Answer: c. Maybe. If you do not know what to do with your life, experimenting with different career options is a good idea. Formal management training is one option. However, MBA training may be more beneficial if one has an idea about how it might be used. Rather than spend money on further education, another option might be to learn as much possible in entry level training by volunteering for additional experiences and on-the-job education.

4. **Which is the better graduate degree?**
   a. MBA
   b. MPH
   c. MS degree

   Answer: a, b, or c. depending on what you want to do with that degree. An MBA is a general business degree that educates people to be a manager in a business. MBAs do not typically focus on health care problems or issues of health care. That can be advantageous if it helps health professionals to think outside the box and examine problems in new ways (e.g., using hotel management techniques to solve hospital service issues). But it can be a disadvantage by teaching topics that may not be particularly relevant to hospital and health-system practice and not educating about critical health care issues (e.g., formulary systems, pharmacoeconomics). A MPH is a good alternative to a MBA because it trains pharmacists in epidemiology and public health. Masters of Science degrees in pharmacy administration or pharmacotherapy are other good options because they can usually be tailored to the career interests of students. Discussion of MS, MBA, and MPH degree programs are beyond the scope of this chapter. Interested individuals can find information about different programs on the Internet or by talking with faculty members at your school.

5. **Which is the better choice regarding when to enter into a graduate program?**
   a. Go straight into a graduate program after pharmacy school
   b. Work for a while before applying to graduate school

   Answer: a or b. Once again, the answer depends on your situation. Many individuals, who wait to go back to graduate school, never do. Life's needs and desires or complacency may get in the way. Then again, working for a while after graduation can help pharmacists identify career opportunities and develop work experience that can be applied to what is learned in graduate school.

6. **Compensation packages in health-system practice are much less than community pharmacy.**
   a. True
   b. False

   Answer: a or b. The answer to this depends upon the geographic location and local job market. Some people automatically assume that chain pharmacies offer better compensation packages, a potentially false assumption. The only way to be sure is to compare them. And if the difference is large, it would be reasonable to ask why it takes so much more money to attract professionals to chain practice. It should be noted that compensation packages (i.e., salary and benefits) are just one consideration when choosing a pharmacy employer. Other important considerations are the potential for professional development and quality of work life.

7. **My parents want me to start working after graduation at a well known community pharmacy chain, but I am thinking about doing a residency. What should I do?**
   a. Listen to your parents—they know what is best for you
   b. Listen to your parents, but make your own decision
   c. Don't listen to your parents about issues related to your career path

Answer: b. Listen to your parents, but make your own decision. Your parents may love you and want the very best for you, but you need to make your own decisions. You are the best person to understand what you want and need in a career.

8. **What is the best way to get into hospital and health-system pharmacy practice?**
   a. Complete a residency
   b. Gain hospital and health-system pharmacy internship experience
   c. Get a MBA
   d. Network with hospital and health-system pharmacists
   e. None of the above

   Answer: e. None of the above. There is no "best" way. The paths to hospital and health-system practice are varied.

9. **I didn't like my initial health-system professional practice experience. Is this what health-system practice is like?**
   a. Yes
   b. No
   c. Maybe
   d. Probably not

   Answer: d. Probably not. Each health-system setting is different, so a bad experience at one setting may not be representative of all practice settings. Do not let a bad experience color your whole opinion of this kind of practice.

10. **Which degree is the highest educational degree possible?**
    e. MPH
    f. MS
    g. MBA
    h. Ph.D.

    Answer: d. The Ph.D. is a research degree that prepares graduates with the ability to conduct complex research and analysis.

Chapter Discussion Questions

1. Is clinical pharmacy the only career path with any future in institutional pharmacy practice?
2. What are the positives and minuses of specializing (e.g., oncology) versus choosing a less specialized area of practice (e.g., ambulatory care)?
3. Will all pharmacists need a residency in the future? Why or why not?
4. What advantages do advanced degrees like the MPH, MS, MBA, and Ph.D. have for one's career?
5. Which is easier, going from community practice to hospital pharmacy or vice versa?

CHAPTER 19

Residency Training

Jill S. Burkiewicz and Carrie A. Sincak

■ ■ ■

Learning Objectives

After completing this chapter, readers should be able to:

1. Summarize the definition and purpose of residency training.
2. Explain the major components of residency training.
3. Identify the benefits of and barriers to pursuing residency training.
4. Identify resources available to research residency training programs.
5. Discuss the process of applying for and securing a residency position.

Key Terms and Definitions

■ **Accreditation:** Recognition and approval granted by ASHP verifying a residency program has maintained and complied with expected standards.
■ **Curriculum vitae (CV):** A detailed account of one's professional experiences commonly used when applying for an academic or professional career.
■ **Postgraduate year one (PGY1) pharmacy residency:** First-year residency program designed to enhance general competencies in medication therapy outcomes for patients within a wide range of therapeutic areas and in managing medication-use systems.
■ **Postgraduate year two (PGY2) pharmacy residency:** Second-year residency program focused in a specific area of practice to be completed after a PGY1 residency. Often called a specialty residency, the program is designed to increase expertise in medication use outcomes for patients in a focused area of practice and promote clinical leadership.
■ **Residency program director (RPD):** Preceptor who oversees the direction and operation of the residency program. The RPD often serves as the resident's primary mentor, or assigns a specific mentor.
■ **Residency:** A focused, organized training program that is systematically designed to build upon the knowledge, skills, attitudes and abilities gained in the doctor of pharmacy degree program.

■ **Resident Matching Program:** Commonly referred to as "The Match." Program aligns residency candidates and programs based on preferences with priority given to the applicant.

■ ■ ■

Introduction

Medication therapy continues to increase in complexity, and pharmacists are continuing to take on larger roles in the management of drug therapy beyond the drug delivery process. Coupled together, these two statements represent why many pharmacists are choosing to pursue additional training after graduating with a doctor of pharmacy degree. Over the last 10 years, the number of residency programs and positions has approximately doubled.[1] Further, the number of pharmacy graduates pursuing residency programs has grown with over 2500 participating in the residency match for first-year positions in 2009.[2]

The profession has envisioned that by 2020, residency training will be a prerequisite to entering into direct patient care practice.[3,4] Pharmacy organizations, including the American College of Clinical Pharmacy[3] and the American Society of Health-System Pharmacists,[4] have concluded that further training beyond a professional degree will be needed for pharmacy graduates to enter clinical practice roles. Leaders in residency training argue that to take responsibility for providing direct patient care to an aging patient population with more chronic diseases, the profession will need more residency trained pharmacists.[5]

This chapter provides an overview of the definition and purpose of residency training and items to ponder when considering further training. For those who have made the decision to pursue a residency, recommendations are provided on how to gather information about residencies and how to apply. It is imperative that each potential applicant spend considerable time and effort reviewing the material relating to residency programs which can be found at ashp.org.

■ ■ ■

Key Point . . .

The profession has envisioned that by 2020, residency training will be a prerequisite to entering direct patient care practice.

. . . So what?

If residency training does become a prerequisite within the next decade, a pharmacy student graduating in the next few years may want to consider this possibility in their career planning.

Postgraduate Year One (PGY1) Residency Programs: Wide Variety

A **residency** is a focused training program that is systematically designed to build upon the knowledge, skills, attitudes and abilities gained in the doctor of pharmacy degree program.[6] A **postgraduate year one (PGY1) pharmacy residency** program is designed to create a 'generalist' with enhanced skills in managing patient medication therapy outcomes within a wide range of therapeutic areas.[6] PGY1 residents learn how to enhance their patient care skills and develop experience in the management of the medication-use system. PGY1 residencies can accomplish these outcomes in a variety of settings including health-systems, community pharmacy or managed care. Even within health-system settings, the broad PGY1 Pharmacy Residency Educational Outcomes[7] (Table 19-1) can be met in a variety of settings that may align more specifically with a student's interest area, such as ambulatory care, home care, community hospitals or large academic medical centers.

Residencies are typically one-year experiences, beginning on July 1st, providing a wide variety of clinical rotations and other learning activities. As part of interprofessional teams, residents learn to work with others in providing direct patient care. Like students, residents complete rotations. However, unlike students, residents are given more direct responsibility for patient care and create a self-development plan under the guidance of a year-long mentor, most commonly the **residency program director**. Individual programs can tailor the residency to the preferences of residents because most residencies have both required and elective rotations. Residencies use a variety of different struc-

> ■ ■ ■
>
> **Key Point . . .**
>
> A PGY1 pharmacy residency program is designed to create a "generalist" with enhanced skills in managing patient medication therapy outcomes within a wide range of therapeutic areas.
>
> **. . . So what?**
>
> A PGY1 residency provides basic training that is broad but not as focused as PGY2 training. A PGY1 residency is good introductory training for institutional practice.

Table 19-1.

Outcomes from Postgraduate Year One (PGY1) Pharmacy Residencies[7]

Required Outcomes

■ Manage and improve the medication-use process.

■ Provide evidence-based, patient-centered medication therapy management with interdisciplinary teams.

■ Exercise leadership and practice management skills.

■ Demonstrate project management skills.

■ Provide medication and practice-related education/training.

■ Utilize medical informatics.

Elective Outcomes

■ Conduct pharmacy practice research.

■ Exercise added leadership and practice management skills.

■ Demonstrate knowledge and skills particular to generalist practice in the home care practice environment.

■ Demonstrate knowledge and skills particular to generalist practice in the managed care practice environment.

■ Participate in the management of medical emergencies.

■ Provide drug information to health care professionals and/or the public.

■ Demonstrate additional competencies that contribute to working successfully in the health care environment.

tures to meet the core outcomes (Table 19-1). While most rotations are concentrated in specific practice settings for a limited time period, such as spending one month with the internal medicine team, some rotation experiences can be longitudinal, such as working with the medication safety committee and related projects throughout the year.

Staffing experiences in the drug-distribution process at the institution are a required element of most residencies. The experience gained as a front-line pharmacist helps the resident to acquire critical knowledge of pharmacy department processes which can help in performing clinical duties.

Teaching is also an important element of many residencies. Most residents help pre-cept pharmacy students, and some residents receive more extensive training in teaching, particularly when enrolled in programs associated with colleges of pharmacy. In addi-tion, some residency programs offer teaching certificate programs and allow residents to participate in classroom-based teaching and assess student learning.[8-10]

All residents also complete a residency project: a focused project identified by the resident and his/her mentor.[7] Typically, the resident formulates the project design, secures any institutional review board (IRB) approvals and implements the project. Like many elements in the residency program, the specifics of the project are sufficiently flexible to meet the interests of the resident. For instance, some projects may emphasize research such as retrospective clinical studies or outcomes studies. Other projects may evaluate aspects of clinical pharmacy practice, such as implementation and evaluation of a new diabetes service. Regardless, all residents share results of the project at regional residency conferences and write a manuscript before completing the residency. Although challeng-ing, completing a multi-month residency project while juggling clinical rotation activities demonstrates to future employers a resident's time management skills, ability to manage a complex research project, and the ability to think and present innovative research.

Postgraduate Year Two (PGY2) Residency Programs: Becoming a Specialist

In contrast to a PGY1 experience, a **post-graduate year two (PGY2) pharmacy residency** program is often called a "spe-cialized" residency.[11] In a PGY2 residency, residents build upon their broad PGY1 training, by focusing on a specific area of practice. Most commonly, specialization occurs in therapeutic areas such as ambula-tory care, critical care, infectious diseases or oncology. However, PGY2 residencies are also available in managed care phar-macy systems, informatics and practice management or health administration (Table 19-2).[12] To meet the needs of con-temporary practice, the types of specialties are continually expanding and undergo-ing revision to remain current. Regardless of whether a pharmacy student knows

■ ■ ■

Key Point . . .

In a PGY2 residency, residents build upon their PGY1 training, but focus on a specific area of practice, such as ambulatory care, critical care, infectious diseases or oncol-ogy.

. . . So what?

Anyone entering a PGY2 residency should have a clear idea of what they want to do with their career and life. Specialization requires individuals to make hard choices about their careers. For instance choos-ing to specialize in ambulatory care may make it harder to change to other practice settings.

Table 19-2.
Types of Postgraduate Year Two (PGY2) Pharmacy Residencies Available[12,a]

- Ambulatory Care
- Cardiology
- Critical Care
- Drug Information
- Geriatrics
- Health-System Pharmacy Administration
- Infectious Diseases
- Informatics
- Internal Medicine

- Medication Use Safety
- Nutrition Support
- Oncology
- Pain Management and Palliative Care
- Pediatrics
- Pharmacotherapy
- Psychiatry
- Solid-Organ Transplant

[a]Types of residencies are expanding; check http://www.ashp.org/Import/ACCREDITATION/ResidencyAccreditation/RegulationsStandards.aspx for the most current list.

where he or she wishes to practice, all PGY2 residencies require completion of a PGY1 pharmacy residency. Select PGY2 programs may also be combined with other programs, such as a fellowship to further research training or a master's degree in administration. In these cases, the program may require additional time to complete these added requirements. Like PGY1 programs, PGY2 programs provide variety in experiences; even within a specialty the resident may rotate to different subspecialty areas. For example, a cardiology resident may have experiences with a cardiovascular surgery team, heart failure team, cardiology intensive care unit and outpatient cardiology clinic. Also similar to PGY1 programs, PGY2 programs require a project and commonly include a staffing component, though these are typically accomplished within the area of specialization.

Benefits and Barriers: Value and Investment in Residency Training

A residency is more than just another year of rotations; it is an intensive, life-changing event that can form the foundation of one's future career path and professional growth. However, the value of the residency is directly proportional to the effort the resident puts into the program. Therefore, potential candidates should assess their readiness to commit to a residency by carefully weighing the benefits of the extra training with any personal sacrifices.

The most obvious sacrifice associated with completing a residency is the lower salary received by a resident in comparison with a practicing pharmacist. The typical salary earned by residents is approximately $35,000 to $45,000, although the exact amount varies based on type of program, type of institution, and geographic salary variations.[13] This means that residents earn $50,000 to $70,000 less (before taxes) during the year of the residency.

Residents also forego some job benefits received by practicing pharmacists, including retirement plans, some insurance coverage, and profit-sharing. On the other hand, most residencies provide health care and other benefits, including travel to professional conferences such as the American Society of Health-System Pharmacists Midyear Clinical Meeting or regional residency conferences.[14] Fortunately, some student loans may be deferred for residents, so individuals should check with their lenders.

Most residents perceive the additional financial sacrifice of residency training as an investment in their future; sound financial management is an essential element in completing a residency without undue stress. Many pharmacists pursue residencies immediately after graduation, hence the salary earned during the residency is typically greater than the salary earned as a pharmacy student. As long as the resident avoids major lifestyle enhancements, the salary and benefits earned during a residency are more than adequate to cover immediate financial needs.

In addition to monetary costs, completing a residency requires a significant commitment of time. While effective time management allows for work-life balance to meet personal and family obligations, students considering a residency are encouraged to discuss this commitment with family and significant others. Another noted psychological barrier to residency training is the trade-off of taking a known job now for an unknown job after graduation.[15] Some pharmacy graduates find it difficult to decline an immediately available, high-paying job to pursue further training. Doing so requires an acceptance that the long-term benefits of residency training will exceed the immediate gains of a high-paying job.

Nevertheless, there are numerous benefits of residency training that continue to attract pharmacy graduates. Some individuals find that residencies provide time to develop clinical maturity.[16,17] Clinical maturity, as defined by Ray, encompasses the development of clinical and professional competence, personally assuming responsibility and accountability, effective problem-solving and communication, and self-confidence without ego.[5,17] It is difficult to develop as a student because although students have some responsibility for patient care, their preceptor ultimately assumes legal and professional accountability for the patient.

> **Key Point . . .**
>
> A residency is not just another year of rotations; it is an intensive, life-changing event that can form the foundation of one's future career path.
>
> **. . . So what?**
>
> Anyone expecting a residency to be like their final year of pharmacy school rotations are likely to be surprised. The intensity of residency rotations are much more and performance expectations much higher. Anyone applying for a residency should be fully committed to getting everything possible from it.

In contrast, a residency provides a bridge between practicing under continued supervision of another pharmacist to the resident's eventual responsibility and autonomy as a manager of drug therapy. This fact is not lost on individuals enrolled in residencies. Residents themselves cite the ability to gain additional experience to develop clinical maturity as a critical factor in their decision to pursue residency training.[15,18]

A case can also be made that the long-term financial and professional benefits of residencies can outweigh the short term costs. Completion of a residency often opens doors both early and late in one's career path. In the short term, many of the best entry level career opportunities in pharmacy require, or at least prefer individuals who have received residency training. In the long run, residency training may be necessary in the future as a requirement to provide direct patient care[3,4] or be a faculty member at a school of pharmacy.[3]

Figure 19-1. Benefits and barriers to residency training.

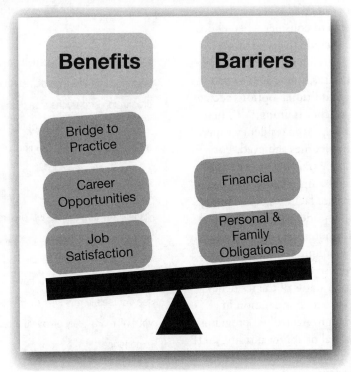

That might explain why residency training has been associated with increased job satisfaction.[19] In a recent survey, pharmacists with post-graduate training reported that their greatest satisfaction came from the opportunity to work with an interdisciplinary team and the ability to perform clinical duties independently. Overwhelmingly, respondents recommended residency training to current students and if faced with a similar opportunity, they would repeat their experience.[20]

For students who are unsure of a particular career path, the PGY1 residency year provides a wide variety of experiences to try in the course of career planning. Regardless of the individual's vision of his/her future, a residency position creates job opportunities, relationships with mentors, networks of colleagues and development of leadership skills.

Residency training may not be right for everyone. Pharmacists wishing to pursue a career in research may be better served with a fellowship, masters degree, or Ph.D. degree with specific training in clinical and translational sciences.[17,21,22] Pharmacists seeking a career involved in the drug distribution systems may find an MBA or additional training in information systems or robotics to be beneficial.[17] However, for students looking to provide direct patient care, residency training is increasingly viewed as a requirement for the future.[3,4] New technology, the increasing complexity of drugs and the aging population mean that the need for specialized clinicians will grow.

Researching Residency Programs

Once the decision to pursue a residency has been made, the next step is to find the specific residency program that is right for the individual student. With approximately 1000 PGY1 and PGY2 residency programs currently available,[1] creating a list of personal needs and desired characteristics of an ideal residency program is a good place to start.

Some factors to consider when choosing a program include the type of institution housing the residency, the program's **accreditation** status, the residency program's size, and additional options such as availability of teacher training.[13,23] These factors can influence the residency experience and final outcomes achieved. For instance, residency training may be completed at hospitals, ambulatory care centers, long term care facilities, community pharmacies, and academic institutions. It is important for potential applicants to understand the unique training experience that each provides.

Accreditation status of the residency is another important consideration in choosing a program. Accredited programs have received a seal of approval from ASHP certifying that they have met core requirements for accreditation.[6,24] Accreditation indicates that the program has achieved thorough training standards and competencies and passed periodic reviews by expert accreditation survey teams. Although accredited residency programs are not necessarily better than many non-accredited programs, accreditation provides an endorsement from ASHP about a program's commitment to excellence in precepting, training, and services.

The size of the program may also be important to the potential applicant. A smaller program might be able to offer more individualized attention, while a larger program might have more resources and better opportunities to network with and learn from other residents.

If teaching or a future career in academia is of interest, one might seek programs that have an affiliation with a college of pharmacy, participate in teaching certificate programs, or provide opportunities to lecture and precept pharmacy students.

Researching the various programs can be overwhelming but ASHP offers a directory of potential PGY1 and PGY2 programs. Each listing provides information including the type of residency offered, accreditation status, contact information of the residency program director, number of positions available, stipend offered, special features of the residency program, institution specific information, and application requirements. Some individual residency programs also maintain an institution-specific residency website with more detailed information about their programs.[13]

Information about residencies can be acquired from other sources too. One valuable resource on residency training is a student's college of pharmacy. Many faculty members have completed residencies and help mentor students (formally or informally) interested in pursuing residency training. State and regional meetings, such as those held by state chapters of ASHP, may also have residency showcases for local programs. These meetings

> ■ ■ ■
>
> **Key Point . . .**
>
> Factors to consider when choosing a program include the type of institution, its accreditation status, the size of the residency program, and additional options such as availability of teacher training.
>
> **. . . So what?**
>
> Before choosing any residency, try to visualize what your life will be like. Think about how each day will unfold, the people with whom you will interact, and what kind of social life you will have. If you can see yourself in this type of environment, you will more likely enjoy your residency experience.

provide students with opportunities to network informally with current and past residents of programs and to meet individuals involved in managing residency programs.

The ASHP Midyear Clinical Meeting in December is the most important networking opportunity for anyone interested in residencies. At this meeting, the Residency Showcase offers applicants an informal opportunity to meet prospective programs throughout the United States and gather more information about programs of interest.

During the Midyear Clinical Meeting, ASHP offers the Personnel Placement Service (PPS) and an online career resource center, CareerPharm™, for pharmacy positions. PPS, the face-to-face component of CareerPharm™, allows potential applicants to interview with various residency programs and potential pharmacy employers at one site, avoiding unnecessary travel.[25] Preliminary interviews at Midyear conducted during PPS are typically followed up with a second on-site interview at the institution for promising candidates. Of note, not all residency programs enroll in PPS, but a majority participate in the Residency Showcase.

> **Key Point . . .**
>
> The ASHP Midyear Clinical Meeting in December is the most important networking opportunity for anyone interested in residencies.
>
> **. . . So what?**
>
> Even if you are unsure if you will be completing a residency, the Midyear Meeting is a good place to see who you will compete with for future pharmacy positions. You will see thousands of young, professionally dressed, and highly motivated individuals who are taking the steps needed to succeed within the profession. After attending the meeting, many pharmacy students step up their career planning efforts.

The Application Process

Table 19-3 illustrates the steps involved and a general timeline for individuals who decide to pursue a residency.[26] The process and timeline delineated in the Table provide some guidance about what is expected in the application process. Although the requirements for an application packet may vary by institution, most programs will request at minimum: a completed application, curriculum vitae, cover letter or letter of intent, official pharmacy school transcripts, and three letters of recommendation.

The term **curriculum vitae (CV)** means the "course of life" in Latin. It is a longer, more detailed record of one's professional activities than a professional resume. A CV is often used when applying for residencies, academic positions, and many other professional opportunities. The CV provides the residency program a thorough overview of an applicant's qualifications and achievements. Items that should be included in a CV are current contact information, educational background, work and rotation experiences, professional and extracurricular activities, honors and awards, presentations given, authored publications, research experiences, volunteer activities, and licenses and certifications. A CV should be well organized, free of errors, actively written, informative, and readable. There are many resources available for CV writing.[27-30]

A letter of intent or cover letter typically accompanies a CV. The letter expresses the applicant's interest in the program and highlights key aspects of the applicant's qualifications for the residency. The letter might mention experiences and skills obtained during phar-

Table 19-3.

Timeline for the Residency Application Process[26]

September	Draft CV and cover letter
October	1. Sign up for ASHP Midyear Clinical Meeting (MCM) (www.ashp.org)
	2. Register for ASHP's Personnel Placement Services (PPS) (www.pps.ashp.org)
November	1. Research programs; see ASHP online residency directory (www.ashp.org)
	2. Develop questions for MCM
	3. Ask references to write letters of recommendation for applications
	4. Sign up with National Matching Services (www.natmatch.com/ashprmp)
December	1. Attend MCM and participate in the Residency Showcase
	2. Fill out applications
January	1. Applications due
	2. Must return agreement to National Matching Services Inc. to register for the Match
February	1. Interview with sites that have extended an invitation
	2. Review instructions for submitting Rank Order Lists and obtaining Match results
March	1. Rank list due to the National Matching Service
	2. Results of the Match are released to applicants and program directors
July	Residency begins

macy school and how the specific program would aid in achieving one's personal goals and objectives. The conclusion of the letter should reiterate interest in the program, inform the reader that the CV is attached, and provide contact information if granted an interview.[27-30]

Letters of recommendation are a critical part of the application process. Three letters are typically requested to be sent to the residency director either directly from the person providing the recommendation or included in the residency application packet provided by the applicant. Recommendation letters supplement the applicant's CV and letter of intent by providing insight from an individual who knows and has worked with the applicant. Applicants should customize the choice of references to fit the position being sought. References can come from pharmacy supervisors, faculty members from schools of pharmacy, and clerkship or rotation preceptors. The best references can accurately attest to the applicant's work ethic, time management skills, people and technical skills, didactic and clinical abilities, as well as any experiences in research or professional activities.

Interviews begin once the application packet is submitted. The interview gives applicants a chance to sell themselves to programs, and it allows the program to learn more about the applicant's goals, reasons for wanting to pursue a residency, interpersonal communication skills, behavioral patterns, and overall fit for their program. The interview also gives the applicant a chance to learn more about the program, potential preceptors, the residency site, and program fit. As with any interview, preparation is important, with preparation resulting in an individualized interview strategy for each unique program. Resources are available to help with interview techniques, questions to ask and to avoid, as well as appropriate attire for the day.[30]

Some residency programs may ask applicants to prepare and give a presentation as part of the interview process. This allows them to evaluate communication and presentation skills of applicants. If asked to present, the applicant should clarify any expectations about the presentation. For example, does the program recommend a topic for presentation or is the choice up to the applicant? No matter what the topic, the applicant should seek help from someone in the program about defined goals and recommendations for the presentation. Often applicants develop, expand, or formalize a lecture, journal club, or case-based presentation previously completed during a rotation experience rather than create an entirely new presentation. Rehearsal of the presentation to a peer or a faculty member is recommended before formal presentation. As with any formal presentation, the applicant should use good presentation procedures including ensuring that everyone in the audience can hear, standing in a way that does not block or face the visuals, and not hiding behind a podium.

Once the interview is complete, it is appropriate to write thank you notes after meeting with residency directors, preceptors, or anyone else interviewed that day. There is some controversy over whether e-mail is acceptable for this type of communication. If time is of the essence, e-mail is acceptable but a hand written thank you note offers a personal touch. Letters or note cards should be sent out quickly after the interview to make a positive impression.

Residency Matching Program

To apply for a PGY1 residency, a candidate must sign up for the **Residency Matching Program**.[31,32] After interviews are complete, the student ranks programs by preference. Both the prospective residents and the residency programs enroll in the National Matching Services Inc. (NMS) which is in charge of operating the matching program. The program helps match residency programs with individuals according to how each ranks the other. NMS attempts to match the candidate to their top ranked choice program, moving down the ranked list until a tentative match is made or all attempts have been exhausted. Details on the match process and examples of the ranking process may be found on the NMS website.

> **Key Point . . .**
>
> To apply for a PGY1 residency, a candidate must sign up for the Residency Matching Program.
>
> **. . . So what?**
>
> Without entering the match, you will not be eligible to apply for the vast majority of residencies available in the U.S.

The residency matching program also provides a matching option for applicant pairs (e.g., spouses) who wish to coordinate their residency program location. Applicant pairs enter the match as a "couple," with greater emphasis for matching being based on a preferred location.

Post-Match

Not all applicants match with their preferred programs during the matching process. Applicants who remain unmatched after the process still can obtain a residency, because a post matching procedure puts unmatched applicants in touch with unmatched programs. Lists of unmatched programs and individuals are distributed and interested individuals and programs directly contact one another during a post-match scramble. Applicants who do not match with their preferred programs in the initial process should not feel discouraged when going through the post-match scramble since residency openings from reputable programs are available due to chance.[31,32]

Summary

Postgraduate residency training programs offer a well-structured, directed, and organized opportunity to strengthen critical thinking and direct patient care skills while gaining invaluable leadership and time management skills. Various options are available for PGY1 training with a specific concentration during PGY2 residency training. Each program is unique in its opportunities and offerings. Various resources are available to assist potential applicants throughout the entire residency process from gathering relevant information to interviewing to sorting preferences for the resident matching program. Residency training offers the possibility to expand one's knowledge, experiences, and skills needed to meet the demands of an ever changing pharmacy career.

Suggested Reading

Fotis MA. Advice for residency candidates going to the midyear clinical meeting. *Am J Health-Syst Pharm.* 2006;63:1787,1791.

Lifshin LS, Teeters JL, Bush CG. ASHP resident matching program: how does it work? *Am J Health-Syst Pharm.* 2004;61:446.

Murphy JE, Nappi JM, Bosso JA, et al. ACCP Position Statement. American College of Clinical Pharmacy's vision of the future: Postgraduate pharmacy residency training as a prerequisite for direct patient care. *Pharmacotherapy.* 2006;26:722-733.

Pierpaoli PG. Residency training: the path to professional and personal dignity [commentary]. *Am J Hosp Pharm.* 1984;41:1849-1851.

Ray MD. Clinical maturity in pharmacy. *Pharmacotherapy.* 2006;26:594-596.

Reinders TP. *The Pharmacy Professional's Guide to Resumes, CVs, and Interviewing.* 2nd ed. Washington, DC: American Pharmacists Association; 2005.

Song A. SOAP note: Why I want to complete a pharmacy practice residency. *Am J Health-Syst Pharm.* 2005;62:2041-2042.

Teeters JL. Pharmacy residency programs: How to find the one for you. *Am J Health-Syst Pharm.* 2004;61:2254-2259.

Tysinger JW. *Resumes and Personal Statements for Health Professionals.* Tucson, AZ: Galen Press, Ltd.; 2007.

References

1. Warner DJ. Future Planning: Is a residency right for you? Available at: http://www.ashp.org/DocLibrary/Midyear08/FuturePlanning.aspx. Accessed June 8, 2009.

2. American Society of Health-System Pharmacists. The Communiqué. Spring 2009, Volume 12, Issue 2. Available at: http://www.ashp.org/DocLibrary/Accreditation/RTP_CommuniqueSpringMay2009.pdf. Accessed June 8, 2009.

3. Murphy JE, Nappi JM, Bosso JA, et al. ACCP Position Statement. American College of Clinical Pharmacy's vision of the future: Postgraduate pharmacy residency training as a prerequisite for direct patient care. *Pharmacotherapy.* 2006;26:722-733.

4. American Society of Health-System Pharmacists. ASHP Policy Positions 1982-2007. Requirement for residency. Policy position 0701. Available at: http://www.ashp.org/DocLibrary/BestPractices/BP_PolPos08.aspx. Accessed June 7, 2009.

5. ASHP REPORTS: Pharmacy residency training in the future: a stakeholders' roundtable discussion. *Am Health-Syst Pharm.* 2005;62:1817-1820.

6. American Society of Health-System Pharmacists. ASHP Accreditation Standard for Postgraduate Year One (PGY1) Pharmacy Residency Programs. Available at: http://www.ashp.org/s_ashp/docs/files/RTP_PGY1AccredStandard.pdf. Accessed June 7, 2009.

7. American Society of Health-System Pharmacists. Required and Elective Educational Outcomes, Goals, Objectives, and Instructional Objectives for Postgraduate Year One (PGY1) Pharmacy Residency Programs. 2nd ed. Effective July 2008. http://www.ashp.org/s_ashp/docs/files/RTP_PGY1GoalsObjectives.doc. Accessed June 7, 2009.

8. Castellani V, Haber SL, Ellis SC. Evaluation of a teaching certificate program for pharmacy residents. *Am J Health-Syst Pharm.* 2003;60:1037-1041.

9. Romanelli F, Smith KM, Brandt BF. Certificate program in teaching for pharmacy residents. *Am J Health-Syst Pharm.* 2001;58:896-868.

10. Carr LS. Teaching as a new practitioner. *Am J Health-Syst Pharm.* 2006;63:1400,1404.

11. American Society of Health-System Pharmacists. ASHP Accreditation Standard for Postgraduate Year Two (PGY2) Pharmacy Residency Programs. Available at: http://www.ashp.org/s_ashp/docs/files/RTP_PGY2AccredStandard.pdf. Accessed June 7, 2009.

12. American Society of Health-System Pharmacists. Residency Accreditation Regulations and Standards. Available at: http://www.ashp.org/Import/ACCREDITATION/ResidencyAccreditation/Regulations-Standards.aspx. Accessed June 7, 2009.

13. American Society of Health-System Pharmacists. Online residency directory. Available at: http://accred.ashp.org/aps/pages/directory/residencyProgramSearch.aspx. Accessed June 12, 2009.

14. Jennings HR, Empey PE, Smith KM. Survey of ASHP-accredited pharmacy residency programs. *Am J Health-Syst Pharm.* 2000;57:2080-2086.

15. Bucci KK, Knapp KK, Ohri LK, et al. Factors motivating pharmacy students to pursue residency and fellowship training. *Am J Health-Syst Pharm.* 1995;52:2696-2701.

16. Ray MD. Clinical maturity in pharmacy. *Pharmacotherapy.* 2006;26:594-596.

17. Haines ST. Making residency training an expectation for pharmacists in direct patient care roles. *Am J Pharm Educ.* 2007;71 (4) Article 71.

18. Fit KE, Padiyara RS, Rabi SM, et al. Factors influencing pursuit of residency training. *Am J Health-Syst Pharm.* 2005;62:2226,2235.

19. Fit KE, Padiyara RS. Impact of post-graduate training on job and career satisfaction of American Society of Health-System Pharmacists members. Paper presented at: Midyear Clinical Meeting of the American Society of Health-System Pharmacists; December 4, 2007; Las Vegas, NV.

20. Komperda KE. Personal communication. Downers Grove: Midwestern University Chicago College of Pharmacy; June 12, 2009.

21. Bauman JL, Evans WE. Pharm.D.-only investigators are critical to the profession: Let's preserve the fellowship as an equally important way to prepare future clinical pharmaceutical scientists [editorial]. *Pharmacotherapy.* 2009;29:129-133.

22. Dowling TC, Murphy JE, Kalus JS, et al. ACCP commentary. Recommended education for pharmacists as competitive clinical scientists. *Pharmacotherapy.* 2009;29:236-244.

23. Nelson T. Selecting the right residency program. *Am J Health-Syst Pharm.* 2005;62:1138-1140.

24. Teeters JL. Pharmacy residency programs: How to find the one for you. *Am J Health-Syst Pharm.* 2004;61:2254-2259.

25. American Society of Health-System Pharmacists. CareerPharm. Available at: http://www.careerpharm.com/. Accessed June 16, 2009.

26. American Society of Health-System Pharmacists. Residency checklist. Available at: http://www.ashp.org/Import/ACCREDITATION/ResidentInfo/ResidencyChecklist.aspx. Accessed June 17, 2009.

27. American College of Clinical Pharmacy. CV preparation tips. Available at: http://www.accp.com/stunet/cv.aspx. Accessed June 10, 2009.

28. American Society of Health-System Pharmacists. Preparing a curriculum vitae. Available at: http://www.ashp.org/Import/ACCREDITATION/ResidentInfo/CurriculumVitae.aspx. Accessed June 10, 2009.

29. Tysinger JW. *Resumes and Personal Statements for Health Professionals.* Tucson, AZ: Galen Press, Ltd.; 2007.

30. Reinders TP. *The Pharmacy Professional's Guide to Resumes, CVs, and Interviewing.* 2nd ed. Washington, DC: American Pharmacists Association; 2005.

31. National Matching Services Inc. Available at: http://www.natmatch.com/ashprmp/. Accessed June 10, 2009.

32. American Society of Health-System Pharmacists. Residency matching program. Available at: http://www.ashp.org/Import/ACCREDITATION/ResidentInfo/FAQs.aspx. Accessed June 10, 2009.

Chapter Review Questions

1. **Stacy is a 4th professional year pharmacy student who has always been interested in critical care. Since she is certain of her area of specialty interest, Stacy can apply for a PGY2 residency program in critical care.**
    a. True
    b. False

    Answer: b. False. Regardless of whether a student is certain of interest in specialty training, all PGY2 residencies require PGY1 residencies to provide a foundation of clinical and practice management skills.

2. **All of the following are REQUIRED components of a PGY1 residency program EXCEPT:**
    a. Staffing experiences in the pharmacy
    b. Completion of a residency project
    c. Core cardiology rotation
    d. Interprofessional interactions
    e. Provision of direct patient care

    Answer: c. Core cardiology rotation. While this is a common rotation for many PGY1 residencies, the exact clinical experiences within a PGY1 residency vary broadly. A PGY1 residency provides experiences in patient care in a broad range of therapeutic areas and each specific residency customizes a plan for each resident based on what the institution can offer and desires of the resident.

3. **A community pharmacy residency is a:**
    a. PGY1 residency
    b. PGY2 residency

    Answer: a. PGY1 residency. While a community residency has its own accreditation standard, it is a type of PGY1 residency designed to be completed after the candidate has completed a professional degree program.

4. **Pharmacy organizations and leaders have proposed that residency training:**
    a. Should be required for all pharmacists by 2015.
    b. Should be required for pharmacists in direct patient care by 2020.
    c. Should be required for pharmacists involved in research by 2020.
    d. Should be required for pharmacists involved in dispensing by 2015.

    Answer: b. Should be required for pharmacists in direct patient care by 2020. Pharmacy organizations including the American College of Clinical Pharmacy and the American Society of Health-System Pharmacists support the requirement for residency training by 2020 for roles where pharmacists are engaged in direct patient care, including where pharmacists have the responsibility for managing drug therapy.

5. **Which of the following is a REQUIRED outcome from a postgraduate year one (PGY1) residency program and therefore a component of all PGY1 programs?**
   a. Conduct pharmacy practice research
   b. Exercise added leadership and practice management skills
   c. Participate in the management of medical emergencies
   d. Provide drug information to health care professionals and/or the public
   e. Provide medication and practice-related education/training

   Answer: e. Provide medication and practice-related education/training. This outcome includes the goal of providing effective medication and practice-related education, training, or counseling to patients, caregivers, health care professionals, and the public. Objectives that support this goal include designing assessment strategies which align with instructional objectives, using preceptor roles, using case-based teaching and using audio-visual and handouts to deliver an effective educational presentation. The other outcomes (a–d) are elective outcomes within PGY1 residency programs.

6. **ASHP accreditation is REQUIRED for all residency programs.**
   a. True
   b. False

   Answer: b. False. Accredited residency programs meet rigorous standards and achieve core outcomes outlined by ASHP. Although it is highly encouraged for all residency programs to apply for and achieve accreditation status, the process is not required. However, it is strongly encouraged and required for all residency programs participating in the match.

7. **Brad is a 4th year pharmacy student in Minnesota who is interested in a PGY1 residency. He was told in order to obtain a residency he had to attend the ASHP Midyear Clinical Meeting (MCM) Residency Showcase. What is the most appropriate answer for Brad?**
   a. Attendance at the MCM Residency Showcase is mandatory to obtain a PGY1 residency.
   b. Attendance at the MCM Residency Showcase is not mandatory but Brad is required to attend a regional residency showcase in Minnesota.
   c. Attendance at the MCM Residency Showcase is not mandatory but the ASHP Personnel Placement Service (PPS) is required.
   d. Attendance at the MCM Residency Showcase is not mandatory but enrollment in the ASHP Resident Matching Program is required.

   Answer: d. The MCM Residency Showcase is not mandatory for students seeking a PGY1 or PGY2 residency. The showcase provides potential applicants the opportunity to learn information and meet current residents and preceptors of various residency programs at one location. The ASHP PPS is also not mandatory for those seeking a residency position. PPS is often utilized for those seeking actual pharmacist positions.

8. **The following components should be considered when choosing a residency program:**
   a. Program setting (institution, community, industry, etc.)
   b. Accreditation status
   c. Size of residency program
   d. Options such as teaching opportunities
   e. All of the above

   Answer: e. All of the above components should be considered when determining the most appropriate residency program that suits the needs and desires of the potential applicant. Other options to consider may be the type of patients, specialty areas available for training, flexibility in scheduling of core requirements and electives, and personal preferences such as location and benefits.

9. **All of the following are REQUIRED during the application process EXCEPT:**
   a. Curriculum vitae (CV)
   b. Letter of intent or cover letter
   c. Presentation during interview
   d. Letters of recommendation
   e. Copy of official transcripts

   Answer: c. During the application process, the majority of residency programs will require a completed application form, CV, cover letter, transcripts, and letters of recommendation. Presentations may be requested by some programs but not all.

10. **Molly has just received notification that she did not match with her preferred list of residency programs. Molly will have to wait to reapply for residency training next year.**
    a. True
    b. False

    Answer: b. False. Participants who did not match within the Matching Program still have an opportunity to secure a residency position during the Post Match period. Applicants who have not matched may contact residency programs who have un-filled positions and vice versa.

Chapter Discussion Questions

1. Compare the benefits of and barriers to pursuing postgraduate residency training.
2. Compare and contrast a postgraduate year one (PGY1) and postgraduate year two (PGY2) residency program.
3. Based on what you have learned about residency training, describe some of the career opportunities that you think may be available post-residency.
4. Where do you think residency training fits in the future of our profession? What do you think the future holds for residency training?
5. What characteristics would influence your selection of one residency program over another?

Index

A

Accounting, 253, 261–62
Accreditation, 1, 11–12, 42, 383, 390
Accrediting body, 39, 40–41, 42
Acuity, 253
Administration error, 99, 102–3
Advanced Pharmacy Practice Experiences (APPEs), 372
Advanced training, 377–78
Adverse drug event (ADE), 99, 105, 203
Adverse drug reaction, 75, 99, 104
    monitoring and reporting, 113–14
Agency for Healthcare Research and Quality, 116
Alerting orders, 113
Allergic drug reactions, 99, 104
American College of Clinical Pharmacy, 48
American Osteopathic Association, Healthcare Facilities Accreditation Program, 43
American Pharmacists Association (APhA), 29, 48
    Pathway Evaluation Program, 367, 370
American Society of Consultant Pharmacists, 48
American Society of Health-System Pharmacists (ASHP), 29–30, 48–51, 116
    Midyear Clinical Meeting and Exhibition, 367, 374
    positions, statements, guidelines, 218–19
Ampul, 299
Ante area, 277, 285
Anteroom, 277
Applications, 352–53
Aseptic technique, 277, 289
ASHP Hilton Head conference, 17, 26–27
Assets, 253, 260–61
Asynchronous CDS, 179, 194
Attitude theory, 321, 329–30
Authentication, 179, 194
Automated dispensing cabinets, 123, 134–35
Automated dispensing devices, 208–10
Automation, 8–9, 203, 204, 223
    cost justification, 220
    history, 205
    impact on manpower, 220–22
    patient safety, 205–6, 216–17
    selection, 219–20, 221

B

Bacterial endotoxins, 279
Balance sheet, 253, 261, 262
Bar code medication administration (BCMA), 203, 205, 212–14, 215
Bar coded medication administration (BCMA), 9, 179, 188
Batch formulas, records, 283
Behavioral interviews, 345, 354
Behavioral theories, 321, 330–31

Benchmarking, 270
Beyond use dating, 292–93
Big L leaders, 321, 325
Biological safety cabinet (BSC), 277, 283
Biometrics, 179, 194
Board certification, 81, 88
Board of pharmacy specialties (BPS), 81, 88
Borrowing pharmaceuticals, 244
Budget, 253, 262
    monitoring, 268
    negotiation, review, approval, 267–68
Buffer area/room, 277, 285

C

Cannula, 299
Capital budget, 253, 263–64
Capital expense, 253, 259
Career path, 368–69
    planning, 369–71
Career plan, developing, 374–76
Carousel dispensing technology (CDT), 203, 210–12
Carrying costs, 236
Case mix index (CMI), 253, 261
Case rate, 253–54, 260
Catholic hospitals, 19
CDS alert, 180, 193
CDS rule, 180, 193
Centers for Disease Control and Prevention, 46
Centers for Medicare and Medicaid Services (CMS), 41, 42, 116
Centralized pharmacy services, 123, 133, 209
Certification, 39, 41–42
Certifying body, 39, 40
Chief executive officer (CEO), 254, 258
Chief financial officer (CFO), 254, 258
Clean room/buffer room, 277, 285, 286
Cleaning, 286–87
Clinical data repository, 180, 193
Clinical decision support (CDS), 180, 192–93
    alert, 172–73
Clinical decision support system (CDSS), 159, 163, 171–72
Clinical decision support-based infusion pumps, 214
Clinical informatics pharmacist, 197–98
Clinical pharmacist, 81, 83
    competencies, 86, 87
    education, training, credentials, 86
    roles of, 88–89
Clinical pharmacy, 81–82, 83–85
    evidence of value, 91–92
    other services, 89–90
Clinical practice guidelines, controlled substances, 152
Clinical-pharmacist-centered model, 5
Closed formulary, 59, 66

Code Federal Regulation (CFR), 143, 145
Cold storage conditions, 278
Community hospital, 3
Competence assessment, 52
Compliance, 39, 42
Components, 278, 282–83
Compounded product handling, 245
Compounded sterile preparation (CSP), 278, 282
Compounding aseptic containment isolator (CACI), 278, 285
Compounding aseptic isolator (CAI), 278, 283
Compounding personnel, 288–91
Compounding verification, 292
Computer-based documentation systems, 159, 163
Computerized prescriber/provider order entry (CPOE), 9, 159, 161, 168–69, 191, 203, 205
    impact assessment, 172–73
    implementing, 169–70
Confidentiality, 180, 194–96
Controlled Substance Act (CSA), 143, 145
Controlled substances, 75, 144
    administration of, 151
    automated storage and distribution devices, 149
    dispensing, record keeping, 212
    disposal of, 149
    electronic prescribing, 150–51
    evaluation of, 151–52
    formulary, 146–47
    handling, 245
    inventory and record requirements, 147–48
    medication orders, 150
    physical security and storage, 148–49
    policies and procedures, 153–54
    procurement, 147
Cost
    control, 255–57
    integration, 269
Cost-base productivity ratios, 271
Credentials, 82, 87–88
Critical factors, 371–72
Critical site, 278
Culture of safety, 107–8
Curriculum vitae (CV), 367, 375, 383, 391

D

Data, 180, 183, 184
    repository, 159–60, 163
    standardization, 160, 167
Decentralized automated dispensing devices, 203–4, 208–9, 210
Decentralized pharmacy services, 123, 133
Deemed status, 39, 42
De-identification, 180, 195
Department standards, 52–53
Diagnosis related group (DRG), 254
Diagnosis-related DUE, 59–60, 72
Didactic curriculum, 373
Direct compounding area (DCA), 278, 283
Direct expense, 254, 257

Direct purchasing, 243
Disinfecting, 286–87
Dispensing, 4
    error, 99, 104
Distributor, recalls and, 241–42
Double entry bookkeeping, 254, 261
Drug
    acquisition, distribution, control, 21–23, 27
    distribution technology, 133–35
    distributional activities, 90–91
    formulary, 59
    misadventures, 99–100, 101
    monograph, 59
    recalls, 241–42
    shortages, 242
    therapy guidelines, 59, 65
    use, rational, 25–26
Drug Enforcement Administration (DEA), 45, 143, 145
Drug use evaluation (DUE), 59, 71–74, 77
Drug wholesaler purchasing, 243–44
Drug-distribution-centered model, 5
Drug-related problems, 100, 101, 104
    consequences, 104, 105
    morbidity, 100, 105
Drug-specific DUE, 60, 72

E

Economic models, 239–40
Economic order quantity (EOQ), 229, 240
Education, 30–31, 65–66
    minimum requirements evolution, 31
Effects analysis, 147
Electrolyte, 299
Electronic health record (EHR), 160, 161–62
    benefits, 164–65
    components, 164
    expansion of, 168
    information content, data issues, 165–67
Electronic medical record (EMR), 160, 161, 229
Electronic medication administration record (eMAR), 204, 212–13
Electronic prescribing (e–prescribing), 150–51, 160, 169
Emergency crash cart, 132
Emotional intelligence, 321, 337–38
Employee termination, 360–61
Employment life-cycle, 347–48
Encryption, 180, 195
Environmental Protection Agency, 46
Environmental testing, 287–88
Epidural, 299
Equal Opportunity Employment Commission (EEOC), 345, 347
Equity, 254
Error of commission, 100, 105–6
Error of omission, 100, 106
Evidence-based, 82, 85
Expense, 254, 258–59
    budget, 265–67
Experience, 372–74

Expired pharmaceuticals, 246–48
External benchmarking, 254, 270
Extravasation, 299

F

Failure modes, 147
Failure modes and effects analysis, 143, 147
Federal Civil Rights Act of 1964, 345, 347
Fellowship, 82, 87
Financial management, 255–57
First air, 278, 283
Fixed expenses, 254, 258, 267
Floor stock, 75
    systems, 123, 125, 126
FOCUS-PDSA, 60
Follower-oriented leaders, 321, 331
Food and Drug Administration, 45
    drug recalls, 241
Formal power, 324
Formulary
    changes, 70
    controlled substances, 146–47
    management, 66–71, 74
    management process, 63
    restrictions, 60, 66–67
    system, 18, 25, 61–62, 230–31
    system maintenance, 64
For-profit hospital, 3
Full time equivalent, 17–18
Functionality, 160, 162

G

Garb, 278, 289–90
General ledger, 254, 262
Generic substitution, 75
Government hospital, 3
Graduate education, 376
Group purchasing organization, 229, 242–43
Guidelines, 39, 40

H

Hazardous drugs, 278
Health care quality measures, 110–
Health Level 7 (HL–7), 160, 167
Health websites, 185
    quality criteria for, 186
Healthcare Facilities Accreditation Program (HFAP),
    40, 42
Health-system board, 60, 62
High risk, 279, 286
HIPAA (Health Insurance Portability and Accountability
    Act), 160, 162
Hiring, 348–49
Hospital pharmacy history, 18–19
    drug product acquisition, distribution, control,
    21–23
    early 1900s, 20
    1800s, 19–20
    50-year perspective, 20–21
    patient safety, 24–25

Hospital transformation, 28
Hospital types, 2–3
Human factors engineering, 204, 222
Human resources
    expense, 265–66
    management, 346–47

I

Idiosyncratic reaction, 100, 104
Income statements, 254, 261–62
Incompatibility, 299
Indirect expense, 254, 259
Infiltration, 299
Informatics, 180, 182
    administrative uses of, 187
    practice applications of, 186–88
Information, 183, 184
    access and use, 189
    retrieval, 185
    security, 180, 194–96
Infusion
    pumps, 307–8
    sites, 305
    therapy documentation, 310
Inpatient care, 10
Institute for Healthcare improvement, 115
Institute of Medicine, 48, 115
Institute of Safe Medication Practices (ISMP), 144
Institutional pharmacy practice, 1,2
Integrate, 204, 207
Integrated health systems, 1, 2
Interface, 180, 186, 188, 204
    types of, 190–92
Internal benchmarking, 254, 271
Internet, 374
Internship, 367, 373
Interoperability, 160, 163
Interpretation error, 100
Interview
    preparation steps, 353–54
    process, 353–55
    screening, 352–53
Intrathecal, 299
Introductory Pharmacy Practice Experiences (IPPEs),
    372
Inventory
    carrying costs, 229
    control, 231–32
    turns, 229, 236–37
Investigational drug
    handling, 245
    orders, 75
ISO Class 5, 279
IV drug delivery systems issues, 314
IV pumps, 308–9

J

Job descriptions, 345, 349
Joint Commission, The, 40, 43, 116
Just-in-time inventory management, 229, 240

K

Knowledge, 180, 183, 184
   source links, 193–94

L

Labeling, 291–92
Labor productivity ratios, 271
Laissez-faire leadership, 321, 323
Laminar air flow workbench (LAFW), 278, 283
Latent injury, 100, 105
Laws, 40, 44–45, 145, 346–47
Leader, 322, 326
   barriers to developing, 338–39
   behaviors of, 330–31
   competencies for institutional pharmacy, 338
   nature of, 328–29
   responses of, 331–33
Leadership, 321–22, 323
   developing abilities, 336–37
   management and, 326–28
   styles, 333–36
   theories, 328
   without formal authority, 325–26
Leapfrog Group, The, 115–16
Liabilities, 254, 261
Little L leaders, 322, 325–26
Low risk, 279, 285

M

Manager, 322, 326
Manufacturer, recalls and, 241–42
Master formula sheet, 284
Media-fill test, 278–79
Medical executive committee, 51, 52, 60, 62
Medication
   administration, 4–5
   administration times, 75
   delivery, 131
   list, 76
   order writing, 74
   orders, 150
   prescribing, dispensing, administering, 74–75
   profile, 124
   purchasing inventory system, 248
   reconciliation, 100, 114–15
   selection, review, 64
Medication administration record (MAR), 123, 129, 130, 180, 189
Medication distribution system
   history, 124–27
   requirements, 137
Medication error, 75, 100, 102, 204
   prevention, 106–7
   types, 106
Medication safety, 101, 107–8, 116
   evaluation, 65
Medication samples, 75
   handling, 246
Medication use
   guidelines, 76–77
   management, 61
   policies, 74–75
   policy and procedures, 76
   process, 3–4, 204, 206, 218
   review, 60
   system future, 136
Medication utilization evaluation (MUE), 64–65, 144
Medications for nursing units, 136
Medium risk, 279, 285
Mentors, 374
Minibag system, 281
Mirror to Hospital Pharmacy, 17, 26, 29
Monitoring, 4–5
   error, 100, 104

N

National Committee for Quality Assurance, 116
National Council for Medication Error Reporting and
   Prevention, 103
National Fire Protection Association (NFPA), 48
National Institute for Occupational Safety and Health,
   45–46
National Integrated Accreditation for Healthcare Organi-
   zations (NIAHO), 40, 42, 43–44
National Quality Forum, 115
Net worth, 254
New product evaluation, 68–70
New program budget, 267
Nonformulary agent, 60
   drug review, 70–71
   item handling, 246
Nonrepudiation, 181, 194–95

O

Occupational Safety and Health Administration, 45
Office for Civil Rights, 46
Office of Inspector General, 46
Open formulary, 60, 66
Operating budget, 254, 263, 264
Order book, 229, 236–37
Order entry rules, 60, 71
Order interpretation, 75
Organization standards, 52–53
Outcome, 100, 112
   assessment, 60
   CDSS alert, 172
   PGY1, 385
Outpatient care, 10–11

P

Packaging, 291–92
Parenteral (injectable), 300
Parenteral administration, 304
   methods of, 306–7
   routes of, 304–6
   set change intervals, 308
Parenteral medication
   nutrition, 300
   preparation, dispensing, 300–302

safety, 310–15
   therapy hazards, 302–4
Pareto ABC analysis, 229–30, 236, 239–40
Par-level systems, 230, 237, 238–39
Patient
   medication profile, 127
   outcomes, optimal, 26
   prescription system, 124, 125–26
   safety, 24–25, 145–46, 280–82
Patient-centered integrated model, 5
PDCA model, 73
PDSA cycle, 109–10
Performance
   evaluation, 52–53
   feedback, 358–60
   motivation, 357–58
   standards, 345, 350–51
Performance improvement (PI), 40, 52–53
Perpetual inventory, 230, 239
Personal health record (PHR), 160, 161–62
Pharmaceutical receiving, storing, 232–34
Pharmacist, 7–8
   advanced training, 377–78
   role in P&T committee, 66
Pharmacotherapy complexity, 146
Pharmacy education, 30–31
Pharmacy informatics, 181, 182
Pharmacy information system, 181, 188, 191
Pharmacy leadership, 12
Pharmacy Quality Alliance, 116
Pharmacy robot, 9
Pharmacy technicians, 8, 234–35
Pharmacy and therapeutics (P&T) committee, 17,
   25–26, 51, 52, 74
   membership, 63–64
   organization, 62–63
   regulatory, accrediting bodies, 66
   responsibilities, 64–66
Pharmacy transformation
   internal factors, 33
   lessons learned, 33
Point-of-care devices, 181, 183
Policies, 75
Policies and procedures, 144
   controlled substance, 153–54
   development, 65
Pop-ups, 60, 71
Portfolio, 367, 375
Position descriptions, 345, 349
Postgraduate residency education, training, 31–32
Postgraduate year one (PGY1) pharmacy residency,
   82, 87–88, 383, 384–86
Postgraduate year two (PGY2) pharmacy residency,
   82, 383, 386–87
   residency types, 387
Potential adverse drug events, 100
Potential injuries, 105
Power, 322, 324–25

Power of attorney, 144, 148
Practice guidelines, 1, 6–7
Practice model, 1–2, 5–6, 12–13
Practice standards, 11–12, 17, 31–33, 257–58
Prescriber-related DUE, 60, 72
Prescribing, 4
   error, 100, 104
Primary engineering control (PEC), 279, 283, 285
Prime vendor contract, 230, 243–44
Priority IV medication safety practices, 312–14
Privileging, 2
Process, 100, 111–12
   improvement, 187–88
Product handling, 234–35
Productivity measurement, 270
Professional associations/organizations, 29–30, 48–51
Professional meetings, 374
Progressive discipline, 345–46, 360
Published formulary, 75–77
Punishment power, 324
Purchasing, 231–32
Pyrogens, 279, 282

Q
Quality assurance, 218
   compounding sterile preparations, 282
   after preparation leaves pharmacy, 293
Quality improvement, 40, 53
   models, 108–9
Quality organizations, 115–16

R
Radiofrequency identification (RFID), 181, 188
Radio frequency (RF) network, 204, 213
Receiving process, 232–33
Recruiting process, 349
Recruitment strategies, 351–52
Refrigerator, 278
Regulations, 2, 40, 44–45, 145, 217, 346–47
Regulatory bodies, 11
Repackaged pharmaceuticals handling, 245–46
Residency, 82, 87, 88, 383, 384
   application process, 391–93
   benefits and barriers, 387–89
   PGY2 types, 387
   researching programs, 389–91
   Residency program director, 383, 385
Resident Matching Program, 384, 393
   Post-match, 393–94
Resume, 367, 375
Retention, 355–56
Return on equity (ROE), 254
Return on investment (ROI), 254, 264
Revenue, 254, 259–60
   analysis, 269
Reward power, 324
Risk levels, 279
Role play interviews, 346, 354
Rules, 40, 44–45

S

Secondary engineering controls, 279, 285–88
Self-administration, 75
Sentinel event, 100, 105
Sharp, 300
Side effects, 100, 104–5
Situation interviews, 346, 354
Situational theories, 322, 331
Smart pumps, 2, 9, 204, 214, 216, 309
Special handling, 244–46
Special information, 77
Special purpose infusion devices, 309–10
Specialized hospital, 3
Standard operating procedures (SOPs), 279, 282, 293–94
Standard precautions, 300
Standards, 40
    organization and department, 52–53
    -setting entities, 47–48
State boards of pharmacy, 46–47
Stock rotation, 230, 233
Stop orders, 60–61, 74, 144, 146
Storage, 292–93
    temperatures/humidity, 234
Storing process, 233–34
Stress interviews, 346, 354
Structure, 100, 110–11, 322, 326
Student organizations, 373
Supply chain management, 204, 206–7
Supply expense, 266–67
Supportive behavior, 322, 331
Surveillance program, controlled substances, 151–52
Survey, 40
    preparation, 44
Synchronous CDS, 181, 194
Systems integration, 188

T

Taper orders, 144, 146
Task-oriented leaders, 322, 331
Teaching hospital, 3
Technology, 8–9, 204
Therapeutic class review, 61, 70
Therapeutic equivalents, 61, 67
Therapeutic interchange, 61, 67, 68

Therapeutic problem solving processes, 85–86
Therapeutic substitution, 75
Time and motion study, 254, 270
Total parenteral nutrition (TPN/hyperalimentation), 300
Traditional interviews, 346, 354
Traffic control, 287
Trait theories, 322, 328–29
Transcribing, 4
Transcription error, 100, 104
Trigger event, 100

U

Unit dose system, 124, 126, 137
    advantages, 127
    delivery models, 133
    drug use control and, 127
    process, 128–33
Unit of use package, 124
Unit-based cabinet, 8–9
United States Pharmacopeia (USP), 47
    Chapter <788> Particulate Matter in Injections, 303
    Chapter <797>, Pharmaceutical Compounding—Sterile Preparations, 279, 280, 294
United States Pharmacopoeia—ISMP Medication Errors Reporting Program, 144, 145
User interface, 160, 163

V

Variable expense, 254, 258–59
Variance
    analysis, 254, 268–69
    cause determination, 269
Vehicle, 300
Verbal orders, 74
Verified Internet Pharmacy Practice Sites (VIPPS), 181, 194–95
VeriSign, 181, 196
Vial, 300
Visionary leadership, 28–29
Volume budget, 254, 264–65

W

Waste disposal, 310
Work volumes, 254, 261
Workflow, 187–88